*Advances
in
Head and Neck
Oncology*

Advances in Head and Neck Oncology

Edited by

K. Thomas Robbins, MD

Department of Otolaryngology—Head and Neck Surgery
University of Tennessee
Memphis, Tennessee

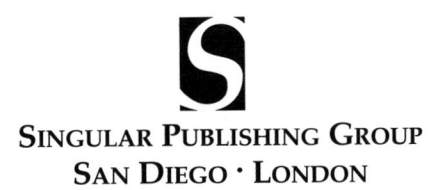

SINGULAR PUBLISHING GROUP
SAN DIEGO · LONDON

Notice: The indications, procedures, drug dosages, and diagnosis and remediation protocols in this book have been recommended in the clinical literature and conform to the practices of the general medical and health services communities. All procedures put forth in this book should be performed only by trained, licensed practitioners. The diagnostic and remediation protocols and the medications described do not necessarily have specific approval by the Food And Drug Administration for use in the disorders and/or diseases and dosages for which they are recommended. Because standards of practice and usage change, it is the responsibility of practitioners to keep abreast of revised recommendations, dosages, and procedures.

Singular Publishing Group, Inc.
401 West "A" Street, Suite 325
San Diego, California 92101-7904

Singular Publishing Ltd.
19 Compton Terrace
London, N1 2UN, UK

© 1998 by Singular Publishing Group, Inc.
Typeset in 10/12 Palatino by So Cal Graphics
Printed in the United States of America by McNaughton & Gunn

Singular Publishing Group, Inc., publishes textbooks, clinical manuals, clinical reference books, journals, videos, and multimedia materials on speech-language pathology, audiology, otorhinolaryngology, special education, early childhood, aging, occupational therapy, physical therapy, rehabilitation, counseling, mental health, and voice. For your convenience, our entire catalog can be accessed on our website at **http//www.singpub.com**. Our mission to provide you with materials to meet the daily challenges of the ever-changing health care/educational environment will remain on course if we are in touch with you. In that spirit, we welcome your feedback on our products. Please telephone **(1-800-521-8545)**, fax **(1-800-774-8398)**, or e-mail **(singpub@mail.cerfnet.com)** your comments and requests to us.

All rights, including that of translation reserved. No part of this publication may be reproduced, stored in a retrieval system, or transmitted in any form or by any means, electronic, mechanical, recording, or otherwise, without the prior written permission of the publisher.

Library of Congress Cataloging-in-Publication Data

Advances in head and neck oncology / [edited by] K. Thomas Robbins.
    p. cm.
  Includes bibliographical references and index.
  ISBN 1-56593-840-2
  1. Head—Cancer. 1. Neck—Cancer. I. Robbins, K. Thomas.
  [DNLM: 1. Head and Neck Neoplasms. WE 707 A244 1998]
RC280.H4A38 1998
616.99'491—dc21
DNLM/DLC
for Library of Congress
97–36322
CIP

CONTENTS

Contributors		vii
Dedication		ix
Acknowledgments		x
CHAPTER 1	**Introductory Overview of** *Advances in Head and Neck Oncology* K. Thomas Robbins, MD	1
CHAPTER 2	**Biology of Upper Aerodigestive Tract Carcinoma** Bruce J. Davidson, MD, FACS, and Stimson P. Schantz, MD, FACS	5
CHAPTER 3	**Hyperfractionated or Accelerated Radiation Therapy for Squamous Cell Carcinoma of the Head and Neck** James T. Parsons, MD, and William M. Mendenhall, MD	25
CHAPTER 4	**The Selective Neck Dissection for Upper Aerodigestive Tract Carcinoma: Indications and Results** Robert M. Byers, MD, and Dianna B. Roberts, PhD	37
CHAPTER 5	**Surgical Approaches to the Nasopharynx** William Ignace Wei, MS, FRCSE, DLO, FACS, and Po Wing Yuen, MS, DLO, FRCSE	47
CHAPTER 6	**Targeted Cisplatin Chemotherapy for Advanced Head and Neck Cancer** K. Thomas Robbins, MD	59
CHAPTER 7	**Endoscopic Resection of Laryngeal Cancer** R. Kim Davis, MD	73
CHAPTER 8	**Supracricoid Partial Laryngectomy** Gregory S. Weinstein, MD, and Ollivier Laccourreye, MD	83
CHAPTER 9	**Advances in Functional Assessment of Patients Treated for Head and Neck Cancer** Gayle Woodson, PhD	99
CHAPTER 10	**Oral Communication After Laryngectomy** R.E. (Ed) Stone, Jr, PhD	105
CHAPTER 11	**Rhabdomyosarcoma of the Head and Neck in Children** Alberto S. Pappo, MD, and William M. Crist, MD	119

CHAPTER 12	**State of the Art Techniques for Mandibular Reconstruction** Wayne B. Colin, DMD, MD, and Bruce H. Haughey, MB, ChB, FRACS, FACS	133
CHAPTER 13	**Quality of Life, Comorbidity, and Cost-Effectiveness in Head and Neck Cancer Treatment** Ernest A. Weymuller, Jr, MD, Frederic W.B- Deleyiannis, MD, MPhil, MPH, Jay F. Piccirillo, MD, FACS, and Bevan Yueh, MD	147
	Index	175

CONTRIBUTORS

Robert M. Byers, MD
Department of Head and Neck Surgery
University of Texas MD Anderson Cancer Center
Houston, Texas

Wayne B. Colin, DMD, MD
Head and Neck Surgical Oncology
Department of Otolaryngology
Washington University School of Medicine
St. Louis, Missouri

William M. Crist, MD
Director, Extramural Program
St. Jude Children's Research Hospital
Memphis, Tennessee

Bruce J. Davidson, MD, FACS
Assistant Professor
Department of Otolaryngology—Head and Neck Surgery
Georgetown University Medical Center
Chief, VAMC
Washington, DC

R. Kim Davis, MD
Beckstrand Professor and Chairman
Division of Otolaryngology—Head and Neck Surgery
Salt Lake City, Utah

Frederic W.-B Deleyiannis, MD, MPhil, MPH
Department of Otolaryngology—Head and Neck Surgery
University of Washington
Seattle, Washington

Bruce H. Haughey, MB, ChB, FRACS, FACS
Associate Professor and Director
Division of Head and Neck Surgical Oncology
Department of Otolaryngology
Washington University School of Medicine
St. Louis, Missouri

Ollivier Laccourreye, MD
Department of Otorhinolaryngology—Head and Neck Surgery
University Paris V
Laënnec Hospital
Assistance Publique des Hopitaux de Paris
Paris, France

William M. Mendenhall, MD
Department of Radiation Oncology
University of Florida College of Medicine
Gainesville, Florida

Alberto S. Pappo, MD
Department of Hematology-Oncology
St. Jude Children's Research Hospital
Memphis, Tennessee

James T. Parsons, MD
Department of Radiation Oncology
University of Florida College of Medicine
Gainesville, Florida

Jay F. Piccirillo, MD, FACS
Department of Otolaryngology—Head and Neck Surgery
Washington University
St. Louis, Missouri

Dianna B. Roberts, PhD
Department of Head and Neck Surgery
University of Texas MD Anderson Cancer Center
Houston, Texas

Stimson P. Schantz, MD, FACS
Head and Neck Surgery Service
Memorial Sloan-Kettering Cancer Center
New York, New York

R.E. (Ed) Stone, Jr, PhD
Department of Otolaryngology
Vanderbilt University Medical Center
Nashville, Tennessee

Gregory S. Weinstein, MD
Associate Professor
Department of Otorhinolaryngology—
Head and Neck Surgery
The University of Pennsylvania Medical Center
Philadelphia, Pennsylvania

Ernest A. Weymuller, Jr., MD
Professor and Chairman
Department of Otolaryngology—Head and Neck Surgery
University of Washington
Seattle, Washington

William Ingnace Wei, MS, FRCSE, DLO, FACS
Department of Surgery
The University of Hong Kong
Queen Mary Hospital
Hong Kong

Gayle Woodson, PhD
Professor of Otolaryngology
University of Tennessee
College of Medicine
Memphis, Tennessee

Po Wing Yuen, MS, DLO, FRCSE
Assistant Professor
Department of Surgery
Tye University of Hong Kong
Queen Mary Hospital
Hong Kong

Bevan Yueh, MD
Assistant Professor
University of Washington
Seattle, Washington

DEDICATION

There are many friends and colleagues with whom I have worked over the years, all of whom have in some way steered my career. However, of greatest influence of all are my teachers and mentors: Wycliffe and Elizabeth Robbins, Frank Wong, Douglas Bryce, John Fredrickson, David Briant, Sir Donald Harrison, Helmuth Geopfert, Robert Byers, Oscar Guillamondegui, Ed Cocke, and Stephen Howell. I would be remiss to omit my best friend and loving wife, Gayle Woodson, who also has been a tremendous colleague. To them I dedicate this book.

ACKNOWLEDGMENTS

I am deeply appreciative of the efforts provided by the authors of each chapter in this book. They have given a significant amount of their valuable time to help me provide a meaningful collection of new and exciting developments in the field of head and neck oncology. Much of their motivation comes through the enjoyment and fulfillment that clinicians and scientists experience through their involvement with head and neck cancer patients. Having devoted 20 years of my own professional life to this cause, I personally witness the devastation and despair that often occurs when patients are confronted by this disease. If we, the authors, can facilitate better care through education and inspire others to join our research commitment to improve the management of these patients, then our efforts through this book will be rewarded.

CHAPTER 1

Introductory Overview of *Advances in Head and Neck Oncology*

K. Thomas Robbins, MD

Head and neck cancer is a disease that afflicts patients in a variety of ways, the worst of which is death from uncontrolled tumor progression at the site of origin, the regional lymphatics, or distant metastases. However, even patients who survive following treatment are frequently left with excessive physical and psychological morbidity related to chronic pain, organ dysfunction, and altered appearance. The multitude of problems that oncologists must deal with in managing these patients necessitates a team approach incorporating many disciplines. Thus there is an ongoing need for head and neck cancer care providers to stay current with management principles and be cognizant of new developments in the field.

The purpose of this book is to highlight 12 areas in the field of head and neck oncology in which significant advances have been made over the past few years. The contributors are experts in their respective fields, which include surgical oncology, medical oncology, radiation oncology, reconstructive surgery, tumor biology, speech-language pathology, and laryngology. The information provided is intended for health care professionals representing all of the disciplines involved in the care of these patients. It is intended to help individual clinicians update their knowledge based on current principles of management as well as to facilitate further multidisciplinary interaction among care providers to further improve the team approach for patients with this disease.

The principles of tumor biology form the basis upon which treatment programs are developed. Therefore, it is important to consider the new developments in this field as they relate to understanding head and neck cancer. Chapter 2 provided by Bruce Davidson, MD, and Stimson Shantz, MD, is extremely current and excellent at focusing in on the relevant issues of a complex maze of information emerging within the broader scope of the biological behavior for solid tumors. Relevant topics include new observations on the effects of chromosomal mutations on carcinogenesis and the mechanisms through which oncogenes and tumor suppressor genes contribute to the process. The role of apoptosis in tumor progression and response to treatment has also come to the forefront and is well summarized. The authors describe how the cyclins are thought to regulate cell growth and relate new observations of how various phases of the cell cycle affect tumor sensitivity to radiation and chemotherapy. P53 expression among head and neck tumors has received a great deal of attention in the literature with contradictory results. This issue is well summarized by Davidson and Shantz. Other topics include retinoids, growth factors, and genes that facilitate metastases.

Hyperfractionated and accelerated fractionated radiation therapy have received a great deal of attention over the past decade primarily because these schedules attempt to capitalize on basic radiobiologic principles for improving the effects of this modality. This topic is reviewed in chapter 3 by James Parsons, MD, and William Mendenhall, MD, investigators who have an extensive experience with this approach, and the reader is provided an updated analysis of treatment results for patients with head and neck cancer managed at the University of Florida. Their work is also compared to others who have conducted both Phase II and Phase III trials. Parsons and Mendenhall also provide an excellent history of the origination of altered fractionations that include split course schedules, prolonged schedules, and various types of multiple daily fractions. This chapter presents a substantial body of evidence indicating that accelerated and hyperfractionated radiation schedules provide improved rates of locoregional control as well as survival advantages. Rebuttal of this philosophy by skeptics has typically been based on the lack of randomized trials comparing programs incorporating multiple daily fractionations to single daily treatments. However, randomized studies have now been completed that support the improved efficacy of the former. The authors present this evidence in stating their case for implementing such schedules into standard practice.

Another topic in head and neck oncology in which there has been a progressive evolution in philosophy is the management of lymph node metastases. Preceded by the descriptions of neck dissection procedures representing modifications of the radical neck dissection, the selective neck dissection evolved from the work of such pioneers as Jesse and Ballentyne. In chapter 4, Robert Byers, a student of these pioneers who has established his own reputation through his extensive analyses of large numbers of patients treated at MD Anderson, presents new data for patients who underwent selective neck dissection from 1985–1990. Results are reviewed according to type of procedure: suprahyoid, supraomohyoid, lateral, and according to whether postoperative radiation therapy was also administered. Analysis was also done according to the site of the primary tumor. The accompanying table displays the results in a manner that allows evaluation of disease control based on all of these parameters. One can also assess how well the selective neck dissection holds up as the only treatment modality for multiple nodal disease. This original work contributes significantly to the soundness of the concept that selective neck dissection is effective for patients with early nodal metastases.

Nasopharyngeal carcinoma is a major health problem in Eastern Asia and is also encountered frequently among Caucasians. It is a disease that continues to be treated primarily with radiation therapy due to its high radiosensitivity. Surgical intervention has been primarily employed to eradicate disease in the regional lymph nodes if there is persistent or recurrent disease following radiation therapy. The feasibility of excising recurrent cancer within the nasopharynx has been explored by skull base surgeons for over a decade. However, major limitations have been obtaining adequate exposure and eradicating disease extending to sites that preclude removal such as the internal carotid artery and cavernous sinus. In this book, chapter 5 on surgical approaches to the nasopharynx by William Wei, MD, from Hong Kong provides us with an overview of the various techniques. He then focuses on the anterolateral approach, a method commonly employed for selected patients at the Queen Mary Hospital in Hong Kong. The data provided are supportive of this treatment strategy for such patients and reinforce the concept that some recurrent nasopharyngeal carcinomas can be successfully removed, provided adequate exposure is obtained. The anterolateral field of view, a technique that requires either removal or transposition of the maxilla, appears to be the best for this purpose.

Targeted chemoradiation is a new concept and one that shows promise for eradicating large bulky carcinomas of the head and neck. It also shows significant potential for organ preservation among patients presenting with T3–T4 lesions of the oropharynx, hypopharynx, and larynx. This treatment program was started 9 years ago at the University of California, San Diego and has since been further developed at the University of Tennessee, Memphis. The research explores the benefits of delivering intra-arterially an unprecedented high dose intensity schedule of cisplatin by combining it with a systemically administered neutralizing agent, sodium thiosulfate. Chapter 6 summarizes the work to date, including survival results, organ preservation effects, quality of life outcomes, toxicity, and ability to tolerate the treatment. The program has now been extended to a national multicenter phase II study and is beginning to be tested at selected international sites.

The management of early laryngeal cancer continues to be an ongoing controversy. With regard to T1 glottic lesions, endoscopic laser resection is a viable alternative to the more traditional approach of radiation therapy, particularly for patients whose disease is confined to the ipsilateral membranous cord. Davis correctly points out in chapter 7 that studies of objective assessment of phonatory function comparing the two treatment modalities are lacking. For T2 glottic lesions, the issue may be better local control following laser resection versus radiation therapy. Davis provides evidence supporting the surgical approach for such lesions with particular emphasis being given to endoscopic techniques. Also covered in this chapter is the method by which early and intermediate supraglottic tumors are removed endoscopically, an approach that has recently received attention based on promising results from Germany. Thus endoscopic laser removal of laryngeal carcinomas is a hot topic among head and neck surgeons and the information provided by Kim Davis, a very reputable head and neck surgeon who has pioneered this approach in the United States, is very timely.

Parallel with the topic of endoscopic removal of laryngeal cancer is the recent awareness of work from France that portions of the larynx can be excised for more advanced glottic and supraglottic tumors without sacrificing the phonatory and respiratory functions of the larynx. In chapter 7 this topic is covered by Greg Weinstein and Ollivier Laccourreye, the latter being the teacher and the former the student from the United States who has made other Americans more aware of this strategy. Together they provide an excellent description of the operation, supracricoid laryngectomy, and the two variations in closure, cricohyoidopexy and cricohyodoepiglottopexy. Data are also provided in support of using this approach for selected patients who are otherwise not suitable candidates for other types of conservation laryngeal procedures and would need a total laryngectomy. As both alternatives provide new expectations for preserving organ function, the winner may ultimately be the patient.

Related to the innovative treatment methods for eradicating laryngeal cancer while preserving the organ itself, or at least the important portions of it, is the need to assess how useful the larynx remains to the patient. Much progress has been made over the past decade in developing assessment methods of laryngeal function including a number of tests for acoustic analysis and measurements of airflow. However, the application of these measures to clinical practice remains only partly successful because laryngeal function, particularly phonation, is dynamic and perceptual. In chapter 9 on functional outcomes following laryngeal preservation, Gayle Woodson addresses this issue in a practical way and outlines which parameters for assessing laryngeal function are relevant following treatment for head and neck cancer. Her observations are based on a series of patients with advanced tumors treated with targeted chemoradiation for whom organ preservation was achieved. With continued evolution of treatment strategies intended to retain the larynx, the observations and conclusions Woodson presents are of paramount importance for developing parallel studies to measure this function.

In contrast to the preceding chapter focusing on the preserved larynx, Ed Stone, PhD, provides an excellent review of the state of the art for managing patients who have lost their larynges. In chapter 10, he correctly points out that much of what we do for these patients has not changed over the past decade, although there are now better devices and more choices. This chapter is quite comprehensive in that all of the techniques within the armamentarium of the speech pathologist are described and put into perspective. Speech rehabilitation continues to play an important role in the management of laryngeal cancer and the material covered in this chapter provides an excellent update for readers.

The management of children with rhabdomyosarcoma is primarily the responsibility of pediatric medical and radiation oncologists. However, the head and neck surgical oncologist is occassionally called upon for help, particularly when there is disease recurrence locally. Treatment programs for pediatric rhabdomyosarcomas have gone through a series of evolutionary changes and improvements over the past decade but very little of this information makes its way into the head and neck oncology literature. Alberto Pappo and William Christ are two of the world's leaders, whose collective experience in this field is extensive. In chapter 11, they provide an excellent chronology of how the treatment for these solid tumors has been refined and made highly effective using combination chemotherapy and radiation therapy.

Management of the mandibular defect following ablative treatment for head and neck cancer has been one of the major challenges for therapists for decades. The development and refinement of free bone transfer using microvascular techniques has had a tremendous impact for effectively overcoming the deficit. In chapter 12, Bruce Haughey, MD, and Wayne Colin, DDS, MD, provide an excellent description of the current methods for repairing the mandibular defect. Subsequent research is needed to address the issues of cost effectiveness and restoration of function and these issues are currently being tackled by these authors and their counterparts at other institutions.

The topics of quality of life, co-morbidity, and cost effectiveness are highly relevant for the final chapter in this book as these parameters underscore some of the more practical concerns that must be raised in prioritizing health care delivery. What difference does it make if a treatment results in a drastic downturn in one's quality of life? Head and neck cancer patients frequently have other major health problems and the therapist must be aware of their impact on treatment outcome. The cost of head and neck cancer management on society is also a key issue, particularly when treatment options are available and there is a limit to society's ability to pay for them. Although research has not progressed sufficiently in the field of head and neck oncology to answer these questions, in chapter 13 the authors very effectively outline new tools that have been developed for this purpose.

The recent advances in head and neck oncology covered in this book are not intended to be all inclusive, instead the chapters that follow highlight some of the substantive issues relevant to health care for this disease. Maintaining an updated education, particularly with state-of-the-art management policies for cancer patients, is an ongoing challenge for health care providers. Hopefully, the ultimate winner will be the patient, who has much to gain.

CHAPTER 2

Biology of Upper Aerodigestive Tract Carcinoma

Bruce J. Davidson, MD, FACS, and Stimson P. Schantz, MD, FACS

In the past decade our understanding of the biology of malignancies has improved, due in large part to the increasing use of molecular biologic techniques in cancer research. Just as the histologic description of tumors can reveal significantly more information about tumor extent and prognosis than does clinical examination alone, molecular biologic investigation allows for a description of tumors at a submicroscopic level. These studies show great potential in improving our understanding of the behavior of cancers and may improve treatment results.

As with other tumor types, researchers have attempted to utilize molecular biologic methods to address basic questions about the biology of head and neck squamous cell carcinoma (HNSCC). This has included efforts to define changes indicative of malignant transformation in aerodigestive epithelium and to identify events associated with tumor development, growth, invasion, and metastasis. These methods promise opportunities in cancer therapy ranging from the use of molecular characteristics to predict treatment response to direct intervention on tumor behavior through gene therapy. This chapter provides an overview of significant advances in molecular biology that have improved our understanding of head and neck squamous cell carcinoma.

PATHOLOGY

The majority of the mucosa of the oral cavity, pharynx, and larynx is stratified squamous epithelium consisting of a basal layer of rounded cells, an intermediate polyhedral layer, and flattened superficial cell layers. This tissue is usually 7–10 layers thick and shows an orderly maturation from deep to superficial layers marked by progressive flattening of the cells and a loss or flattening of the nuclei. Mitoses are rare and are confined to the basal layer.

In contrast to normal aerodigestive epithelium, squamous cell carcinoma reveals a loss of cellular maturation and invasion of this abnormal epithelial tissue through the underlying basement membrane into soft tissues. Cells reveal a variation in size and shape and enlarged hyperchromatic nuclei. Mitoses are common. Tumors may vary from well differentiated squamous cell carcinomas with evidence of keratin formation (seen as onion-like deposits known as keratin pearls) and few mitoses to poorly differentiated tumors exhibiting no recognizable squamous features. The leading edge of well differentiated tumors is often rounded (a "pushing border") whereas that of poorly differentiated tumors may show diffuse infiltration into surrounding soft tissues. Most head and neck squamous cell carcinomas are characterized as moderately or poorly differentiated tumors.

Intraepithelial Neoplasia

Abnormal characteristics may be seen in mucosa without the presence of basement membrane invasion. These findings fall under the broad heading of intraepithelial neoplasia and constitute a spectrum of changes from normal mucosa to frank invasion. Pathologic findings include a loss of normal epithelial maturation. Cellular and nuclear pleomorphism may be seen in suprabasal cell layers with the degree of dysplasia determined by the amount of epithelium that is affected. Mild dysplasia may show such changes through the lower third of the epithelium and essentially normal maturation in the upper two thirds. In the superficial layers there is a flattening of the cells and nuclear changes and mitoses are absent. Severe dysplasia, on the other hand, involves almost the entire epithelium.

At the most advanced end of the spectrum of intraepithelial neoplasia is carcinoma in situ. This describes epithelia showing features consistent with invasive carcinoma except that the basement membrane remains intact. No evidence of maturation is seen between the basal and superficial layers of the epithelium. Nuclei and mitotic figures may be seen throughout the entire thickness of the epithelium.

Although the pathologic finding of intraepithelial neoplasia is considered premalignant, whether such atypia progresses to invasive carcinoma and how this transformation occurs is not well defined. Oral leukoplakia is a clinical finding that may herald the development of invasive carcinoma, but most large series estimate the risk of transformation to invasive carcinoma at under 10%.[1] We can obtain a histologic sampling of mucosa and assess the degree of atypia at a point in time, further defining the risk of transformation. When dysplasia is noted on biopsy, the risk of malignant transformation is 10–14%.[2,3] Although these estimates of malignant potential are based on follow-up of clinically apparent or pathologically assessed lesions, efforts to determine the precise molecular events underlying this transformation continue and are discussed below.

CARCINOGENESIS

The distinguishing features of squamous cell carcinoma, like all carcinomas, are (1) malignant transformation, (2) uncontrolled growth, (3) local invasion, and (4) regional or distant metastases. The first two may be seen in intraepithelial neoplastic lesions. Regional or distant metastases follow the development of local invasion and are seen in about 50% of head and neck squamous cell carcinomas.[4] Given that local invasion defines carcinoma, most cancer treatment addresses invasive and metastatic lesions and does not focus on the process of transformation. However, carcinoma begins with malignant transformation or, more precisely, with exposures or inherent susceptibility leading to such transformation. A better appreciation of malignant transformation is essential to understanding carcinogenesis.

The study of chemical carcinogenesis has defined the process of malignant transformation as two steps: initiation and promotion. Many chemical agents have been defined as acting by one or both mechanisms to induce carcinomas. The process of initiation describes the onset of permanent DNA damage which (1) evades repair by the cellular host defense, (2) is not so severe that cell death is caused by the DNA damage, and (3) is passed on to progeny of the cell.

Promotion is caused by chemicals that stimulate cellular proliferation or alter differentiation. This is thought to increase the rate of further mutations by increasing cell turnover and may speed up the clonal selection process.

Mutations that develop may, of course, be silent if no vital genes are affected, but mutations significant for the development of carcinoma will affect genes important in determining cell behavior. These include genes regulating cell cycle control, intrinsic DNA repair processes, and differentiation machinery. These mutations may influence DNA integrity, proliferation, and differentiation and result in malignant transformation and uncontrolled cell growth. Other genes play a role in invasion and metastases. These include those instrumental in cell adhesion and motility, angiogenesis, and evasion of host immune defense systems. The multiple changes noted above may require several mutations or mutations of genes with multiple functions to lead to cancer. No single mutational event appears adequate to result in carcinoma. However, for the development of invasive squamous cell carcinoma, it has been statistically estimated that only 6–10 mutations are required.[5]

Current models of head and neck carcinogenesis have attempted to describe a sequence of mutations that accompany transformation, invasion, and metastasis[6] (see Table 2–1). The precise order of these mutations is not proven and may not be critical, but specific mutations are found more frequently and are presumably more essential in the development of HNSCC.

Oncogenes and Tumor Suppressor Genes

Genes whose protein product is overexpressed or excessively active due to a mutation may be associated with tumor development. These mutated genes are defined as oncogenes. Many of the genes documented to be oncogenes are important in normal cell cycle regulation and when overexpressed will allow cell cycle progression.

TABLE 2–1. Model of genetic alterations in HNSCC development

Progression	Chromosome Alteration[6]	Tumor Suppressor/Oncogene Correlate
Normal Mucosa ↓		
	9p loss	p16 loss/dysfunction
Hyperplasia ↓		
	3p loss	?
	17p loss	p53 loss/mutation
Dysplasia ↓		
	11 gain	cyclin D1 overexpression/amplification
	14q loss	?
	13q loss	Retinoblastoma loss/mutation
Carcinoma in situ ↓		
	6p loss	?
	8p loss	?
	4q loss	?
Invasive carcinoma		

Genes that are associated with tumor development when exhibiting mutations that result in a lack of expression or activity are referred to as tumor suppressor genes. That is, in their normal state, these genes suppress the development of tumors. These genes are also important regulators of the cell cycle, allowing inhibition of cell division when cellular conditions are not appropriate or when DNA repairs are required. Abnormal function of these genes removes this cell cycle regulation, resulting in uncontrolled proliferation and potential loss of DNA integrity.

One method used to indicate the deletion of a tumor suppressor gene detects the loss of heterozygosity at a segment of the genome. When a loss of genetic material is detected in a tumor but not in normal tissue of the same individual, the segment lost is suspected to harbor a tumor suppressor gene. The loss of multiple areas of the genome has been correlated with early recurrence and poor prognosis in HNSCC.[7,8] This may imply a lack of growth control due to loss of multiple tumor suppressor genes.

TUMOR KINETICS

The growth of a tumor is determined by the proportion of cells dividing and the rate of cell division adjusted for the rate of cell death. There is a complex interplay of various factors that may influence these rates. Inherent characteristics of the tumor will be perhaps the most influential factors, but external factors, such as the presence of growth factors and oxygenation, play a significant role as well.

The proportion of tumor cells dividing determines, in part, the rate of tumor growth. The rate of DNA synthesis and cell division will also influence the rate of tumor growth. The following section describes measures of tumor proliferation and various molecular alterations that may influence proliferation.

The rate of cell death negatively impacts on tumor growth. Cell death may occur from necrosis or from apoptosis. Necrosis is seen after a cell is exposed to toxic stimuli or hypoxia. The result is loss of cellular membrane integrity, followed by swelling and lysis of the cell. The disintegrating cell induces an inflammatory response, distinctly different from apoptosis.

Apoptosis describes a genetically programmed sequence of events that results in cell death without induction of an inflammatory reaction. The hallmarks of apoptosis include DNA fragmentation, chromatin condensation, and breakup of the nuclear and cytoplasmic membranes with resulting formation of membrane-bound cellular fragments. These fragments, called apoptotic bodies, are then phagocytosed by adjacent cells or by macrophages.[9] The lack of cellular lysis prevents an inflammatory reaction from being induced.

Apoptosis is essential for normal development, acting as a system to allow sculpting of the organism. It also appears to act as a defense mechanism against viral infections by allowing the death of infected cells in an effort to prevent further dissemination of the virus to the rest of the organism. In terms of cancer development, apoptosis is protective when resulting in sacrifice of cells in which genetic aberrations exceed the cellular capabilities for DNA repair. Given this protective function, it is not surprising that cancers and viruses exhibit mechanisms for inhibiting apoptosis and thus increasing their own growth potential and survival. It has emerged recently that apoptosis is an important mechanism of tumor cell death after radiotherapy and chemotherapy.[10] We will discuss specific issues regarding apoptosis and HNSCC later.

PROLIFERATION

The proportion of cells cycling can be measured using proliferation markers Ki-67, proliferating cell nuclear antigen (PCNA), or flow cytometric methods. Immunohistochemical (IHC) staining for Ki-67 indicates the proportion of cells in cycle (ie, all phases except G0 stain positive). Immunostaining for PCNA reveals cells in late G1, S, and early G2. PCNA has shown correlation with flow cytometric assessment of S-phase fraction.[11] These IHC methods and flow cytometry can provide an estimate of the proportion of cells cycling at a single point in time.

Other methods of estimating proliferation include measurement of tritiated thymidine, iododeoxyuridine (IdUrd), and 5'-bromodeoxyuridine (BrdUrd) incorporation. These methods are considerably more complicated than immunohistochemical methods, but have the advantage of allowing calculations of tumor doubling time (T_{pot}) by measuring not only the proportion of cells cycling, but the rate of DNA synthesis. These methods thus allow assessment of the factors that impact positively on tumor kinetics. Unfortunately, no measure of apoptosis or necrosis is factored into these calculations of T_{pot}, so the resulting assessment may overestimate doubling time.

Proliferation assessment using PCNA has been shown to be a useful marker of malignant transformation. A series of mucosal biopsies showing various degrees of atypia were shown to demonstrate increased PCNA expression in the basal layer of normal epithelium of patients with head and neck squamous cell carcinoma (HNSCC) when compared to normal mucosa from nonsmokers. In the cancer patients, this staining extended to suprabasal layers in normal mucosa adjacent to tumors and PCNA staining increased as tissue progressed from normal epithelium to dysplasia to HNSCC. This increase was seen in labeling index as well as intensity of staining.[12]

Assessment of proliferation in tumors is complicated by the fact that proliferation appears to correspond to local tumor oxygenation. This is indicated by the concentration of proliferating cells surrounding tumor vessels in HNSCC.[13] An inverse relationship between Ki-67 staining and intercapillary distance has also been shown in esophageal carcinoma.[14] This relationship between vascular density (and presumably oxygenation) and proliferation may be a factor that explains data showing increased radioresponsiveness in oral cancers having high PCNA labeling indices.[15]

When more biologic measures of proliferation (using IdUrd) are used and T_{pot} calculated, tumors that have short doubling times appear to be more radioresistant.[16] However, the radioresistance of these fast growing tumors may be overcome by accelerated fractionation radiotherapy.[16,17] Thus, although tumors with an increased proportion of proliferating cells may be more vulnerable to treatment with radiotherapy, those with rapid doubling times (a calculation based on the proportion of cells dividing *and* the rate of DNA synthesis) may require more intensive treatment schedules to overcome tumor cell repopulation.

Further complicating our understanding of the role of proliferation markers and tumor behavior are data showing that metastatic disease in larynx carcinoma is correlated with increased expression of PCNA and MIB1 (Ki-67).[18] Whether metastatic potential is mechanistically related to increased proliferation is not known.

Internal Regulation of Proliferation—Cell Cycle Control

Cell cycle regulation is determined by the interplay of positive and negative forces on the cell cycle. The majority of this regulation occurs in G1, as preparations for DNA synthesis (S-phase) are underway. The decision to proceed with cell division occurs near the G1-S interface with an irreversible point beyond which division will occur regardless of the presence of growth factors or other cellular nutrients. Although cell cycle regulation in a normal cell will be controlled by such mechanisms as contact inhibition or a lack of adequate growth factors, malignant cells appear less sensitive to these influences. Oncogenes and tumor suppressor genes are critical components in the regulation of the cell cycle and most appear to act during G1.

Cyclin D1

The cyclin D1 protein is one member of a family of proteins that contribute to cell cycle regulation. Cyclins can be broadly characterized as mitotic or G1 cyclins depending on the cell cycle phase in which they exert their predominant effect. Cyclin D1 is one of several G1 cyclins and is essential for cellular progression through late G1. It has an affinity for PCNA, cyclin dependent kinase (CDK4), and p21 and with these proteins regulates phosphorylation of Rb. This phosphorylation of Rb releases Rb-regulated cell cycle inhibition.

Overexpression of cyclin D1 has been associated with an acceleration of G1[19] and cyclin D1 induces malignant transformation in concert with both Ha-ras[20] and adenovirus E1A[21] oncogenes. Overexpression of cyclin D1 protein or mRNA has been shown in a diverse array of tumor types including HNSCC[22,23], breast cancer[24,25], esophageal cancers,[26] and mantle cell lymphomas.[27] In HNSCC, the mechanism underlying this overexpression appears to be amplification of the cyclin D1 gene although other mechanisms may also play a role.[23,28] Cyclin D1 is coded for by the CCND1 gene located at chromosome 11q13 tumors, an area known to be involved in translocations in certain lymphomas (also resulting in cyclin D1 overexpression)[27] and amplifications in HNSCC and other carcinomas.[29]

Although the logical effect of cyclin D1 overexpression in cancers would be to increase cell cycle progression, cyclin D1 and tumor proliferation are not consistently correlated. Proliferation measured by PCNA has shown a correlation with CCND1 amplification.[30] Unfortunately, the interaction between cyclin D1 and PCNA in Rb phosphorylation may show a flaw in attempting to estimate proliferation using PCNA. Using Ki-67 labeling index as a measure of proliferation, we compared CCND1 gene amplification to proliferation in a group of 43 HNSCC tumors and did not find correlation (Davidson, unpublished data). Comparison between cyclin D1 protein expression and labeling index measured by IdUrd has also shown no correlation.[31] However, the same study reported a correlation between cyclin D1 expression and apoptosis, a relationship suggesting perhaps an as yet undefined role for cyclin D1 in the apoptotic pathway of cell death.[31]

Clinical correlation with cyclin D1 overexpression or with 11q13 or CCND1 amplification contributes to our understanding of the causes and consequences of this molecular alteration (see Table 2–2). We have

TABLE 2-2. Clinical correlation with cyclin D1 amplification in HNSCC

Clinical Correlation	Reference
HNSCC	
Tobacco exposure	23,32
Poor differentiation	22
Diffuse invasion pattern	22
Hypopharynx primary site	22
Larynx Cancer	
T4 primary disease	33
Nodal metastases	33
Decreased survival	34

shown a correlation between tobacco exposure and CCND1 amplification and cyclin D1 mRNA overexpression in HNSCC.[23] Others have described supporting data using another genetic probe from chromosome band 11q13.[32] This may describe one molecular pathway linking risk factor exposure to transformation.

The relationships between tumor behavior and CCND1 amplification and/or expression have also been investigated. These include correlation with hypopharynx primary site, poor tumor differentiation, and diffusely infiltrative growth pattern for a diverse group of head and neck tumors.[22] In studies looking at larynx cancer alone, correlation has been shown between CCND1 amplification and T4 primary disease and nodal disease.[33] Others have noted that decreased overall survival in larynx cancer was associated with advanced T stage and with CCND1 amplification in both univariate and multivariable analyses.[34]

Thus CCND1 amplification has been correlated with increased proliferation as measured by PCNA in HNSCC tumors. However, no correlation with Ki-67 or IdUrd has been shown. Whether any one molecular abnormality can be found to show correlation with overall tumor proliferation is doubtful given the variety of mutations that each tumor possesses. The correlation between CCND1 and site, invasion pattern, grade, and survival are noteworthy, but do not appear to follow directly from any effect of cyclin D1 overexpression on proliferation. The recently described association between CCND1 amplification and apoptosis raises further questions about the effects of cyclin D1 overexpression in HNSCC. Although this molecular abnormality mechanistically would appear to relate to proliferation, the clinical correlation that has emerged raises questions about tumor differentiation, invasion, and apoptosis. How these various factors relate to cyclin D1 is an area that merits further investigation.

p53

The tumor suppressor gene p53 has received a great deal of attention in the past decade. First thought to act as an oncogene, p53 was later shown to perform a regulatory function at the G1-S transition by controlling a cell cycle checkpoint. Cellular injury induced by radiotherapy and other insults triggers p53 activation and a cell cycle block allowing DNA repair (or apoptosis if cellular damage is severe). The importance of normal p53 function is underscored by the fact that it is the single most commonly identified mutation among all cancers. Individuals with an inherited mutation of one p53 allele (Li-Fraumini syndrome) are at high risk of developing sarcomas, breast cancer and other tumors.[35] Although these patients with an inherited p53 mutation constitute a small fraction of cancer patients, acquired p53 mutations would appear to be common in many tumor types. In patients with HNSCC, p53 mutations have been found in 42–69% of tumors.[36,37]

Dysfunction of p53 may be caused by mutation of the gene resulting in a truncated or altered protein with loss of cell cycle checkpoint activities. Other mechanisms of p53 dysfunction may be posttranslational as the E6 protein of human papilloma virus (HPV) has shown the ability to block p53 protein function and accelerate p53 degradation.

The majority of investigations looking at p53 abnormalities in HNSCC have utilized IHC staining for the p53 protein. The normal protein has a short half-life so detection of p53 protein by IHC is assumed to represent a mutated version of the protein. Unfortunately, the correlation between p53 overexpression and p53 mutations as detected by molecular methods is weak with significant false positive and false negative assessments using IHC methods.[38]

Both p53 overexpression[39-41] and mutations[42] have been reported in premalignant lesions with overexpression reported in 31–50% and p53 mutations noted in 19%. p53 overexpression by IHC has been investigated in laryngeal lesions as a marker for risk of progression to invasive cancer. A series of patients with multiple laryngeal biopsies were assessed for markers of progression. The biopsies of patients who later progressed to cancer were compared with biopsies from a control group who did not develop cancer. Atypia, p53 staining, cyclin D1 staining, and epidermal growth factor receptor staining were all noted to predict transformation. Although assessment of atypia is a standard pathologic practice, about one third of patients who progressed to cancer had no atypia on earlier biopsies. Thus, p53 and these other markers may have a role as adjuvant measures of malignant potential.[43]

Although a significant proportion of HNSCC tumors demonstrate abnormal p53 expression and/or p53 mutations, the effects of p53 dysfunction on tumor cell behavior are not well defined. This may be because of the dual functions of p53 as a cell cycle checkpoint regulator and as a component of the apoptotic pathway. Because a loss of checkpoint control might allow uncontrolled cell cycling, the correlation between p53 abnormalities and increased proliferation has been investigated. Several studies have compared p53 expression by IHC to proliferation markers. Although correlations with PCNA[44,45] and with Ki-67[46] have been reported, others have failed to show correlations with PCNA.[46,47] No correlation between p53 expression and S-phase fraction[46,48] or IdUrd[47] has been shown; and in a study using BrdUrd to estimate labeling index and T_{pot}, no correlation with p53 expression was seen.[49] Likewise, no correlation has been shown between p53 mutations in HNSCC and assessment of proliferation with PCNA or IdUrd.[50] Thus, the majority of evidence would not support a correlation between p53 abnormalities and tumor proliferation.

As with cyclin D1, the correlation between p53 and risk factor exposure has been investigated. p53 overexpression[51] and p53 mutations[42] have both been correlated with history of tobacco use. Alcohol use has also been correlated with these p53 abnormalities. The prevalence of p53 mutations in HNSCC tumors from individuals with no risk factor exposure is <5%, but rises to 33% in individuals with tobacco-only exposure and to 58% in individuals with tobacco and alcohol exposures.[42]

Despite extensive investigations to determine the clinical significance of p53 abnormalities on HNSCC behavior, little correlation with respect to natural history and prognosis has been shown (see Table 2–3). A reported association between p53 mutations and stage IV HNSCC tumors[52] has not been

TABLE 2–3. Clinical correlation with p53 mutation in HNSCC

Clinical Correlation	Reference
Tobacco exposure	37
High T stage	52
Radioresistance (for p53 expression if labeling index<20%)	56
Increased locoregional recurrence (for patients treated with radiotherapy)	53

verified by others.[53] Likewise, a trend associating p53 mutations with poorly differentiated tumors[54] has not been supported by other work.[53]

Comparisons of p53 abnormalities and radiation sensitivity have led to conflicting results. No correlation was shown between p53 expression and local control in patients treated with accelerated fractionation radiotherapy.[49] Similarly, analysis of p53 mutations in a series of HNSCC cell lines also failed to show correlation with radiation sensitivity.[55] In contrast, however, a group of patients treated with conventional radiotherapy with or without brachytherapy showed decreased radiotherapy response in patients with low (<20%) Ki-67 labeling index and increased p53 expression using both univariate and multivariable analyses.[56] Radioresistance was indicated by a decreased likelihood of local control. HNSCC tumors in patients treated with primary or adjuvant radiotherapy have been assessed for p53 mutations and shown a correlation between mutations and an increased likelihood of locoregional failure. Although the overall survival was no different between the groups, locoregional failure was seen in 48% of tumors with p53 mutations and only 26% of those with wild-type p53.[53]

In summary, p53 has functional implications for cell cycle control, but this does not appear to be reflected in altered proliferation. p53 overexpression and p53 mutations appear in a subset of premalignant lesions and in about half of all HNSCC tumors. They are associated with tobacco and alcohol exposure and thus again describe a pathway linking risk factor exposure to malignant transformation. No correlation between p53 abnormalities and the natural history of HNSCC tumors can be shown, but response to conventional radiotherapy may be correlated with p53 abnormalities. This may reflect the apoptotic pathway functions of p53 and the importance of apoptosis in radiotherapy response rather than any direct effect of p53 on tumor behavior.

9p21

A region of the genome shown to be altered frequently in HNSCC is 9p21. This area shows loss of heterozygosity in about 70% of HNSCC tumors and in a similar proportion of lesions showing severe dysplasia and carcinoma in situ.[57] This suggests that loss of genes at 9p21 is a very early molecular event in carcinogenesis. Loss of heterozygosity is usually indicative of a tumor suppressor gene in the region, so an effort has been ongoing to identify such a gene. The gene considered most likely to be involved has been the putative tumor suppressor gene p16/MTS1/CDKN2. This protein acts as an inhibitor of cyclin D-CDK interaction with the Rb protein, thus indirectly controlling cell cycle progression. The gene has been shown to block S-phase entry and inhibit tumor proliferation in vitro and in vivo.[58] Low expression or mutation of p16 has been suggested to allow uncontrolled cell growth by removing this inhibition.

While frequent LOH was shown at 9p21 in allelotype analyses and MTS1 was mutated in 44% of HNSCC cell lines, few primary tumors showed these mutations.[59] Sequencing analysis of MTS1 in primary tumors has also failed to show frequent mutations of this gene.[60] This may indicate that other mechanisms may be contributing to p16 dysfunction. Homozygous deletions have been detected in a significant number of these tumors.[61] Another possible mechanism is through codominant tumor suppression with mutation of only one allele required for loss of p16 function. Another possible mechanism is through hypermethylation of a 5' CpG island resulting in a lack of gene transcription.[62] Still, an alternative explanation is that another, as yet undiscovered, 9p21 tumor suppressor gene exists.[63]

Correlation between 9p21 deletion and clinical behavior of tumors has been suggested. 9p deletion has been associated with poor prognosis in acute lymphoblastic leukemia[64] and aggressive biologic behavior in bladder cancer.[65] In HNSCC, loss of heterozygosity at 9p21 has correlated with an increased recurrence rate.[66] The pattern of loss at 9p21 suggests that a tumor suppressor gene other than MTS1 may determine this association.

External Regulation of Proliferation—Growth Factors and Signaling Pathways

In normal cells, proliferation is controlled by external cellular signals. These include contact inhibition and the influence of growth factor stimulation as well as extracellular growth inhibitors. Tumor cells have acquired the ability to proliferate despite these stimuli. Examples of factors that are critical to extracellular-intracellular signaling in head and neck cancers are TGF-α, TGF-β (a growth inhibitor), EGFR, and HER2/neu/erbB2.

EGFR and TGF-α

EGFR is a 170 kilodalton glycoprotein which is found at the cellular membrane of many tumor tissues. It spans the membrane exhibiting an extracellular binding domain and an intracellular domain with tyrosine kinase activity. Ligands that bind to the extracellular domain include EGF and TGF-α. Binding of these ligands to EGFR results in tyrosine kinase activity and stimulates cellular growth and proliferation. TGF-α has been found in a variety of tumors including HNSCC.[67,68] Increased TGF-α is usually accompanied by increased EGFR expression and this has suggested an autocrine regulatory mechanism for these two proteins.[68]

Increased expression of EGFR and TGF-α mRNA has been shown in tumor tissue and in the normal mucosa of patients with HNSCC when compared to normal mucosa from patients without HNSCC.[69] This suggests that increased expression of EGFR and TGF-α is an early marker of carcinogenesis. A moderate upregulation of EGFR has been shown in normal tissue adjacent to HNSCC with a further upregulation upon transition from dysplasia to invasive carcinoma demonstrating a two-step process in EGFR dysregulation.[70] Immunohistochemical staining to localize the cells of origin of EGFR and TGF-α have shown them to be localized primarily to the epithelium in "normal" mucosa from HNSCC patients and at the advancing margins of HNSCC tumor tissue.[71]

The impact of these two proteins on tumor behavior is not clearly elucidated. A correlation between EGF and EGFR levels and PCNA has been reported in laryngeal lesions.[72] Cancers with elevated expression of both EGF and EGFR show significantly higher PCNA labeling implying higher proliferation levels.[72] Higher EGFR expression was seen in tumors classified as T3–4 and stages III–IV compared to less advanced tumors. This may reflect the clinical impact of EGFR expression on tumor proliferation, but data supporting such an effect are lacking.

EGFR expression has been correlated with survival in a prospective trial in which approximately two thirds of the patients were treated with cisplatin and 5-fluorouracil.[73] Here increased expression was seen in tumors when compared to normal mucosa of cancer patients. No correlation was seen between chemotherapy response and EGFR espression. In multivariate analysis, EGFR and stage were independent predictors of overall survival whereas EGFR alone correlated with relapse-free survival.[73]

HER2/neu/c-erbB-2

C-erbB-2 shows significant homology to EGFR and like EGFR is a transmembrane glycoprotein with tyrosine kinase activity. Significant correlations are emerging between c-erbB-2 expression and aggressive growth characteristics. In particular, an increase in metastatic potential has been suggested and is discussed below.

DIFFERENTIATION

Normal mucosa of the head and neck is stratified squamous epithelium, whereas malignant mucosa exhibits various degrees of squamous differentiation. Altered differentiation is thus a component of malignant transformation and efforts have focused on assessing the changes that occur. Once malignant transformation has occurred, tumor differentiation can be classified and most HNSCC meet criteria for moderately or poorly differentiated squamous cell cancer. Although these tumors show variations in degree of differentiation, there does not appear to be a correlation between differentiation and proliferation or calculated tumor doubling time.[74] In support of this, verrucous carcinoma, a well-differentiated HNSCC, has been shown to have a high labeling index and short tumor doubling time.[74] This is particularly interesting when one considers that verrucous carcinomas usually follow a relatively noninvasive course and are considered radioresistant.[75]

Cytokeratins

Markers of differentiation include cytokeratins, involucrin, and transglutaminase. Cytokeratins (CK) are a family of intermediate filaments that are markers of squamous differentiation. The family consists of at least 19 members and the pattern of expression appears to correlate with the type of epithelial differentiation.[76] CK 1 and 19 appear to be markers of carcinogenesis in head and neck aerodigestive mucosa[77] with CK 19 associated with dysplasia.[78] CK 16 has been associated with increased proliferation.[79] An increase in CK 16 and 19 has been shown in the "normal" mucosa of HNSCC patients when compared to normal controls.[80] Low CK 13 expression has been correlated with resistance to growth inhibition from retinoic acid treatment.[81]

Analysis of CK 8 and 18 in a diverse array of squamous cell carcinomas has noted variable expression of these cytokeratins depending on the tissue of origin. Tumors developing through squamous metaplasia of nonsquamous epithelium (eg, lung) tend to show more intense expression than those developing from preexisting squamous epithelium (eg, floor of mouth).[82] In all sites, these CK 8 and 18 are maximally expressed at the invasion front of squamous cancers and at areas of tumor-stroma contact indicating that these cytokeratins are influenced by paracrine effects.[82]

Retinoids

Retinoids have emerged as promising chemopreventive agents due in part to their ability to control cell differentiation. Retinoids show the ability to inhibit abnormal squamous differentiation in cultured keratinocytes and squamous cell carcinoma.[83,84] 13-cis retinoic acid has shown clinical efficacy in preventing malignant transformation of aerodigestive tract mucosa as demonstrated by fewer second primary malignancies in HNSCC patients treated with this retinoid after curative treatment of an initial primary cancer.[85,86]

The activity of retinoids is mediated through nuclear retinoid receptors. These receptors are classified as RARs or RXRs and further identified by #, *, and ♦ subtypes. RAR-* appears to play a significant role in the malignant transformation of HNSCC. In-situ hybridization of head and neck mucosal tissues ranging from normal to malignant has been performed for various retinoic acid receptor (RAR) mRNA transcripts. RAR-# and RAR-* are more frequently expressed in normal mucosa than in malignant mucosa, but this difference is significant only for RAR-*. Expression of RAR-* mRNA can be detected in the mucosa of all normal volunteers, 70% of the normal mucosa from patients with head and neck squamous cell cancer, 56% of the dysplastic mucosa from these cancer patients, and 36% of the tumor specimens.[87] This decreased expression of RAR-* may play a functional role in the development of head and neck squamous cell carcinoma. Treatment of premalignant oral lesions with isotretinoin is associated with upregulation of RAR-* expression and correlation is seen between this expression and clinical response.[88] Thus, a reduction in RAR-■ expression can be correlated with malignant transformation and prevention of transformation using isotretinoin may occur through upregulation of RAR-■ expression.

APOPTOSIS

In terms of cancer treatment, apoptosis has emerged as a major cause of cell death after radiotherapy or chemotherapy.[10] Appreciation of the importance of apoptosis as a mechanism in tumor control has led to attempts to predict apoptotic potential. Two genes that appear to play a major role in regulation of apoptosis are bcl-2 and p53. The possibility of stimulating apoptosis in HNSCC is being investigated using gene therapeutic methods.

bcl-2

Bcl-2 was initially identified as a putative oncogene in follicular lymphomas with 14:18 translocations.[89] It was later shown to be the first gene implicated in apoptosis regulation.[90] It acts as a negative regulator of apoptosis through two mechanisms. It shows the ability to prolong survival of noncycling cells as well as prevent apoptosis in cells in cycle.[90] Bcl-2 does not appear to have any direct effects on proliferation. Apoptotic repression by bcl-2 expression has been suggested to be related to regulation of calcium transport or through antioxidant pathways associated with increased thiol levels.[10]

As noted previously for cyclin D1 and p53 abnormalities, correlation between tobacco exposure and bcl-2 has been reported. Bcl-2 protein overexpression measured by IHC has also been correlated with increased pack-years of smoking and 9 of 10 nonsmokers were bcl-2 negative.[91] This correlation adds yet another molecular linkage between tobacco exposure and HNSCC (see Table 2–4).

Whether there is any clinical significance to bcl-2 overexpression in carcinoma is not yet clear. In surgically treated esophageal squamous cell carcinoma, a correlation with poorly differentiated tumors has been shown, but a relationship to survival has not.[92] In surgically treated non-small cell lung cancer (NSCLC), correlation between increased bcl-2 expression and improved survival has been reported.[93,94]

In contrast to these series, bcl-2 has been correlated with decreased survival in patients treated with radiotherapy for HNSCC.[95] By both univariate and multivariable analyses, bcl-2 overexpression was

TABLE 2–4. Clinical correlation with bcl-2 in HNSCC

Clinical Correlation	Reference
Risk Factors	
Tobacco exposure	91
Radiotherapy	
Decreased disease-free survival	95
Decreased overall control	95
Accelerated fractionation radiotherapy	
Increased local control	96
Increased overall survival	96

associated with decreased overall and disease-free survival, suggesting perhaps a radioprotective effect of apoptosis repression through bcl-2 expression.[95] In contrast, however, bcl-2 expression has been associated with improved local control and survival in HNSCC patients treated with accelerated fractionation radiotherapy.[96] The strength of this association, however, may be limited by the fact that most cases with increased bcl-2 expression were N0, diploid, and fast growing.[96] Thus, although the function of bcl-2 is to repress apoptosis, and apoptosis is a significant mechanism of chemotherapeutic or radiotherapeutic cell killing, the clinical findings noted above would imply contradictory effects of bcl-2 overexpression on radiosensitivity in HNSCC.

p53 in Apoptosis

While p53 has been discussed above with respect to cell cycle regulation and G1 arrest, a second function of p53 is to stimulate apoptosis in cells that have been irradiated or otherwise undergone significant DNA damage. G1 arrest and induction of apoptosis through p53-dependent pathways appear to be independent events and may be related to the environmental and intracellular conditions at hand (reviewed in [97]). Investigations of chemosensitivity using a variety of agents and cell lines have shown sublethal doses of chemotherapy to result in G1 arrest, whereas lethal doses are associated with apoptosis. This would imply that cellular response (arrest or apoptotic death) is dependent on the degree of DNA damage.[98] In addition, p53-independent apoptosis may occur; however, transgenic animals with absence of both p53 alleles are unable to carry out apoptosis or G1 arrest.[99,100]

In support of a relationship between p53 status and radioresponsiveness, data reported above correlate p53 mutations in HNSCC with decreased locoregional control in patients treated with primary or adjuvant radiotherapy.[53] An increase in locoregional recurrences may be the result of defective apoptotic cell death in these p53 mutated tumors.

The clinical significance of p53 apoptosis appears to be emerging from studies designed to increase apoptosis in HNSCC through transfection of tumor cells with wild-type p53. Growth suppression of HNSCC from wild-type p53 transfection has been shown in vitro and in vivo and the predominant mechanism appears to be apoptosis.[101] This has been tested in vivo as a way to treat microscopic residual carcinoma[102] and is currently being investigated in a phase I trial of refractory HNSCC. Wild-type p53 transfection using transferrin-liposomal complexes or adenoviral vectors has also been shown to increase the radioresponsiveness of HNSCC cell lines.[103,104] Translation of this work to clinical investigations is underway.

INVASION AND METASTASIS

Normal epithelial cellular behavior requires cellular adhesion and migration, both for fetal development and wound healing, but invasion of basement membrane and underlying vasculature and lymphatic channels is distinctive of the disordered cellular behavior seen in malignancy. The basement membrane consists of type IV collagen, laminin, and proteoglycans and its breakdown is essential as part of the invasion process. Basement membrane breakdown involves a number of hydrolases including urokinase and several collagenases.

Urokinase

Urokinase-type plasminogen activator controls the synthesis of plasmin from zymogen plasminogen. Plasmin, a serine protease, acts on basement membrane in two ways. It is able to degrade laminin, one component of the basement membrane, and plasmin also activates type IV collagenases, further contributing to basement membrane breakdown. Urokinase-type plasminogen activator is produced in cutaneous and oral squamous cell carcinoma[105,106] and has been associated with poorly differentiated, but not well-differentiated, carcinoma.[107] The importance of urokinase on tumor cell invasion has been suggested by the ability of urokinase-directed antibodies to block migration of oral cancer cells through a matrix-coated filter in vitro.[106]

Collagenase

The collagenase family is a group of metalloproteinases (MMP) that demonstrate various activities. MMP-2 and MMP-9 are type IV collagenases; other members of this family (eg, MMP-1) show type I collagenase activity. A subgroup of this family of enzymes are the stromolysins, which show activity against several components of the basement membrane.

Type IV Collagenase

MMP-9. MMP-9 is a 92 kilodalton type IV collagenase that may contribute to basement membrane breakdown. Evidence for its involvement in HNSCC includes the presence of MMP-9 mRNA and protein in oral cavity carcinoma.[108] An inhibitor of MMP-9, TIMP-2, can block invasion in vitro.[108] MMP-9 expression and collagenase activity have been shown to be induced by a soluble protein derived from fibroblasts. This paracrine pathway may explain why MMP-9 expression is greatest in tumor cells found at the tumor-stromal interface.[109]

MMP-2. MMP-2 is a 72 kilodalton enzyme which, like MMP-9, also shows the ability to degrade type IV collagenase. Unlike MMP-9, however, this enzyme is synthesized in peritumor stromal cells rather than in tumor cells.[110] This reveals the interaction between tumor cells and stromal cells that may exist in vivo. Specifically, tumor cells may take advantage of existing collagenase cascades to allow basement membrane breakdown and invasion. Presumably these intercellular cascades are present in normal cells to allow the cooperation between cells necessary for fetal development or wound healing. Malignant tumors have developed mechanisms for utilizing these cascades for basement membrane invasion.

Type I Collagenase

In addition to the capability to invade basement membrane, tumor cells require the ability to degrade fibrillar collagen, which comprises the extracellular matrix of the interstitial space. The presence of type I collagenase mRNA has been found in 80% of HNSCC tumors, but rarely in normal mucosa.[111] This collagenase mRNA was found to be expressed primarily in the stromal cells at the leading edge of tumors,[112,113] with expression in scattered HNSCC tumor cells as well.[113]

Stromolysin

The stromolysin family of collagenases shows overlap with the metalloproteinases and shows broad activity against components of the basement membrane. MMP-3, also known as stromolysin-1, can degrade type IV collagen, laminin, proteoglycans, and fibronectin and also can activate procollagenase. Although stromolysin-1 has not been identified in HNSCC,[113] stromolysin-2 and -3 have been found. Stromolysin-2 has been investigated in HNSCC revealing expression in over 50% of tumors.[111] High expression of stromolysin-2 correlated with increased expression of type I collagenases and was associated with increased local invasion.[111] In situ hybridization studies of HNSCC tumors have shown detectable stromolysin-2 expression in tumor cells as well as in stromal cells adjacent to tumor.[114]

Stomolysin-3 is found in 95% of HNSCC tumors. Unlike stromolysin-2, however, expression of stromolysin-3 is confined to peritumor stromal cells. This pattern of expression suggests paracrine pathways of intercellular signaling between tumor cells and surrounding stroma. Tumors with increased expression of this stromolysin mRNA show increased local invasion.[113]

c-erbB-2

Although urokinase and the collagenases noted above appear to be involved in tumor invasion, other proteins have been correlated to metastasis. C-erbB-2 is a transmembrane protein that appears to be linked to metastatic potential. It is variously known as c-erbB-2, her-2, and neu and shows significant homology to EGFR. This transmembrane protein also demonstrates tyrosine kinase activity suggesting a role in intracellular signaling. C-erB-2 promotes multiple adhesion and invasion steps of the metastatic cascade. Clayman has demonstrated increased chemotaxis in vitro of cells transfected to overexpress c-erbB-2.[115] These same transfects showed increased growth rate and increased lymph node metastases in a nude mouse model. Urokinase and MMP-9 induction were demonstrated in this model, implicating involvement of other members of the metastatic cascade

Several studies have attempted to define clinicopathologic findings in HNSCC with respect to c-erbB-2 expression. Xia has shown an inverse correlation between c-erb-2 expression in oral cavity squamous cell carcinoma and survival.[116] This same study showed a correlation with nodal positivity and metastatic disease. Others have failed to show clinical correlation between c-erbB-2 expression and clinical features.[117,118] However, in a series of low T stage, node negative oral carcinomas, Clayman showed direct correlation between c-erbB-2 expression and the risk of death from disease.[115]

SUMMARY

We have attempted here to describe advances in our understanding of the biology of HNSCC. Through molecular biologic investigations, the mechanisms of malignant transformation were described. These include dysregulation of PCNA, TGF-#, EGFR, and loss of tumor suppressor activity at 9p21. Other molecular events such as cyclin D1 amplification, p53 mutations, and bcl-2 overexpression appear to occur later but are correlated with history of tobacco exposure. With the exception of cyclin D1 and c-erbB-2, most molecular events do not directly correlate with staging or prognostic information.

The process of apoptosis has been the focus of significant investigation and has emerged as perhaps the most important factor in radiation and chemotherapy sensitivity in HNSCC. The molecular events associated with apoptotic potential, p53 mutation, and perhaps bcl-2 overexpression are emerging as significant events in the molecular characterization of HNSCC due to their impact on radiation and chemotherapy sensitivity. Finally, molecular advances in the field of gene therapy show great potential for allowing us to manipulate the apoptotic potential of tumors and improve disease control.

REFERENCES

1. Pindborg JJ, Renstrup G, Joist O, Roed-Petersen B. Studies in oral leukoplakia: a preliminary report on the period prevalence of malignant transformation on leukoplakia based on a followup study of 248 patients. *JADA*. 1968;76:767–771.
2. Mincer HH, Coleman SA, Hopkins KP. Observations on the clinical characteristics of oral lesions showing histologic epithelial dysplasia. *Oral Surg*. 1972;33:389–399.
3. Silverman S, Gorsky M, Lozada F. Oral leukoplakia and malignant transformation—a follow-up study of 257 patients. *Cancer*. 1984;53:563–568.
4. Parker SL, Tong T, Bolden S, Wingo PA. Cancer statistics, 1997. *CA Cancer J Clin*. 1997;47:5–27.
5. Renan MJ. How many mutations are required for tumorigenesis? Implications from human cancer data. *Mol Carcinog*. 1993;7:139–146.

6. Califano J, van der Riet P, Westra W, et al. Genetic progression model for head and neck cancer: implications for field cancerization. *Cancer Res.* 1996;56:2488–2492.
7. Lydiatt WM, Davidson BJ, Shah JP, Schantz SP. The relationship of loss of heterozygosity to tobacco exposure and early recurrence in head and neck squamous cell carcinoma. *Am J Surg.* 1994;168:437–440.
8. Li X, Lee NK, Waber Y, Schweitzer C, Cheng Q, Nisen PD. Allelic loss at chromosomes 3p, 8p, 13q and 17p associated with poor prognosis in head and neck cancer. *JNCI.* 1994;86:1524–1529.
9. Wyllie AH, Kerr JFR, Currie AR. Cell death: the significance of apoptosis. *Int Rev Cytol.* 1980;68:251–306.
10. Meyn RE, Stephens LC, Milas L. Programmed cell death and radioresistance. *Cancer Metastasis Rev.* 1996;15:119–131.
11. Garcia RL, Coltrera MD, Gown AM. Analysis of proliferative grade using anti-PCNA/cyclin monoclonal antibodies in fixed embedded tissues. Comparison with flow cytometric analysis. *Am J Path.* 1989;134:833–838.
12. Shin DM, Voravud N, Ro JY, Lee JS, Hong WK, Hittelman WN. Sequential increases in proliferating cell nuclear antigen expression in head and neck tumorigenesis: a potential biomarker. *JNCI.* 1993;85:971–978.
13. Edstrom SSF, Gustafsson B, Stenman G, Lyden E, Stein H, Westin T. Proliferative pattern of head and neck cancer. *Am J Surg.* 1991;162:412–416.
14. Porschen R, Classen S, Piontek M, Borchard F. Vascularization of carcinomas of the esophagus and its correlation with tumor proliferation. *Cancer Res.* 1994;54:587–591.
15. Gunzl H, Horn H, Schuke R, Donath K. Prognostic value of PCNA and cytokeratins for radiation therapy of oral squamous cell carcinoma. *Eur J Cancer Oral Oncol.* 1993;29b:141–145.
16. Begg AC, Hofland I, Moonen L, et al. The predictive value of cell kinetic measurements in a European trial of accelerated fractionation in advanced head and neck tumors: an interim report. *Int J Rad Onc Biol Phys.* 1990;19:1449–1453.
17. Horiot JC, Begg AC, Le Fur R, et al. Present status of EORTC trials of hyperfractionated and accelerated radiotherapy on head and neck carcinoma. *Recent Results Cancer Res.* 1994;134:111–119.
18. Franchi, A, Gallo, O, Boddi, V, Santucci, M. Prediction of occult neck metastases in laryngeal carcinoma: role of proliferating cell nuclear antigen, MIB-1, and E-cadherin immunohistochemical determination. *Clin Cancer Res.* 1996;2:1801–1808.
19. Quelle DE, Ashmun RA, Shurtleff SA, et al. Overexpression of mouse D-type cyclins accelerates G1 phase in rodent fibroblasts. *Genes and Dev.* 1993;7:1559–1571.
20. Lovec H, Sewing A, Lucibello FC, Muller R, Moroy T. Oncogenic activity of cyclin D1 revealed through cooperation with Hares: link between cell cycle control and malignant transformation. *Oncogene.* 1994;9:323–326.
21. Hinds PW, Dowdy SF, Eaton EN, Arnold A, Weinberg RA. Function of a human cyclin gene as an oncogene. *Proc Natl Acad Sci.* 1994;91:709–713.
22. Williams ME, Gaffey MJ, Weiss LM, Wilczynski SP, Schuuring E, Levine PA. Chromosome 11q13 amplification in head and neck squamous cell carcinoma. *Arch Otolaryngol Head Neck Surg.* 1993;119:1238–1243.
23. Davidson BJ, Lydiatt WL, Abate MP, Schantz SP, Chaganti RSK. Cyclin D1 abnormalities and tobacco exposure in head and neck squamous cell carcinoma. *Head Neck.* 1996;18:512–521.
24. Schuuring E, Verhoeven E, Van Tinteren H, et al. Amplification of genes within the chromosome 11q13 region is indicative of poor prognosis in patients with operable breast cancer. *Cancer Res.* 1992;52:5229–5234.
25. Buckley MF, Sweeney KJE, Hamiltin JA, et al. Expression and amplification of cyclin genes in human breast cancer. *Oncogene.* 1993;8:2127–2133.
26. Jiang W, Kahn SM, Tomita N, Zhang Y, Lu S, Weinstein B. Amplification and expression of the human cyclin D gene in esophageal cancer. *Cancer Res.* 1992;52:2980–2983.
27. Rosenberg CL, Wong E, Petty EM, et al. PRAD1, a candidate BCL1 oncogene: mapping and expression in centrocytic lymphoma. *Proc Natl Acad Sci.* 1991;88:9638–9642.
28. Gaffey MJ, Iezzoni JC, Meredith SD, et al. Cyclin D1 (PRAD1, CCND1) and glutathione-S-transferase pi gene expression in head and neck squamous cell carcinoma. *Hum Pathol.* 1995;26:1221–1226.
29. Lammie GA, Fantl V, Smith R, et al. D11S287, a putative oncogene on chromosome 11q13, is amplified and expressed in

squamous cell and mammary carcinomas and linked to BCL1. *Oncogene.* 1991;6:439–444.
30. Callender T, ElNaggar AK, Lee MS, Frankenthaler R, Luna MA, Batsakis JG. PRAD-1 (CCND1)/Cyclin D1 oncogene amplification in primary head and neck squamous cell carcinoma. *Cancer.* 1994;74:152–158.
31. Kotelnikiv VM, Coon JS, Mundle S, et al. Cyclin D1 expression in squamous cell carcinomas of the head and neck and in oral mucoas in relation to proliferation and apoptosis. *Clin Cancer Res.* 1997;3:95–101.
32. Volling P, Jungehulsing M, Jucker M, Stutzer H, Diehl V, Tesch H. Coamplification of the hst and bcl1 oncogenes in advanced squamous cell carcinomas of the head and neck. *Eur J Cancer.* 1993;29A:383–389.
33. Jares P, Fernandez PL, Campo E, et al. PRAD-1/Cyclin D1 gene amplification correlates with messenger RNA overexpression and tumor progression in human laryngeal carcinomas. *Cancer Res.* 1994;54:4813–4817.
34. Bellacosa A, Almadori G, Cavallo S, et al. Cyclin D1 gene amplification in human laryngeal squamous cell carcinomas: prognostic significance and clinical implications. *Clin Cancer Res.* 1996;2:175–180.
35. Levine AJ, Momand J, Finlay WM. The p53 tumor suppressor gene. *Nature.* 1991;351:453–456.
36. Ahomadegbe JC, Barrois M, Fogel S, et al. High incidence of p53 alterations (mutation, deletion, overexpression) in head and neck primary tumors and metastases; absence of correlation with clinical outcome. Frequent protein overexpression in normal epithelium and in early non-invasive lesions. *Oncogene.* 1995;10:1217–1227.
37. Brennan JA, Boyle JO, Koch WM, et al. Association between cigarette smoking and mutation of the p53 gene in squamous cell carcinoma of the head and neck. *N Engl J Med.* 1995;332:712–717.
38. Xu L, Chen YT, Huvos AG, et al. Overexpression of p53 protein in squamous cell carcinomas of head and neck without apparent gene mutation. *Diagnostic Mol Pathol.* 1994;3:83–92.
39. Girod SC, Pape HD, Krueger GR. p53 and PCNA expression in carcinogenesis of the oropharyngeal mucosa. *Eur J Cancer B Oral Oncol.* 1994;30b:419–423.
40. SC, Kramer C, Knufermann R, Krueger GRF. p53 expression in the carcinogenesis in the oral mucosa. *J Cell Biochem.* 1994;56:444–448.
41. Sauter ER, Cleveland D, Trock B, Ridge JA, Klein-Szanto AJP. p53 is overexpressed in fifty percent of preinvasive lesions of head and neck epithelium. *Carcinogenesis.* 1994;15:2269–2274.
42. Boyle JO, Hakim J, Koch W, et al. The incidence of p53 mutations increases with progression of head and neck cancer. *Cancer Res.* 1993;53:4477–4480.
43. Uhlman DL, Adams G, Knapp D, Aeppli DM, Niehan G. Immunohistochemical staining for markers of future neoplastic progression in the larynx. *Cancer Res.* 1996;56:2199–2205.
44. Gorgoulis V, Zoumpoulis V, Rassidakis G, et al. Molecular analysis of p53 gene in laryngeal premalignant and malignant lesions: p53 protein immunohistochemical expression is positively related to proliferating cell nuclear antigen labelling index. *Virchows Arch.* 1995;426:339–344.
45. Nishioka H, Hiasa Y, Hayashi I, Kitahori Y, Konishi N, Sugimura M. Immunohistochemical detection of p53 oncoprotein in human oral squamous cell carcinomas and leukoplakias: comparison with proliferating cell nuclear antigen and correlation with clinicopathologic findings. *Oncology.* 1993;50:426–429.
46. Frank JL, Bur ME, Garb JL, et al. p53 tumor suppressor oncogene expression in squamous cell carcinoma of the hypopharynx. *Cancer.* 1994;73:181–186.
47. Nylander K, Stenling R, Gustafsson H, Zackrisson B, Roos G. p53 expression and cell proliferation in squamous cell carcinomas of the head and neck. *Cancer.* 1995;75:87–93.
48. Nadal A, Campo E, Pinto J, et al. p53 expression in normal, dysplastic and neoplastic laryngeal epithelium. Absence of a correlation with prognostic factors. *J Path.* 1995;175:181–188.
49. Wilson GD, Richman PI, Dische S, et al. p53 status of head and neck cancer: relation to biologic characteristics and outcome of radiotherapy. *Br J Cancer.* 1995;71:1248–1252.
50. Nylander K, Nilsson P, Mehle C, Roos G. p53 mutations, protein expression and cell proliferation in squamous cell carcinomas of the head and neck. *Br J Cancer.* 1995;71:826–830.

51. Field JK, Zoumpourlis V, Spandidos DA, Jones AS. p53 expression and mutations in squamous cell carcinoma of the head and neck: expression correlates with the patients' use of tobacco and alcohol. *Cancer Detect Prevent.* 1994;18:197–208.
52. Nagai MA, Miracca EC, Yamamoto L, Kowalski LP, Brentani RR. TP53 mutations in upper aerodigestive squamous cell carcinomas from a group of Brazilian patients. *Am J Surg.* 1995;170:492–494.
53. Koch WM, Brennan JA, Zahurak M, et al. p53 mutation and locoregional treatment failure in head and neck squamous cell carcinoma. *JNCI.* 1996;88:1580–1586.
54. Sakai E, Rikimaru K, Ueda M, et al. The p53 tumorsuppressor gene and ras oncogene mutations in oral squamouscell carcinoma. *Int J Cancer.* 1992;52:867–872.
55. Brachman DG, Beckett M, Graves D, Haraf D, Vokes E, Weischelbaum RR. p53 mutations increases with progression of head and neck cancer. *Cancer Res.* 1993;53:3667–3669.
56. RaybaudDiogene H, Fortin A, Morency R, Roy J, Monteil RA, Tetu B. Markers of radioresistance in squamous cell carcinomas of the head and neck: a clinicopathologic and immunohistochemical study. *J Clin Oncol.* 1997;15:1030–1038.
57. van der Riet P, Nawroz H, Hruban RH, et al. Frequent loss of chromosome 9p21-22 early in head and neck cancer progression. *Cancer Res.* 1994;54:1156–1158.
58. Jin X, Nguyen D, Zhang W, Kyritsis AP, Roth JA. Cell cycle arrest and inhibition of tumor cell proliferation by the p16INK4 gene mediated by an adenovirus vector. *Cancer Res.* 1995;55:3250–3253.
59. Zhang S, KleinSzanto JP, Sauter ER, et al. Higher frequency of alterations in the p16/CDKN2 gene in squamous cell carcinoma cell lines than in late primary tumors of the head and neck. *Cancer Res.* 1994;54:5050–5053.
60. Cairns P, Mao L, Merlo A, et al. Rates of p16 (MTS1) mutations in primary tumors with 9p loss. *Science.* 1994;265:416.
61. Cairns P, Polasick TJ, Eby Y, et al. Frequency of homozygous deletion at p16/CDKN2 in primary tumor human tumors. *Nature Genetics.* 1995;11:210–212.
62. Merlo A, Herman JG, Mao L, et al. 5' CpG island methylation is associated with transcriptional silencing of the tumour suppressor p16/CDKN2/MTS1 in human cancers. *Nature Med.* 1995;7:686–692.
63. Lydiatt WM, Murty VVVS, Davidson BJ, et al. Homozygous deletions and loss of expression of the CDKN2 gene occurs frequently in head and neck squamous cell carcinoma cell lines but infrequently in primary tumors. *Genes Chromosom Cancer.* 1995;13:94–98.
64. Heyman M, Grander D, Brondum-Nielsen K, Liu Y, Soderhall S, Einhorn S. Deletions of the short arm of chromosome 9, including the interferon-alpha/beta genes, in acute lymphocytic leukemia. Studies on loss of heterozygosity, parental origin of deleted genes and prognosis. *Int J Cancer.* 1993;54:748–753.
65. Orlow I, Lianes P, Lacombe L, Dalbagni G, Reuter VE, Cordon-Cardo C. Chromosome 9 allelic losses and microsatellite alterations in human bladder tumors. *Cancer Res.* 1994;54:2848–2851.
66. Lydiatt WM, Davidson BJ, Schantz SP, Caruana S, Chaganti RSK. 9p21 deletion correlates with recurrence in head and neck cancer. *Head Neck.* 1997;(In press).
67. Todd R, Donoff BR, Gertz R, et al. TG-Falpha and EGF-receptor mRNA in human oral cancers. *Carcinogenesis.* 1989;10:1553–1556.
68. Derynck R, Goeddel DV, Ullrich A, et al. Synthesis of messenger RNAs for transforming growth factoralpha and beta by human tumors. *Cancer Res.* 1987;47:707–712.
69. Grandis JR, Tweardy DJ. Elevated levels of transforming growth factoralpha and epidermal growth factor receptor messenger RNA are early markers of carcinogenesis in head and neck cancer. *Cancer Res.* 1993;53:3579–3584.
70. Shin DM, Ro JY, Hong WK, Hittelman WN. Dysregulation of epidermal growth factor receptor in premalignant lesions during head and neck tumorigenesis. *Cancer Res.* 1994;54:3153–3159.
71. Grandis JR, Melhem MF, Barnes EL, Tweardy DJ. Quantitative immunohistochemical analysis of transforming growth factoralpha and epidermal growth factor receptor in patients with squamous cell carcinoma of the head and neck. *Cancer.* 1996;78:1284–1292.
72. Wen QH, Nishimura T, Miwa T, Nagayama I, Furukawa M. Expression of EGF, EGFR

and PCNA in laryngeal lesions. *J Laryngol Otol.* 1995;109:630–636.
73. Dassonville O, Formento JL, Francoual M, et al. Expression of epidermal growth factor receptor and survival in upper aerodigestive tract cancer. *J Clin Oncol.* 1993;11:1873–1878.
74. Dische S, Saunders MI, Bennett MH, Wilson GD, McNally NJ. Cell proliferation and differentiation in squamous cancer. *Radiother Oncol.* 1989;15:19–23.
75. Ferlito A, Recher G. Ackerman's tumor (verrucous carcinoma) of the larynx. *Cancer.* 1980;46:1617–1620.
76. Moll R, Franke WW, Schiller D. The catalog of human cytokeratins: patterns of expression in normal epithelial cells. *Cell.* 1982;31:11–24.
77. Linberg K, Rheinwald JG. Suprabasal 40kd keratin (K19): expression as immunohistological marker of premalignancy in oral epithelium. *Am J Pathol.* 1989;134:419–426.
78. Cintorino M, Petracca R, Vindigni C, Tripodi SA, Leoncini P. Topography-related expression of individual cytokeratins in normal and pathological (non-neoplastic and neoplastic) human oral mucosa. *Virchows Arch.* 1990;417:419–426.
79. Van Der Velden LA, Schaafsma E, Manni JJ, Ramaekers FCS, Kuypers W. Cytokeratin expression in normal and (pre)malignant head and neck epithelia: an overview. *Head Neck.* 1993;15:133–146.
80. Bongers V, Snow GB, De Vries N, Braakhuis BJM. Potential early markers of carcinogenesis in the mucosa of the head and neck using exfoliative cytology. *J Pathol.* 1996;178:284–289.
81. Kim SY, Berger D, Yim SO, Sacks PG, Tainsky MA. Coordinate control of growth and cytokeratin 13 expression by retinoic acid. *Mol Carcinog.* 1996;16:6–11.
82. Schaafsma HE, Van Der Velden LA, Manni JJ, et al. Increased expression of cytokeratins 8, 18 and vimentin in the invasion front of mucosal squamous cell carcinoma. *J Pathol.* 1993;170:77–86.
83. Gudas LJ, Sporn MB, Roberts AB. *The Retinoids: Biology, Chemistry, and Medicine*, New York: Raven Press; 1994:443.
84. Borden EC, Lotan R, Levens D, Young CW, Waxman S. Differentiation therapy of cancer: laboratory and clinical investigations. *Cancer Res.* 1993;53:4109–4115.
85. Benner SE, Pajak TF, Lippman SM, Earley C, Hong WK. Prevention of second primary tumors with isotretinoin in patients with squamous cell carcinoma of the head and neck: long-term follow-up. *JNCI.* 1994;86:140–141.
86. Hong WK, Lippman SM, Itri LM, et al. Prevention of second primary tumors with isotretinoin in squamouscell carcinoma of the head and neck. *N Engl J Med.* 1990;323:795–801.
87. Xu X, Ro JY, Lee JS, Shin DM, Hong WK, Lotan R. Differential expression of nuclear retinoid receptors in normal, premalignant, and malignant head and neck tissues. *Cancer Res.* 1994;54:3580–3587.
88. Lotan R, Xu XC, Lippman SM, et al. Suppression of retinoic acid receptor beta in premalignant oral lesions and its upregulation by isotretinoin. *N Engl J Med.* 1995;332:1405–1410.
89. Tsujimoto Y, Croce CM. Analysis of the structure, transcripts and protein products of bcl-2, the gene involved in human follicular lymphoma. *Proc Natl Acad Sci.* 1986;83:5214–5218.
90. Vaux DL, Cory S, Adams JM. Bcl-2 gene promotes haemophilus cell survival and cooperates with c-myc to immortalize pre-B cells. *Nature.* 1988;335:440–442.
91. Gallo O, Bianchi S, Porfirio B. Bcl-2 overexpression and smoking history in head and neck cancer. *JNCI.* 1995;87:1024–1025.
92. Sarbia M, Bittinger F, Porschen R, et al. bcl-2 expression and prognosis in squamous-cell carcinomas of the esophagus. *Int J Cancer.* 1996;69:324–328.
93. Ritter JH, Dresler CM, Wick MR. Expression of bcl-2 protein in stage T1N0M0 non-small cell lung carcinoma. *Hum Pathol.* 1995;26:1227–1232.
94. Pezzella F, Turley H, Kuzu I, et al. bcl-2 protein in non-small cell lung carcinoma. *N Engl J Med.* 1993;329:690–694.
95. Gallo O, Boddi V, Calzolari A, Simonetti L, Trovati M, Bianchi S. Bcl-2 protein expression correlates with recurrence and survival in early stage head and neck cancer treated by radiotherapy. *Cancer Res.* 1996;2:261–267.
96. Wilson GD, Grover R, Richman PI, Daley FM, Saunders MI, Dische S. Bcl-2 expression correlates with favourable outcome in head and neck cancer treated by accelerated radiotherapy. *Anticancer Res.* 1996;16(4c):2403–2408.

97. Hale AJ, Smith CA, Sutherland LC, et al. Apoptosis: molecular regulation of cell death. *Eur J Biochem.* 1996;236:1–26.
98. Wu GS, El-Diery WS. Apoptotic death of tumor cells correlates with chemosensitivity, independent of p53 or bcl-2. *Clin Cancer Res.* 1996;2:623–633.
99. Lowe S, Schmitt E, Osborne B, Jacks T. p53 is required for radiation-induced apoptosis in mouse thymocytes. *Nature.* 1993;362:847–849.
100. Clarke A, Purdie C, Harrison D, Morris R, Bird C. Thymocyte apoptosis induced by p53-dependent and independent pathways. *Nature.* 1993;362:849–852.
101. Liu TJ, Zhang WW, Taylor DL, Roth JA, Goepfert H, Clayman GL. Growth suppression of human head and neck cancer cells by the introduction of a wildtype p53 gene via a recombinant adenovirus. *Cancer Res.* 1994;54:3662–3667.
102. Clayman GL, El-Naggar AK, Roth JA, et al. In vivo molecular therapy with p53 adenovirus for microscopic residual head and neck squamous carcinoma. *Cancer Res.* 1995;55:1–6.
103. Xu L, Pirollo KF, Chang EH. Transferrin-liposome-mediated p53 sensitization of squamous cell carcinoma of the head and neck to radiation in vitro. *Human Gene Ther.* 1997;8:467–475.
104. Pirollo KF, Hao Z, Rait A, et al. p53 mediated sensitization of squamous cell carcinoma of the head and neck to radiotherapy. *Oncogene.* 1997;14:1735–1746.
105. Sappino A, Belin D, Huarte J, Hirschel-Scholz S, Saurat J, Vassalli J. Differential protease expression by cutaneous squamous and basal cell carcinomas. *J Clin Invest.* 1991; 88:1073–1079.
106. Clayman G, Wang SW, Nicolson GL, et al. Regulation of urokinase-type plasminogen activator expression is squamous cell carcinoma of the oral cavity. *Int J Cancer.* 1993; 54:73–80.
107. Miller SJ, Jensen PJ, Dzubow LM, Lazarus GS. Urokinase plasminogen activator is immunocytochemically detectable in squamous cell but not basal cell carcinomas. *J Invest Dermatol.* 1992;98:351–358.
108. Juarez J, Clayman G, Nakajima M, Tanube KK, Saya H, Nicolson GL. Role and regulation of expression of 92-kDa type IV collagenase (MMP-9) in 2 invasive squamous cell carcinoma cell lines of the oral cavity. *Int J Cancer.* 1993;55:10–18.
109. Lengyel E, Gum R, Juarez J, et al. Induction of M(r) 92,000 type IV collagenase expression in a squamous cell carcinoma cell line by fibroblasts. *Cancer Res.* 1995;55:963–967.
110. Pyke C, Palkiaer E, Huhtala P, Hurskainen T, Dano K, Tryggvason K. Localization of messenger RNA for Mr 72,000 and 92,000 type IV collagenase in human skin cancers by in situ hybridization. *Cancer Res.* 1992;52: 1336–1341.
111. Muller D, Breathnach R, Engelman A, et al. Expression of collagenase-related metalloproteinases genes in human lung or head and neck tumors. *Int J Cancer.* 1991;48: 550–556.
112. Gray ST, Wlikins RJ, Yun K. Interstitial collagenase gene expression in oral squamous cell carcinoma. *Am J Pathol.* 1992;141:301–306.
113. Muller D, Wolf C, Abecassis J, et al. Increased stromolysin 3 gene expression is associated with increased local invasion in head and neck squamous cell carcinomas. *Cancer Res.* 1993;53:165–169.
114. Polette M, Clavel C, Muller D, Abecassis J, Binninger I, Birembaut P. Detection of mRNAs encoding collagenase I and stromolysin 2 in carcinomas of the head and neck by in situ hybridization. *Invasion Metastasis.* 1991;11:76–83.
115. Clayman GL, Liu TJ, El-Naggar AK, Goepfert H. HER-2/neu oncogene as a regulator of aggressive phenotypic behavior in head and neck squamous cell carcinoma. In: Shah JP, Johnson JT, eds. *Proceedings of the 4th International Conference on Head and Neck Cancer.* Arlington, Va: Society of Head and Neck Surgeons; 1996:493–501.
116. Xia W, Lau Y, Zhang H, et al. Strong correlation between c-erbB-2 overexpression and overall survival of patients with oral squamous cell carcinoma. *Clin Cancer Res.* 1997; 3:3–9.
117. Craven JM, Pavelic ZP, Stambrook PJ, et al. Expression of c-erbB-2 gene in human head and neck carcinoma. *Anticancer Res.* 1992; 12(6B):2273–2276.
118. Field JK, Spandidos DA, Yiangnisis M, Gosney JR, Papadimitriou K, Stell PM. C-erbB-2 expression in squamous cell carcinoma of the head and neck. *Anticancer Res.* 1992;12(3):613–619.

CHAPTER 3

Hyperfractionated or Accelerated Radiation Therapy for Squamous Cell Carcinoma of the Head and Neck

James T. Parsons, MD, and William M. Mendenhall, MD

In the United States, radiation therapy for mucosal lesions of the head and neck is most often delivered with a continuous course of irradiation consisting of five 1.8- to 2-Gy fractions per week administered Monday through Friday. Deviations from this schedule have usually been done for one of three reasons:

1. Convenience. From a practical standpoint, both patient and physician want treatment to be completed in as short a time as is consistent with good results. Until the late 1970s, most clinical investigations of altered fractionation involved delivery of a reduced number of large-dose fractions, administered once, twice, or thrice weekly, or occasionally even single-dose therapy. Such treatment, known as "hypofractionation,"[1] is less expensive, results in less interruption of normal daily activities, and reduces the workload in a busy radiation therapy department.

Various methods have been devised through the years to mathematically equate these abbreviated treatment schedules with conventional fractionation schemes. The most commonly used method was the nominal standard dose (NSD) formula of Ellis.[2] Other investigators developed new fractionation schemes that produced equivalent acute reactions to those produced by conventional schemes on the assumption that late effects and tumor control would also be equivalent.

The majority of these fractionation schemes, whether devised mathematically or by matching acute reactions, have produced a high incidence of late complications.[3-12]

Despite the description of the dissociation between acute and late effects by Coutard in 1934,[13] this concept received little attention until the 1980s. It is now known that, as the size of the dose per fraction is reduced, there is a differential sparing of tissues responsible for late effects relative to those responsible for acute effects.[14] This greater sensitivity to changes in dose per fraction for late-effects tissues is believed to be due to differences in the shapes of the dose survival curves for late- versus acute-effects tissues. The curves for late-effects tissues are "curvier" and their #/∎ ratios are consistently lower than those of acute-effects tissues. If the dose survival characteristics of tumor cells resemble those of acutely responding normal cells, and if late injury in normal tissues is dose-limiting, then a therapeutic gain would result from reducing the dose per fraction. This is the rationale for hyperfractionation.[3]

2. *Patient comfort.* Large-volume treatment at 1.8–2 Gy per fraction, five fractions per week, to 60–75 Gy generally produces considerable mucositis. Several investigators have reported treatment results after irradiation with schemes designed to minimize acute side effects.

Andrews[5] reported National Cancer Institute (NCI) treatment results in patients with head and neck squamous cell carcinoma who received approximately 9000 R over 14 weeks (6 Gy per week) with three fractions per week. Such protracted treatment schedules produce little or no mucositis. Although a few early cancers were controlled at the NCI with this schedule, failure to control moderately advanced and advanced cancers was nearly uniform.

At the University of California, San Francisco, in the late 1950s, emphasis was placed on low daily doses for early vocal cord cancer to avoid acute mucosal reactions.[14,15] A dose of 1.6–1.8 Gy per fraction was administered to total doses of 55–70 Gy. With these protracted schedules, local failure rates (T1, 24%; T2, 53%) were twice those usually reported. In their updated series, local control was achieved in 98% of patients who received >2 Gy per fraction.[16]

Split-course irradiation, which was used routinely at the University of Florida between 1969 and 1974, also limits acute toxicity. Tumor control by split-course techniques was poor compared with tumor control by continuous-course techniques.[17] Overgaard and others have shown that .5–.6 Gy per day are required to overcome the adverse effects of such treatment protraction.[18] Split-course irradiation has not been shown to decrease late effects, which are dependent on total dose and dose per fraction.

The explanation for lower control rates after split-course or excessively protracted continuous-course irradiation is accelerated repopulation of clonogenic cells during the treatment course. The time factor is of extreme importance in radiotherapy and is the rationale for accelerated fractionation.

3. *Improvement in therapeutic ratio.* During the last 15 years, hyperfractionation and accelerated fractionation have been used with increasing frequency in an attempt to exploit basic radiobiologic principles to improve the efficacy of radiation therapy. Hyperfractionated radiotherapy refers to the delivery of a large number of smaller than conventional fractional doses in an overall treatment time that is similar to conventional; hyperfractionation is usually accomplished by delivering more than one fraction per day. The total dose is generally higher than that delivered by conventional schemes. If the total dose is not increased over that conventionally used, the potential therapeutic advantage of hyperfractionation is lost. The rationale is to exploit the differential sensitivity to changes in dose per fraction between acute- and late-effects tissues, thereby resulting in an increased rate of tumor control while keeping the rate of complications at an acceptable level.[19]

Accelerated fractionation refers to shortening the overall treatment duration, using conventional (1.8–2 Gy) dose fractions. Total dose is similar to or slightly less than conventional dose. Acceleration may be accomplished in a variety of ways, for example by treating a patient six or seven times per week instead of five.[20] Alternatively, it may be accomplished by using multiple fractions per day.

The regenerative response of tumors during irradiation is thought to be an important determinant of tumor control in a significant number of patients. Accelerated fractionation significantly shortens the overall duration of treatment, thereby reducing the time available for regeneration of clonogenic tumor cells during the treatment course. Because the ability of an acutely responding tissue (such as skin or mucous membrane) to withstand a course of fractionated treatment depends on its regenerative response during treatment, acute tolerance becomes a limiting factor.

Clinical Experience with Multiple Fractions per Day

The idea of irradiating head and neck cancers with more than one fraction per day is not new. From 1920 to 1926, at the Fondation Curie in Paris, France, Coutard[21] routinely treated patients with cancer of the oropharynx, hypopharynx, and larynx twice a day whenever the overall duration of the treatment course was less than 20 days because he thought that the tolerance was better than with once-a-day treatment. This short-duration, twice-a-day schedule was used only for early cancers. Between 1927 and 1933, Coutard and Baclesse[13] extended the overall treatment time by using markedly reduced doses per fraction, two fractions per day, and with this approach, were able to cure a number of advanced lesions that up to that time had not been cured.

From the 1940s through the 1960s, the vast majority of radiotherapy patients around the world were treated with one fraction per day. In the early 1970s, hyperfractionation was suggested as a means of improving the therapeutic ratio.[22-24]

Figure 3–1 and Tables 3–1 to 3–5[24-44] describe time-dose schemes for conventional (once-a-day) irradiation schemes commonly used in the United States and Canada and report on 13 accelerated and 7 hyperfractionation schemes. Note that in Figure 3–1 all of the accelerated and hyperfractionated schemes deliver a greater total dose per unit time than do any of the conventional programs.

Table 3–1 shows conventional time-dose schemes for five regimens commonly used in the United States (Figure 3–1, starred data points 1–5), representing treatment at 64.8–75.6 Gy at 1.8 Gy per fraction or 66–70 Gy at 2 Gy per fraction. The Canadian schemes (starred data points 6 and 7) are 50 Gy over 4 weeks or 55 Gy over 5 weeks.

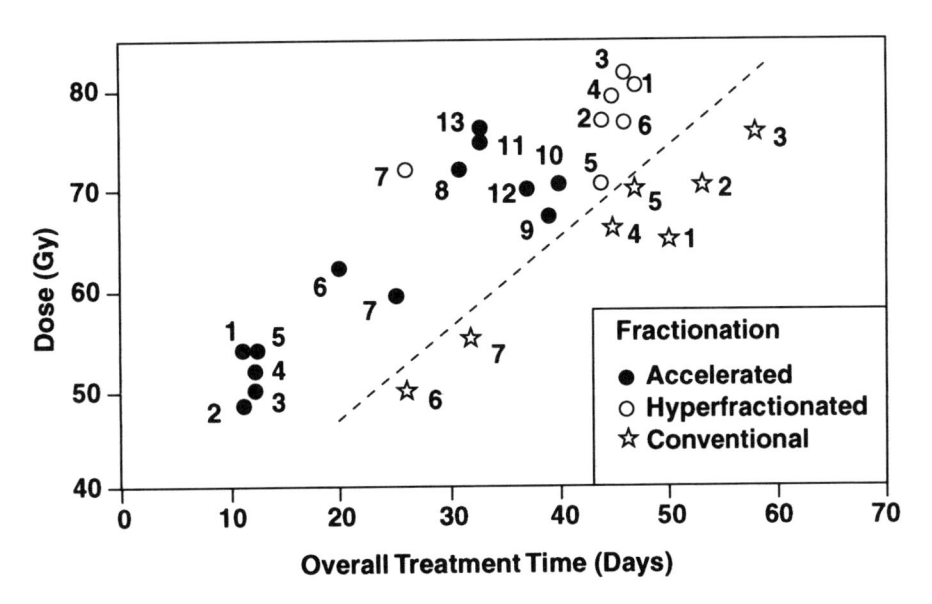

FIG 3–1. Total dose versus overall treatment time for 7 conventional fractionation schemes in the United States (starred data points 1–5) or Canada (stars 6 and 7); 13 accelerated schemes (black circles); and 7 hyperfractionated schedules (open circles). Refer to Tables 3–1 to 3–5 for specific time-dose data. The dashed line (- - - -) is for reference only and illustrates the time-dose differences between the conventional and modified schemes.

Table 3–1. "Conventional" fractionation schedules for head and neck squamous cell carcinoma

	Fractionation Scheme*	Total Dose (Gy)	Treatment Scheme	Dose (Gy) per Fraction
United States	1	64.8	Once a day	1.8
	2	70.2	Once a day	1.8
	3	75.6	Once a day	1.8
	4	66	Once a day	2.0
	5	70	Once a day	2.0
Canada	6	50	Once a day	2.5
	7	55	Once a day	2.3

* Fractionation schemes correspond to starred data points 1–7 in Fig 3–1.

Table 3–2. Very accelerated fractionation radiotherapy for head and neck cancer with low total dose given over 1.5 weeks

Study Number*	Institution	Total Dose (Gy)	Treatment Scheme (interfraction interval)	Dose (Gy) per Fraction
1	Parma, Italy[25]	54	3 times a day (4 hr)	2.0
2	University of Amsterdam[26]	48.6	3 times a day (4 hr)	1.8
3	Portsmouth, UK[27]	50	3 times a day (3 hr)	~2.0
4	Florence, Italy[28]	52	3 times a day (4 hr)	2.0
5	Northwood, England CHART[45]†	54	3 times a day (6 hr)	1.5

* Study numbers correspond to black circle data points 1–5 in Fig 3–1.
† CHART = continuous, hyperfractionated accelerated radiotherapy.

The accelerated schemes form three "clusters." The first data "cluster" (Fig 3–1, black circle data points 1–5) represents treatment at a very accelerated rate. All five trials were conducted in Europe. Table 3–2[24-28] shows the fractionation details. The overall treatment times were approximately 1.5 weeks and all used three fractions per day, mostly with 1.8- to 2-Gy fractions. Total doses were limited to approximately 50–54 Gy because of severe acute reactions. Several investigators reported frequent hospitalization in the postirradiation period. Four of the five trials reported low tumor control rates due to low total dose. Only the CHART[45] program has reported improved rates of tumor control.[16]

The second cluster of accelerated schemes (Fig 3–1, black circles 6 and 7) is also very accelerated (Table 3–3).[29-31] Both treatment programs deliver an intermediate radiation dose (approximately 60 Gy) in an overall treatment time of 3–3.5 weeks. The treatments were mostly at 1.75 Gy twice a day or 1.8 Gy thrice daily. Both schedules produce very severe acute side effects, often requiring total parenteral nutrition or hospitalization. Sepsis, pneumonitis, or other life-threatening complications have been reported in some patients.

In order to achieve higher doses via acceleration (Fig 3–1, the third cluster, black circles 8–13) the degree of acceleration is reduced

Table 3–3. Very accelerated fractionation to intermediate total dose (approximately 60 Gy in 3–3.5 weeks)

Study Number*	Institution	Total dose (Gy)	Treatment Scheme (interfraction interval)	Dose (Gy) per Fraction
6	Institut Gustave Roussy, France[29]	62.0	Twice a day (9–10 hr)	Mostly 1.75
7	Wellington Hospital, New Zealand[30,31]	59.4	3 times a day (4 hr)	1.8 (3 days per week)

* Study numbers correspond to black circles data points 6 and 7, Fig 3–1.

to prevent excessive mucosal toxicity (Table 3–4).[32-37] This has been accomplished by (1) using split-course irradiation as at Massachusetts General Hospital[33,46] or in EORTC 22851;[47] or (2) using concomitant boost irradiation as at MD Anderson Cancer Center,[34,48] Medical College of Virginia,[35] and The Netherlands,[36] such that the dose intensity is limited to the terminal portion of the treatment and is restricted to a reduced volume of tissues; or (3) using the weekly dose escalation schedule of the University of Wisconsin (the so-called HARDE regimen), which also displaces the period of highest dose intensity to the final weeks of treatment.[37]

The hyperfractionated schedules (Fig 3–1, open circles 1–7) all use continuous-course irradiation, mostly at 1.1–1.2 Gy per fraction twice a day (Table 3–5).[38-44] The doses are generally higher than conventional doses. All of the schedules provide a modest (approximately 1 week) reduction in overall treatment time compared with conventionally fractionated schedules delivering a similar dose.

TREATMENT RESULTS

Accelerated Fractionation

The clearest retrospective evidence for a benefit of accelerated fractionation comes from Wang et al., who in the past used approximately 65 Gy (1.8 Gy once a day) or, more recently, approximately the same total dose (67.2 Gy) in an overall treatment time that was shorter by 10 days (1.6 Gy twice a day). Tumor control rates were significantly higher with the accelerated schedule.[33,46,49-52] Late effects were reportedly the same for each of the two schedules.

There are two reported randomized trials comparing accelerated and conventional fractionation. At the Medical College of Virginia,[35] 74.8 Gy (administered via a three-fractions-per-day concomitant boost schedule) was compared with 70 Gy in 35 fractions over 7 weeks (2 Gy once a day). Acute reactions were more severe in the concomitant boost arm. Fifteen-month actuarial local control rates significantly favored the concomitant boost arm (66% vs. 31%, $p = 0.03$).

Dische and Saunders[53] reported on 918 patients treated between April 1990 and March 1995 at 11 cancer centers for squamous cell carcinoma of the head and neck. Patients were randomized to CHART (continuous hyperfractionated accelerated radiotherapy), consisting of 54 Gy given as 1.5-Gy fractions three times per day over 12 consecutive days (no weekend interruptions); or continuous-course once-a-day irradiation, consisting of 66 Gy in 33 fractions once a day over 45 days. There was a significant improvement in 3–year control at the primary site ($p = 0.024$) but no difference in control of nodal disease. Early mucosal reactions appeared earlier and were more troublesome in the three-times-a-day arm; there was no difference in late morbidity.

Hyperfractionation

The clearest retrospective evidence for a benefit of hyperfractionation comes from the University of Florida[39,54,55] where doses of

Table 3–4. Moderately accelerated fractionation with high total dose (67–76 Gy) over 5–6 weeks

Study Number*	Institution	Treatment Technique	Scheme	Total Dose (Gy)	Dose (Gy) per Fraction
8	EORTC 22851[32]	Split course	3 times a day	72	1.6
9	Massachusetts General Hospital[33]	Split course	Twice a day	67.2	1.6
10	MD Anderson Cancer Center[34]	Concomitant boost	Twice a day	70.5	1.5–1.8
11	Medical College of Virginia[35]	Concomitant boost	3 times a day	74.8	1.8; 1.5
12	Nijmegen, Netherlands[36]	Concomitant boost	Twice a day	70	2.0
13	University of Wisconsin, HARDE[37]†	Weekly dose escalation	Twice a day	76	1.2 (2 wk); 1.4 (2 wk); 1.6 (2 wk); (Saturday 2.0 ÷ 4)

* Study numbers correspond to black circles data points 8–13 in Fig 3–1.

† HARDE = hyperfractionated accelerated radiotherapy with dose escalation.

Table 3–5. Hyperfractionation

Study Number*	Institution	Treatment Scheme (interfraction interval)	Total Dose (Gy)	Dose (Gy) per Fraction
1	EORTC 22791[38]	Twice a day (4–6 hr)	80.5	1.15
2	University of Florida[39]	Twice a day (4–6 hr)	76.8	1.2
3	RTOG 83–13[40]	Twice a day (6 hr)	81.6	1.2
4	New Delhi, India[41]	Twice a day (6 hr)	79.2	1.2
5	National Cancer Institute, Brazil[42]	Twice a day (6 hr)	70.4	1.1
6	MD Anderson Hospital[43]	Twice a day (6 hr)	76.6	1.1–1.2
7	Reims, France[44]	8 per day (2 hr)	72	0.9

* Study numbers correspond to open circle data points 1–7 in Fig 3–1.

74.4–81.6 Gy at 1.2 Gy per fraction twice a day have been used for moderately advanced and advanced squamous cell carcinoma of the larynx, hypopharynx, and oropharynx since March 1978. Until 1989, a 4-hour interfraction interval was used; subsequently, a 6-hour interval has been used.

Tables 3–6 and 3–7[39,56] show comparative results between once-a-day versus twice-a-day irradiation for these sites. Results for each substage and tumor site favor the hyperfractionated groups. Severe acute reactions were noted in 66 of 419 patients (16%), necessitating nasogastric or percutaneous

TABLE 3-6. Hyperfractionation for cancer of the larynx and hypopharynx at the University of Florida[39]

	Local Control		
Stage	Once a Day	Twice a Day	p value
T2	124/170 (73%)	61/67 (91%)	0.02
T3	20/46 (43%)	59/88 (67%)	0.007
T4	2/17 (12%)	4/12 (33%)	0.17

Source: Adapted from Parsons JT, Mendenhall WM, Stringer SP, Cassisi NJ, Million RR. Twice-a-day radiotherapy for squamous cell carcinoma of the head and neck: the University of Florida experience. Head Neck 1993;15:87–96. (Table 3, p 90)

Table 3-7. Hyperfractionation for oropharyngeal cancer (base of tongue, soft palate, tonsillar region) at the University of Florida[56]

	Local Control		
Stage	Once a Day	Twice a Day	p value
T1	27/33 (82%)	13/13 (100%)	0.12
T2	72/92 (78%)	57/66 (86%)	0.14
T3	39/61 (64%)	55/73 (75%)	0.11
T4	7/24 (29%)	19/36 (53%)	0.06

Source: Adapted from Fein DA, Lee WR, Amos WR, Hinerman RW, Parsons JT, Mendenhall WM, Stringer SP, Cassisi NJ, Million RR. Oropharyngeal carcinoma treated with radiotherapy: a 30-year experience. Int J Radiat Oncol Biol Phys. 1996;34(2):289–296. (Table 3, p 291)

gastrostomy feeding in 41 patients (nasogastric feeding was recommended in 9 others but was refused), unplanned split-course irradiation in 5 patients (1%), temporary tracheostomy in 3 patients; or requiring hospitalization for hydration (8 patients). There were 18 (4%) severe complications of irradiation, including 11 soft tissue, cartilage, or bone necroses; 1 esophageal stricture; 3 patients who experienced severe laryngeal fibrosis (2 required tracheotomy, 1 underwent arytenoidectomy); and 3 patients who required a permanent gastrostomy for swallowing dysfunction. Complications were related to increasing T stage, primary site, and irradiation dose. There was a 2% incidence of severe complications among 194 patients with oropharyngeal carcinomas and a 6% incidence among 217 patients with hypopharyngeal or laryngeal lesions. There were no severe complications in the oropharyngeal group below 79.2 Gy and no severe complications in the laryngeal or hypopharyngeal patients below 76.8 Gy. Of 102 patients who underwent planned unilateral neck dissection after irradiation, there were 7 (7%) wound complications (4 closed spontaneously and 3 required reoperation).

There are four reported randomized trials comparing hyperfractionation with conventional fractionation.

The first (and largest) trial was EORTC 22791,[38] which randomized 356 patients with T2–T3 N0–N1 squamous cell carcinoma of the oropharynx (excluding base of tongue) to 80.5 Gy over 7 weeks using 1.15-Gy fractions twice a day (4–6 hours between fractions) versus 70 Gy in 2-Gy fractions once a day also over 7 weeks. Acute reactions were more severe in the twice-a-day arm. Late reactions were equal. The 5-year rates of local control were 59% and 40% ($p = 0.02$) for the twice-a-day and once-a-day arms, respectively. Five-year survival rates were marginally significant (40% vs. 30%, $p = 0.08$) in favor of the twice-a-day arm.

Pinto et al[42] (Rio de Janeiro, Brazil) randomized 112 patients with stage III–IV squamous cell carcinoma of the oropharynx to 66 Gy in 33 fractions (2 Gy once a day) versus 70.4 Gy in 64 fractions (1.1 Gy twice a day with a minimum 6-hour interfraction interval) at the National Cancer Institute in Brazil. Both arms were completed in 6.5 weeks. Acute and late effects were equal. Primary site control was achieved in 84% of the twice-a-day patients compared with 64% of the once-a-day patients ($p = 0.02$). Overall survival at 3.5 years favored the twice-a-day arm ($p = 0.03$).

Datta et al[41] (New Dehli, India) randomized 212 patients with T2–T3 N0–N1 oral cavity, oropharyngeal, or laryngeal squamous cell carcinomas between 66 Gy in 33 fractions (2 Gy once a day) and 79.2 in 66 fractions (1.2 Gy twice a day with a 4–6 hour interfraction interval). Two-year survival (71% vs. 45%) and disease-free survival (63% vs. 33%) both significantly favored the twice-a-day group ($p < 0.005$). Acute reactions were more severe in the twice-a-day patients. Late reactions were equivalent.

Cummings et al[57] recently reported a randomized trial of hyperfractionation conducted at the Princess Margaret Hospital (Toronto). Three hundred thirty-six patients were randomized between their conventional fractionation schedule (51 Gy at 2.55 Gy per fraction over 4 weeks) and a hyperfractionated derivative of that schedule (58 Gy in 1.45-Gy fractions twice a day, also over 4 weeks). Results show benefit for some but not all subsets of patients.

CONCLUSIONS

Efficacy

Evidence from both retrospective and randomized trials points to improved therapeutic ratio with these modified fractionation schedules. Given that irradiation is effective treatment for head and neck primary squamous cell carcinoma, it should not be surprising that higher doses of irradiation given more intensively would be more effective in providing tumor control. Most observers have noted no increase in late toxicity with the various regimens. It is concluded that these schedules yield an improved therapeutic ratio.

Caution with Regard to Late (delayed) Toxicity of Accelerated Fractionation

Several notes of caution are in order with regard to accelerated fractionation.

Conventional wisdom holds that late effects are dependent on total dose and dose per fraction, with little dependence on overall treatment time as long as the interval between fractions is sufficient to allow repair of sublethal injury. When insufficient intervals are allowed between successive fractions (currently most investigators recommend a minimum of 6 hours), it is believed that incomplete repair of sublethal injury leads to an increased rate of late severe complications. Following are some data regarding interfraction intervals of 4, 2, 6, and 8 hours, respectively. In 1986, Vanuytsel and colleagues[58] reported on 91 patients with prostate cancer who received 2 Gy three times a day with one or two splits in the treatment course (60 Gy was administered over 5–7 weeks). The interfraction interval was 4 hours. The authors reported a

21% incidence of severe (grade 4–6) complications. A recent update[47] of the series reported 51% and 14% 5-year actuarial rates of genitourinary and gastrointestinal complications, respectively.

When acceleration is extraordinarily aggressive, the usually observed dissociation between acute and late effects disappears. Nguyen and colleagues[59] delivered 72 Gy over 3.5 weeks (90 Gy per fraction, 8 fractions per day at 2-hour intervals over 5 days for a total of 36 Gy in 1 week, followed by a 2-week interruption, after which the same dose was repeated). Extensive mucosal necrosis was noted in 23% of patients within the first 6 months, and 22% developed severe complications after 6 months. A follow-up article showed late complications in 70% of patients.[44] In such instances, late effects (ie, necrosis) evolve directly from acute effects, and the occurrence of late effects directly correlates with the severity of acute effects. Such late effects are termed "consequential late" effects[60] or "acute necroses."

Two further observations prove that our understanding of late effects after accelerated schemes is imperfect. Saunders and colleagues[61] reported four unexpected cases of radiation myelitis after CHART (1.5 Gy three times a day with 6-hour interfraction intervals). The total doses (Table 3–8)[61] were within a range generally considered acceptable.

Nyman and Turesson[62] reported on late effects after accelerated fractionation with either 4- or 8-hour interfraction intervals. Patients with breast cancer were treated with bilateral parasternal irradiation to a total dose of 50 Gy in 25 fractions. Each patient served as her own control. The right parasternal field received treatment at 24-hour intervals over 5 weeks. The left parasternal field received 2 Gy twice a day with 4- or 8-hour interfraction intervals over 2.5 weeks. Late effects were compared using telangiectasia (#/▪ ratio of 3.9) as an end point. Based on our current knowledge of the time that it takes to repair sublethal injury, it was not surprising that patients with 4-hour interfraction intervals had more severe late effects than those with 24-hour intervals. The surprise finding was that the 8-hour interfraction interval group also had more severe late injury than the 24-hour group and, in fact, the severity of their late reactions was equal to the 4-hour group (Fig 3–2).[62] These data indicate that even 8 hours may be insufficient for complete repair between fractions.

The effect of inadequate interfraction interval is magnified in a three-fractions-per-day regimen, because there may be interaction not only between the first and second, and second and third fractions, but also between the first and third fractions if the intervals are too short.

Table 3–8. Incidence of radiation myelitis according to spinal cord dose after CHART* in head and neck cancer[61]

Spinal Cord Dose (Gy)	No. of Patients	No. Myelitis (%)
<30 – 37.5	26	0
40 – 42.5	36	2 (6%)
42.5 – 45	10	1 (10%)
45 – 47.5	2	1 (50%)

*CHART = continuous, hyperfractionated accelerated radiotherapy.

Source: Adapted from Saunders MI, Dische S, Grosch EJ, Fermont DC, Ashford RFU, Maher EJ, Makepeace AR. Experience with CHART. Int J Radiat Oncol Biol Phys. 1991;21:871–878. (Table 5, p 875)

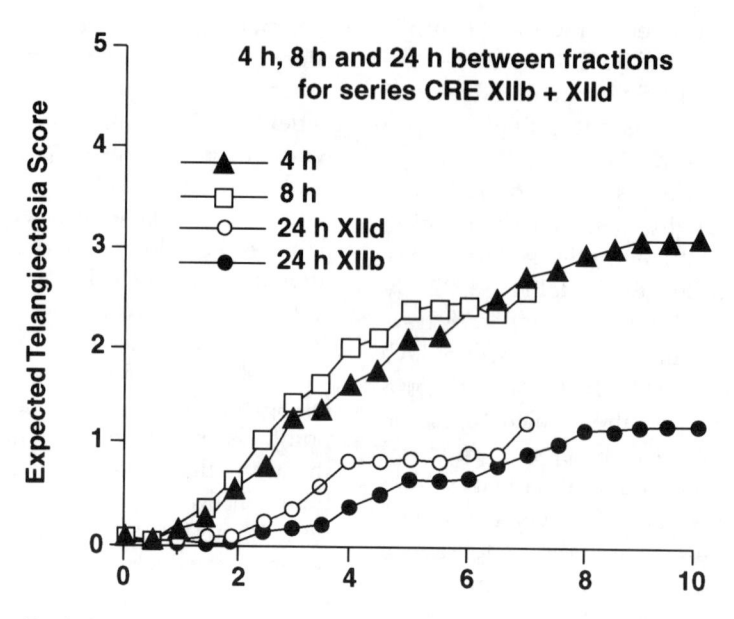

FIG 3–2. Severity of telangiectasia according to time and fractionation schedule. (Adapted from: Nyman J, Turesson I. Does the interval between fractions matter in the range of 4–8 h in radiotherapy? A study of acute and late human skin reactions. *Radiother Oncol.* 1995;34:171–178. (Fig 4, p 175)[62] (Reprinted with permission.)

REFERENCES

1. Cox JD. Large-dose fractionation (hypofractionation). *Cancer.* 1985;55(9 Suppl):2105–2111.
2. Ellis F. Dose, time and fractionation: a clinical hypothesis. *Clin Radiol.* 1969;20:1–7.
3. Thames HD Jr, Withers HR, Peters LJ, Fletcher GH. Changes in early and late radiation responses with altered dose fractionation: implications for dose-survival relationships. *Int J Radiat Oncol Biol Phys.* 1982;8:219–226.
4. Withers HR, Thames HD Jr, Flow BL, Mason KA, Hussey DH. The relationship of acute to late skin injury in 2 and 5 fraction/week gamma ray therapy. *Int J Radiat Oncol Biol Phys.* 1978;4:595–601.
5. Andrews JR. Dose-time relationships in cancer radiotherapy: a clinical radiobiology study of extremes of dose and time. *Am J Roentgenol Radium Ther Nucl Med.* 1965;93:56–74.
6. Rubenfeld S. Experiences with a rapid irradiation technic in oral carcinoma. *Radiology.* 1953;60:724–731.
7. Atkins HL. Massive dose technique in radiation therapy of inoperable carcinoma of the breast. *Am J Roentgenol Radium Ther Nucl Med.* 1964;91:80–89.
8. Edelman AH, Holtz S, Powers WE. Rapid radiotherapy for inoperable carcinoma of the breast: benefits and complications. *Int J Radiat Oncol Biol Phys.* 1965;93:585–599.
9. Singh K. Two regimes with the same TDF but differing morbidity used in the treatment of stage III carcinoma of the cervix. *Br J Radiol.* 1978;51:357–362.
10. Bennett MB. The treatment of stage III squamous carcinoma of the cervix in air and hyperbaric oxygen. [Abstract]. *Br J Radiol.* 1978;51:68
11. Dische S, Martin WMC, Anderson P. Radiation myelopathy in patients treated for carcinoma of bronchus using a six fraction regime of radiotherapy. *Br J Radiol.* 1981;54:29–35.
12. Handa K, Edoliya TN, Pandey RP, Agarwal YC, Shina NA. Radiotherapeutic clinical trial of twice per week vs. five times per week in oral cancer. *Strahlentherapie.* 1980;156:626–631.
13. Coutard H. Principles of x-ray therapy of malignant diseases. *Lancet.* 1934;227:1–8.
14. Woodhouse RJ, Quivey JM, Fu KK, Sien PS, Dedo HH, Phillips TL. Treatment of carcinoma of the vocal cord: a review of 20 years experience. *Laryngoscope.* 1981;91(7):1155–1162.

15. Buschke F, Vaeth JM. Radiation therapy of carcinoma of the vocal cord without mucosal reaction. *Am J Roentgenol Radium Ther Nucl Med.* 1963;89:29–34.
16. Le QT, Krieg RM, Quivey JM, Fu KK, Meyler TS, Stuart AA, Phillips TL. Influence of fractionation and time on local control to T1 and T2 glottic carcinoma. [Abstract]. *Int J Radiat Oncol Biol Phys.* 1996;36(Suppl 1):234
17. Parsons JT, Bova FJ, Million RR. A re-evaluation of split-course technique for squamous cell carcinoma of the head and neck. *Int J Radiat Oncol Biol Phys.* 1980;6(12):1645–1652.
18. Overgaard J, Hjelm-Hansen M, Johansen LV, Andersen AP. Comparison of conventional and split-course radiotherapy as primary treatment in carcinoma of the larynx. *Acta Oncol.* 1988;27:147–152.
19. Fletcher GH. Keynote address: the scientific basis of the present and future practice of clinical radiotherapy. *Int J Radiat Oncol Biol Phys.* 1983;9(7):1073–1982.
20. Lipsett JA, Desai K, Pezner R, Vora N, Chong LM, Archambeau JO. Acute normal tissue tolerance to 7 day per week accelerated fractionation. *Int J Radiat Oncol Biol Phys.* 1984;10(7):1049–1052.
21. Coutard H. Roentgen therapy of epitheliomas of the tonsillar region, hypopharynx and larynx from 1920–1926. *Am J Roentgenol Radium Ther.* 1932;28:313–331.
22. Withers HR. Cell renewal system concepts and the radiation response. In: Vaeth JM, ed. *Frontiers of Radiation Therapy and Oncology.* Baltimore: Karger, Basel, and University Park Press; 1972:93–107.
23. Backstrom A, Jakobsson PA, Littbrand B, Wersall J. Fractionation scheme with low individual doses in irradiation of carcinoma of the mouth. *Acta Radiol Ther Phys Biol.* 1973;12:401–406.
24. Jakobsson A, Littbrand B, Backstrom A. Andrat fraktioneringsschema vid behandling av skivepitelkancer i munhala. [Abstract]. *Nord Med.* 1971;28:1253.
25. Peracchia G, Salti C. Radiotherapy with thrice-a-day fractionation in a short overall time: clinical experiences. *Int J Radiat Oncol Biol Phys.* 1981;7:99–104.
26. Gonzalez DG, Breur K, Schueren EVD. Preliminary results in advanced head and neck cancer with radiotherapy by multiple fractions a day. *Clin Radiol.* 1980;31:417–421.
27. Svoboda VHJ. Further experience with radiotherapy by multiple daily session. *Br J Radiol.* 1978;51:363–369.
28. Olmi P, Cellai E, Chiavacci A, Fallai C. Accelerated fractionation in advanced head and neck cancer: results and analysis of late sequelae. *Radiother Oncol.* 1990;17(3):199–207.
29. Bourhis J, Fortin A, Dupuis O, et al. Very accelerated radiation therapy: preliminary results in locally unresectable head and neck carcinomas. *Int J Radiat Oncol Biol Phys.* 1995;32(3):747–752.
30. Gray AJ. Treatment of advanced head and neck cancer with accelerated fractionation. *Int J Radiat Oncol Biol Phys.* 1986;12(1):9–12.
31. Lamb DS, Spry NA, Gray AJ, Johnson AD, Alexander SR, Dally MJ. Accelerated fractionation radiotherapy for advanced head and neck cancer. *Radiother Oncol.* 1990;18(2):107–116.
32. Horiot JC, Le Fur R, Schraub S, van den Bogaert W, van Glabbeke M, Pierart M, Begg AC. Status of the experience of the EORTC cooperative group of radiotherapy with hyperfractionated and accelerated radiotherapy regimes. *Semin Radiat Oncol.* 1992;2(1):34–37.
33. Wang CC. Local control of oropharyngeal carcinoma after two accelerated hyperfractionation radiation therapy schemes. *Int J Radiat Oncol Biol Phys.* 1988;14(6):1143–1146.
34. Ang KK, Peters LJ. Concomitant boost radiotherapy in the treatment of head and neck cancers. *Semin Radiat Oncol.* 1992;2(1):31–33.
35. Johnson CR, Schmidt-Ullrich RK, Arthur DW, Huang DT, Duffy EW. Standard once-daily versus thrice-daily concomitant boost accelerated superfractionated irradiation for advanced squamous cell carcinoma of the head and neck: preliminary results of a prospective randomized trial. [Abstract]. *Int J Radiat Oncol Biol Phys.* 1995;32(Suppl 1):162
36. Kaanders JHAM, van Daal WAJ, Hoogenraad WJ, van der Kogel AJ. Accelerated fractionation radiotherapy for laryngeal cancer, acute, and late toxicity. *Int J Radiat Oncol Biol Phys.* 1992;24:497–503.
37. McGinn CJ, Harari PM, Fowler JF, Ford CN, Pyle GM, Kinsella TJ. Dose intensification in curative head and neck cancer radiotherapy-linear quadratic analysis and preliminary assessment of clinical results. *Int J Radiat Oncol Biol Phys.* 1993;27:363–369.
38. Horiot JC, Le Fur R, N'Guyen T, et al. Hyperfractionation versus conventional fractionation in oropharyngeal carcinoma: final analysis of a randomized trial of the EORTC cooperative group of radiotherapy. *Radiother Oncol.* 1992;25:231–241.

39. Parsons JT, Mendenhall WM, Stringer SP, Cassisi NJ, Million RR. Twice-a-day radiotherapy for squamous cell carcinoma of the head and neck: the University of Florida experience. *Head Neck*. 1993;15(2):87–96.
40. Fu KK, Pajak TF, Marcial VA, et al. Late effects of hyperfractionated radiotherapy for advanced head and neck cancer: long-term follow-up results of RTOG 83-13. *Int J Radiat Oncol Biol Phys*. 1995;32(3):577–588.
41. Datta NR, Choudhry AD, Gupta S, Bose AK. Twice a day versus once a day radiation therapy in head and neck cancer. [Abstract]. *Int J Radiat Oncol Biol Phys*. 1989;17(Suppl 1):132
42. Pinto LHJ, Canary PCV, Araujo CMM, Bacelar SC, Souhami L. Prospective randomized trial comparing hyperfractionated versus conventional radiotherapy in stages III and IV oropharyngeal carcinoma. *Int J Radiat Oncol Biol Phys*. 1991;21:557–562.
43. Garden AS, Morrison WH, Ang KK, Peters LJ. Hyperfractionated radiation in the treatment of squamous cell carcinomas of the head and neck: a comparison of two fractionation schedules. *Int J Radiat Oncol Biol Phys*. 1995;31(3):493–502.
44. Nguyen TD, Panis X, Froissart D, Legros M, Coninx P, Loirette M. Analysis of late complications after rapid hyperfractionated radiotherapy in advanced head and neck cancers. *Int J Radiat Oncol Biol Phys*. 1988;14(1):23–25.
45. Saunders MI, Dische S, Fowler JF, et al. Radiotherapy employing three fractions on each of twelve consecutive days. *Acta Oncol*. 1988;27(2):163–167.
46. Wang CC, Montgomery W, Efird J. Local control of oropharyngeal carcinoma by irradiation alone. *Laryngoscope*. 1995;105:529–533.
47. Lievens Y, Vanuytsel L, Rijnders A, van Poppel H, van der Schueren E. The time course of development of late side effects after irradiation of the prostate with multiple fractions per day. *Radiother Oncol*. 1996;40:147–152.
48. Ang KK, Peters LJ, Weber RS, Maor MH, Morrison WH, Wendt CD, Brown BW. Concomitant boost radiotherapy schedules in the treatment of carcinoma of the oropharynx and nasopharynx. *Int J Radiat Oncol Biol Phys*. 1990;19:1339–1345.
49. Wang CC, Blitzer PH, Suit HD. Twice-a-day radiation therapy for cancer of the head and neck. *Cancer*. 1985;55(9 Suppl):2100–2104.
50. Wang CC. Improved local control of advanced oropharyngeal carcinoma following twice-daily radiation therapy. [Abstract]. *Am J Clin Oncol*. 1985;8(1):22
51. Wang CC, Suit HD, Blitzer DP, Blitzer PH. Twice-a-day radiation therapy for supraglottic carcinoma. *Int J Radiat Oncol Biol Phys*. 1986;12(1):3–7.
52. Wang CC. The enigma of accelerated hyperfractionated radiation therapy for head and neck cancer. *Int J Radiat Oncol Biol Phys*. 1988;14(1):209–210.
53. Dische S, Saunders MI. Randomised multicentre trial of CHART versus conventional radiotherapy in head and neck cancer—interim results and implications. [Abstract]. *Int J Radiat Oncol Biol Phys*. 1996;36(Suppl 1):234
54. Parsons JT, Cassisi NJ, Million RR. Results of twice-a-day irradiation of squamous cell carcinomas of the head and neck. *Int J Radiat Oncol Biol Phys*. 1984;10(11):2041–2051.
55. Parsons JT, Mendenhall WM, Million RR, Cassisi NJ, Stringer SP. Twice-a-day irradiation of squamous cell carcinoma of the head and neck. *Semin Radiat Oncol*. 1992;2(1):29–30.
56. Fein DA, Lee WR, Amos WR, et al. Oropharyngeal carcinoma treated with radiotherapy: a 30-year experience. *Int J Radiat Oncol Biol Phys*. 1996;34(2):289–296.
57. Cummings BJ, Keane TJ, Pintilie M, et al. A prospective randomized trial of hyperfractionated versus conventional once daily radiation for advanced squamous cell carcinomas of the larynx and pharynx. [Abstract]. *Int J Radiat Oncol Biol Phys*. 1996;36(Suppl 1):235.
58. Vanuytsel L, Ang KK, Vandenbussche L, Vereecken R, van der Schueren E. Radiotherapy in multiple fractions per day for prostatic carcinoma: late complications. *Int J Radiat Oncol Biol Phys*. 1986;12(9):1589–1595.
59. Nguyen TD, Demange L, Froissart D, Panis X, Loirette M. Rapid hyperfractionationed radiotherapy. Clinical results in 178 advanced squamous cell carcinomas of the head and neck. *Cancer*. 1985;56:16–19.
60. Peters LJ, Ang KK, Thames HD, Jr. Accelerated fractionation in the radiation treatment of head and neck cancer. A critical comparison of different strategies. *Acta Oncol*. 1988;27(2):185–194.
61. Saunders MI, Dische S, Grosch EJ, Fermont DC, Ashford RFU, Maher EJ, Makepeace AR. Experience with CHART. *Int J Radiat Oncol Biol Phys*. 1991;21:871–878.
62. Nyman J, Turesson I. Does the interval between fractions matter in the range of 4–8 hr in radiotherapy? A study of acute and late human skin reactions. *Radiother Oncol*. 1995;34:171–178.

CHAPTER 4

The Selective Neck Dissection for Upper Aerodigestive Tract Carcinoma: Indications and Results

Robert M. Byers, MD, and Dianna B. Roberts, PhD

In 1906, Dr. George Crile published an article in *JAMA* describing a surgical technique which would become known as the radical neck dissection.[1] It was popularized by Dr. Hayes Martin as *the* oncologic procedure for treating metastatic disease in the lymph nodes of the neck and is still today regarded as the "gold standard" to which all other therapies are compared. However, in the late 1960s and early 1970s, men such as Suárez[2] from Argentina, Ballantyne[3] from the United States, and Bocca[4] from Italy began to explore surgical alternatives that would be oncologically sound but preserve important functional and cosmetic anatomical structures in the neck. These variations in the surgical procedures were categorized as modified radical neck dissections and were refined and perfected so that today these procedures are standardized and can be incorporated in training programs throughout the world. The most recent classification of neck dissections suggests that the lymphadenectomies can be divided into comprehensive and selective types.[5] The comprehensive procedures remove node levels I–V. These include the classic radical neck dissection, the modified radical neck dissection, and the functional neck dissection. The only difference among them is whether they preserve either the sternocleidomastoid muscle, the internal jugular vein, the XIth cranial nerve, or all three structures. The selective neck dissection uses the level of nodes in the neck and their relative risks of containing metastatic disease depending on the site of the primary cancer in the upper aerodigestive tract as a means to define the extent of the lymphadenectomy. The nomenclature is somewhat arbitrary but the dissections are recognizable as independent procedures.

This chapter will focus only on the varieties of selective neck dissections, their appropriate use, how they can be incorporated in a multidisciplinary therapeutic approach, and the results when they are selected to treat a patient with occult or obvious cancer in the neck. Also, the level of nodes at risk depending on the primary cancer site is defined.

RESULTS

To support the concepts and principles proposed in this chapter we have reviewed the medical records of patients (468) operated on at the University of Texas MD Anderson Cancer Center between the years of 1985–1990 for squamous carcinoma of the upper aerodigestive tract in which a selective neck dissection was part of their treatment. In reviewing the charts of the patients, the following information was obtained: site and stage of primary, type of selective neck dissection, unilateral or bilateral, initially with or subsequent to the treatment for the primary, elective or therapeutic, number of nodes removed, number of pathologically positive nodes, location in the neck of the clinically and pathologically positive nodes, level of nodes removed, anatomic structures removed, presence of extracapsular disease, and the use of postoperative radiation therapy. Regional control was correlated with these parameters. Regional failure was categorized as within the dissected side of the neck, outside the dissected field but on the same side of the neck, or in the opposite undissected side of the neck. The regional failure was included in the analysis and correlated with the parameters as long as the primary remained controlled.

We have elected to group the results by type of dissection with or without postoperative radiation therapy and the regional failure by primary site and N-stage with and without postoperative radiation therapy (Table 4–1).

I. Suprahyoid Dissection with Postoperative Radiation Therapy

Thirteen patients had a submaxillary triangle dissection. Three patients had bilateral dissections. One patient failed regionally within the dissected area. Two patients had a unilateral dissection only with no regional failures. Eight patients had a suprahyoid dissection in combination with another type of neck dissection: two with a supraomohyoid, two with an anterior or lateral dissection, and four with a modified radical neck dissection. Two patients failed in the neck, but the recurrences were outside of the dissected area.

II. Suprahyoid Dissection Without Postoperative Radiation Therapy

Twenty-two patients had a submaxillary triangle dissection. Three were bilateral with no regional failures. Five patients had a unilateral dissection only with no regional failures. Fourteen patients had a suprahyoid dissection in combination with another type of neck dissection; 10 with a supraomohyoid neck dissection and no regional recurrences; 2 with an anterior or lateral neck dissection and no regional recurrences; and 2 with a modified radical neck dissection and no recurrences.

III. Supraomohyoid Dissection with Postoperative Radiation Therapy

One hundred and twenty-five patients had this type of selective dissection combined with radiation therapy. Thirty-three had a bilateral dissection with two regional failures (6%). Both of these regional recurrences were outside of the dissected neck. Thirty-three patients had a supraomohyoid dissection in combination with some other type of neck dissection with six regional failures, none of which were on the side of the supraomohyoid dissection. Ninety-two patients had a unilateral dissection with 17 recurrences (18%). Three were in the dissected area; 2 on the same side but outside the dissected area and 12 were in the contralateral undissected side of the neck. Thus, 14 recurrences were the result of a geographic miss or doctor error in choosing the proper extent of the surgery. The recurrence rate in the dissected area was 3% (3/125).

Table 4–1. Supraomohyoid selectve neck dissection (no combinations)

Unilateral	RR*/No	RR/N1	RR/N2	Primary Site	RR/N2	RR/N1	RR/No	Bilateral
29 without XRT+	0/24	0/4	1/1	Oral tongue	0/1	0	0/1	2 with XRT
15 with XRT	1/3	1/8	2/4		0	0/2	0/1	3 without XRT
8 without XRT	0/6	0	0	Floor of mouth	0	3/5	0/8	13 without XRT
5 with XRT	0/1	2/3	0/1		1/4	0/3	0/1	8 with XRT
3 without XRT	0/3	0	0	Buccal mucosa	0	0	0	0
1 with XRT	0	0	1/1		0	0	0	0
15 without XRT	1/12	1/2	0/1	Lower gum/	0/1	0	0/1	2 without XRT
15 with XRT	0/6	0/1	0/8	retromolar trigone	0/1	0	0	1 with XRT
4 without XRT	0/4	0	0	Palate/faucial arch	0	0	0	0
3 without XRT	0/1	0	0/2		0	0	0	0
1 without XRT	0/1	0	0	Base of tongue	0	0	1/1	1 without XRT
4 with XRT	0/1	0/1	0/2		0/1	0/1	0	2 wtih XRT
2 without XRT	0	0/2	0	Tonsil	0	0	0	0
4 with XRT	0/1	0	1/3		0	0	0	0
4 with XRT	0/2	1/1	0/1	Pyriform sinus	0	0	0/1	1 without XRT
					0	0/1	0/1	2 with XRT
1 with XRT	0	1/1	0	Vocal cord/ transglottic	0	0/2	0/2	4 with XRT
6 with XRT	0/2	0/3	1/1	Supraglottic	0	0/1	0/1	2 without XRT
				larynx	0/5	0/5	1/3	13 with XRT
1 with XRT	0/1	0	0	Lip and other	0	0	0/1	1 without XRT
					0	0	0/1	1 with XRT

*RR: Regional recurrence
+XRT: Radiation therapy

IV. Supraomohyoid Dissection Without Postoperative Radiation Therapy

There were 105 patients in this group. Twenty-three had bilateral dissections with four regional recurrences (17%). Two were within the dissected area and two were outside of it. Sixty-two patients had a unilateral dissection with three regional recurrences (5%). One was on the same side of the neck, but outside the dissected area and two were in the contralateral undissected side of the neck. Twenty patients had a supraomohyoid neck dissection with various combinations of other types of neck dissections. There was one regional recurrence which was outside of the dissected area. Thus, six of the recurrences were outside of the dissection. Consequently, only 2%

(2/105) of the failures could be considered a fault of the operation.

V. Anterior or Lateral Neck Dissection with Postoperative Radiation Therapy

Seventy-seven patients had an anterior or lateral neck dissection (level II–IV). Thirty-three were bilateral with three regional recurrences all within the dissected area (8.6%). There were 42 unilateral dissections alone or in combination with some other neck dissection. There were nine regional recurrences in this group (21%) of which two were on the same side of the anterior or lateral neck dissection. Thus, the recurrence rate within the dissected area was 6.5% (5/77).

VI. Anterior or Lateral Neck Dissection Without Postoperative Radiation Therapy

This group consisted of 54 patients. Twenty-four had a bilateral dissection. There were three regional recurrences (12.5%) all within the dissected area. Thirty patients had a unilateral dissection alone or in combination with some other type of neck dissection. Four of these patients had a regional recurrence (13%) of which none were on the side of the anterior or lateral neck dissection. The recurrence rate within the dissected area was 5.5% (3/54).

If you break down the operations by the site of primary (Table 4–1), the usual sites for a selective neck dissection include the oral tongue, floor of mouth, lower gum, retromolar trigone, pyriform sinus, and larynx. The sites of lower lip, hard palate, soft palate, tonsil, faucial arch, oro/hypopharyngeal wall, base of tongue, and buccal mucosa had too few patients to have any meaningful analysis. The larynx was divided into vocal cord, supraglottic, and transglottic. The overall regional failure above the clavicle with the primary controlled using the supraomohyoid neck dissection for any N-stage with or without postoperative radiation is 14/122 (11%) for oral cavity primaries and 2/21 (9.5%) for oropharynx primaries.

Oral Tongue

The most common operation for oral tongue was a supraomohyoid neck dissection. Most of the supraomohyoid neck dissections (35) were unilateral. In the patients without radiation therapy (32), there was one regional recurrence (3%). In the patients with postoperative radiation (23) there were four regional failures (17%).

Floor of Mouth

The selective operations for floor of mouth primaries varied. Thirty-three patients were treated with surgery only. There were nine unilateral supraomohyoids with two regional failures. There were 13 bilateral supraomohyoids with one regional failure. There were six combinations of suprahyoid and supraomohyoid with no regional failures. There were three supraomohyoids plus a modified radical neck dissection with no regional failures and two supraomohyoid neck dissections with a lateral neck dissection with no regional failures. Twenty-three patients had at least a unilateral supraomohyoid and postoperative radiation therapy. Seven patients were treated with a unilateral supraomohyoid and three patients developed a regional failures. Eleven patients had bilateral supraomohyoids with one regional failure. Seven patients had a combination of dissections: two with a suprahyoid and no regional failure, one with a lateral dissection which failed in the neck, two with a modified radical neck dissection and one regional failure, and two patients had a suprahyoid and a modified radical neck dissection with no regional failures. In summary, 33 patients were treated with surgery only with a 6% regional failure (3/33). Twenty-five patients had postoperative radiation with a 24% regional recurrence (6/25).

Lower Gum/Retromolar Trigone

Twenty-six patients had selective neck dissections, most common, a supraomohyoid and no postoperative radiation. There were four regional failures (15%). Nineteen patients had postoperative radiation with no regional failure.

Pyriform Sinus

Six patients had no postoperative radiation with no regional failures. Most patients had a bilateral levels II–IV dissection. Twenty-four patients had postoperative radiation. Most patients also had bilateral levels II–IV dissections. There were two regional failures (4%).

Larynx (Supraglottic, Glottic, Transglottic)

Twenty four patients received postoperative radiation. The most common selective neck dissection was the bilateral anterior or lateral. Three patients had a regional recurrence (12.5%). Sixty-six patients had postoperative radiation. Again, the most common neck dissection was the bilateral anterior or lateral. Five patients had a regional recurrence (7.5%).

Results Based on Neck Stage

If a selective neck dissection is performed electively (183 patients) and pathologically positive nodes are found (65 patients), the regional failure in the neck with postoperative radiation is 12.8% (6/47); without postoperative radiation it is 33% (6/18). If an elective supraomohyoid neck dissection (110 patients) is performed and pathologically positive nodes are found (39 patients), the regional failure in the neck is 17% (5/29) with postoperative radiation and 30% (3/10) without postoperative radiation. If a selective neck dissection for clinically N1 (54 patients) is performed and pathologically positive nodes are found (33 patients), the regional failure in the neck with postoperative radiation is 22% (6/27) and without postoperative radiation 33% (2/6). If a supraomohyoid neck dissection is performed for a clinically N1 neck (37 patients) and pathologically positive node(s) are found (23 patients), the regional failure in the neck with postoperative radiation is 25% (5/20) and without postoperative radiation 33% (1/3). If a selected neck dissection for a clinically N2 neck (16 patients) is performed and pathologically positive node(s) are found (10 patients), the regional failure in the neck with postoperative radiation is 43% (3/7) and without postoperative radiation 0/3. In most of these clinical settings, the numbers are small, but one can easily see that the use of postoperative radiation in patients with positive nodes reduces the incidence of regional failure.

CLINICAL CONSIDERATIONS

First, let me emphasize that these selective procedures are not "grandiose node pluckings." The extent of the surgical dissection and its thoroughness is no different than with the comprehensive procedures in the area of highest risk for nodal disease. Anatomic structures not obviously involved with cancer are preserved. Those that are suspected to be involved should be removed. The surgeon must decide if the patient should be treated initially with surgery or radiation therapy. If the primary is best treated with radiotherapy and the neck is clinically N0, no surgery is required. If the neck has significant metastatic disease present precluding successful radiation therapy alone, then the surgeon must decide when to resect the neck, either before or after radiation therapy.[6] This decision can be made based on several factors. One, if the patient needs to be put under a general anesthesia for a biopsy of the primary and/or dental extractions prior to beginning radiation therapy, then it would be appropriate to remove the mass first before radiation. If, on the other hand, the patient does not need any prior anesthesia, then the radiation can be given and the surgeon can remove the residual disease in the neck approximately 5 weeks after completion of the radiotherapy. If surgery is the best initial treatment for the primary and the neck is N0 clinically, the surgeon must determine if an elective neck dissection is justified. If, in order to resect the primary cancer the neck must be entered, then a selective neck dissection is appropriate, which one depends on the site of the primary. If the primary cancer can be adequately resected without entering the neck, then the surgeon must decide whether to include a lymphadenectomy or not. The oral cavity is really the only primary site where this dilemma is applicable. This decision will usually be based on the stage or thickness of the primary. If the risk for occult nodal disease is sufficiently great (20% or more) as it is with oral tongue cancer regardless of the T-stage or if the floor of mouth or tongue primary is 4 mm or greater in thickness where the incidence may approach 40%, then an elective supraomohyoid neck dissection is indicated, either unilateral or bilateral depending if the lesion is midline. This neck dissection can be part of a pull-through procedure or separate from the intraoral resection.

The basis for this conceptual approach is that every node in the neck is not at the same risk for involvement depending on where the primary is located. For instance, if the cancer is located in the base of tongue, pharyngeal wall, or pyriform sinus, the retropharyngeal nodes are at more risk than the submental nodes. Experience has taught us that the suboccipital, the buccinator, and the external jugular nodes are not at risk for metastasis from cancers arising in the upper aerodigestive tract. The lower posterior cervical nodes are rarely, if ever, involved with squamous carcinomas of the oral cavity. Submaxillary (level I) nodes are rarely, if ever, involved with squamous carcinoma of the glottis, supraglottic larynx, or pyriform sinus. This concept depends on the ability of the surgeon to predict the nodal levels at risk for occult disease and, thereby, selectively remove only those nodes while preserving all of the uninvolved structures within the neck. A patient whose neck is staged clinically N0 does not need a comprehensive dissection if the primary is in the lateral oral tongue. In fact, a patient whose neck is N0 clinically should never need a radical neck dissection as the initial elective procedure regardless of the primary cancer site. Removing node levels I–IV is sufficient. A squamous carcinoma of the larynx does not need bilateral comprehensive neck dissections. Removal of levels II–IV bilaterally is sufficient. If no pathologically positive nodes are discovered or only one positive node with no extracapsular extension is found, no postoperative radiotherapy treatment is necessary. If multiple subclinical, pathologically positive nodes are found or extracapsular extension is present, then postoperative radiation is indicated. Levels I and V are left undisturbed and this, obviously, decreases operating time. Under these circumstances, a selected neck dissection is not just a "staging" procedure. It is as therapeutic as any other type of dissection and provides worthwhile information for subsequent counseling. If the neck contains an obviously clinically positive node in the first echelon of drainage for a particular primary, then the choice of a selective neck dissection is also appropriate. If all nodal groups at risk are included, all gross disease removed, only one node is pathologically positive with no extracapsular extension, the operation is also definitive. Obviously if the patient has clinically positive nodes in multiple levels, a comprehensive neck dissection is a better choice although, even in this circumstance, a radical neck dissection is not mandatory. The goal of the neck dissection is only to remove all the gross disease. If the patient has a single, large node (over 3 cm) infiltrating the structures in the neck, a selective neck dissection can also be performed. This requires the surgeon to only remove the gross disease in the immediate region of the nodal disease. This demands that the surgeon accept the principle of combined therapy and the effectiveness of radiation to treat subclinical microscopic disease.

As the goal of the selected dissection is to remove the "big potatoes," any given procedure may not exactly fit any of the described operations. Therefore, it is very important to record, in the operative note, the nodal groups removed and the structures preserved. If this requires removing the paraspinous muscles, the digastric muscle, the strap muscles, the phrenic nerve, and sympathetic nerves, cranial nerves VII, X, XI, XII, the external carotid artery, internal jugular vein and sternocleidomastoid muscle, the surgeon and patient are prepared to proceed. Removal of the internal or common carotid or both internal jugular veins is usually not appropriate. This decision should be made preoperatively, but occasionally must be made intraoperatively. Ironically, a selective neck dissection can actually be more radical than the classic radical dissection in this circumstance, but only as it encompasses the extent of the local disease. If the mass is in level II, there is no need to dissect the lower part of level V and the lower jugular nodal area of level IV. On the left side of the neck, this means that the thoracic duct is not in jeopardy.

The types of selected neck dissection useful for squamous carcinoma of the upper aerodigestive tract can be labeled as suprahyoid, supraomohyoid, and anterior or lateral. The suprahyoid contains the submandibular and the submental nodes (level I). There is only one submental triangle of nodes, but a right and left submaxillary triangle of nodes. This operation is seldom used as a definitive procedure because level II (the subdigastric nodes) are not included. It is most often used as a procedure to remove a large nodal metastasis adherent to the horizontal ramus of the mandible in the upper submaxillary triangle area from a primary in the oral cavity in which the need for postoperative radiation has already been determined preoperatively and the scope of the operation is to only remove the gross disease. Occasionally, a supraomohyoid dissection is appropriate as a bilateral procedure for squamous carcinomas in the anterior floor of mouth, lower lip, and anterior lower gum for staging or to remove the submaxillary glands whose drainage has been compromised by resection of Wharton's ducts.

The supraomohyoid is the most often used selected neck dissection. This was very adequately described by Medina et al in 1989.[7] There is some controversy concerning the extent of the procedure. Specifically, how far posterior to the internal jugular vein is it necessary to go in removing the nodes in levels II and III and how far inferior on the internal jugular vein is necessary to remove level III or IV? The omohyoid muscle travels across the neck from a low in the posterior cervical region to a high where it inserts into the hyoid bone within the anterior carotid triangle. Where it crosses the internal jugular vein is usually considered the lowest level of nodes included. However, with certain primaries in the lateral oral tongue and retromolar trigone/lower gum level IV nodes are also at risk. Consequently, if a supraomohyoid dissection is considered for treatment of these primary sites, the omohyoid muscle should be transected and nodes in levels I, II, III, and IV should be removed. In order to get a good clean out of these nodal groups, it is necessary to go above, under, and below the spinal accessory nerve before it enters the sternocleidomastoid muscle. It is also important to extend the dissection beyond the internal jugular vein posteriorly to the roots of the cervical plexus. This allows for a comprehensive removal of the jugular chain of nodes because it is sometimes very difficult to arbitrarily decide which nodes to remove and which to preserve. Actually, the only nodes that are not included are the nodes in the lower posterior cervical triangle. The spinal accessory is not disturbed as it leaves the sternocleidomastoid muscle in the posterior triangle and enters the trapezius muscle. To do this operation well, it takes about two and a half hours. It is essential that the node(s) under the anterior belly of the digastric muscle and lateral to the mylohyoid muscle be included. This node is particularly at risk for cancers arising in the floor of mouth. The node(s) along the facial vessels under the marginal branch of the VIIth nerve are usually at risk from skin cancers of the mid face and nasal vestibule, but cancers of the lower lip can drain to these nodes also. Care must be taken to dissect the nodes from around this branch of the facial nerve. These nodes are called prevascular, and if you use the technique of ligating the facial vessels and reflecting them superiorly in order to preserve the marginal branch of the VIIth nerve, the nodes will also be preserved. The supraomohyoid dissection is indicated for all primaries in the oral cavity, especially the oral tongue and some selected sites in the oropharynx. Base of tongue cancers are probably better treated with a comprehensive dissection. The most cosmetic incision to use is one that starts in the submental area and runs posteriorly parallel to and two finger breadths below the horizontal ramus of the mandible to the level of the earlobe and then gently curves downward toward the lateral one third of the clavicle along the posterior border of the sternocleidomastoid muscle.

The anterior or lateral selective neck dissection is usually reserved for the larynx and hypopharynx primaries. The nodes at highest risk for cancers in this region are the ones in levels II–IV and the paratracheal and retropharyngeal nodes. The retropharyngeal nodes are also potentially involved with cancers in the oropharynx and can be included with a supraomohyoid dissection; however, they are more often at risk for cancers of the hypopharyngeal wall and pyriform sinus. The anterior or lateral selective dissection also is most often performed bilaterally because most cancers of the supraglottic larynx and hypopharynx drain to the nodes in both sides of the neck. This is what is meant when the term "widefield laryngectomy" is used. In an N0 neck, this can be accomplished with very little additional operating time. The nodes along the internal jugular vein from the posterior belly of the digastric muscle to the clavicle are swept medially after opening the fascial plane along the anterior border of the sternocleidomastoid muscle and retracting it laterally. The paratracheal nodes are also included if the tumor extends subglottically. There is no need to dissect the posterior cervical triangle nodes (level V). When palpable nodes are present, the anterior or lateral node dissection is still feasible; however, occasionally some of the sternocleidomastoid muscle must be removed as well as the internal jugular vein if the nodal disease involves them. Because it may be possible to preserve both external jugular veins, removing both internal jugular veins may not result in a prohibitive morbidity; however, usually one or the other internal jugular vein can be saved. It is usually a good idea to approach the least involved side first. When there are very enlarged nodes bilaterally or unilaterally, the same concept applies as it did with the supraomohyoid dissection— use surgery to remove the gross disease and combine it with radiation therapy for any residual microscopic disease in the neck. It is not necessary to include level I nodes except sometimes if there is preepiglottic space invasion, exposure above the hyoid is facilitated by removing the tissue in the submental triangle.

SUMMARY

The indications for a selective neck dissection can be stated in relation to the pre-op status of the neck and the site of the primary. The N0 neck requires an operation to encompass the occult disease in the nodes at risk depending on the patterns of drainage. The N+ neck requires all gross disease removed as well as the suspected occult disease in the nodes at highest risk. The reason for this is that occasionally the clinically N+ neck turns out to be pathologically N0 and if all nodes at risk have not been removed, complete pathologic information is missing. Consequently no further treatment may be necessary if the other nodes were also negative. In addition, the N+ neck may reveal one single pathologically positive node with no extracapsular extension and if all nodes at risk are included and are negative, again no further treatment is necessary. The need for adjunctive radiotherapy is determined by the findings when the neck specimen is examined by the pathologist. However, the use of radiotherapy postoperatively can be suspected preoperatively if the patient has multiple clinically positive nodes or a large mass with obvious connective tissue invasion. When the correct selective neck dissection is chosen, performed appropriately and competently, the procedure is oncologically sound and much better from a functional and cosmetic point of view than the more radical procedures. If a radical neck dissection was performed and the patient did not require postoperative radiation therapy, then a selective neck dissection was probably possible and certainly preferable.

ACKNOWLEDGMENTS

The authors gratefully thank Sylvia S. Aguirre for her effort in preparing this manuscript.

REFERENCES

1. Crile G. Excision of cancer of the head and neck: with special reference to the plan of dissection based on one hundred and thirty-two operations. *JAMA*. 1906;47:1780–1785
2. Suárez O. El problema de las metástasis linfáticas y alejadas del cáncer de laringe e hipofaringe. *Rev Otorrinolaryngol*. 1963;23:83–99
3. Ballantyne AJ, Guinn GA. Reduction of shoulder disability after neck dissection. *Am J Surg*. 1966;112:662–665
4. Bocca E, Pignataro O. A conservation technique in radical neck dissection. *Ann Otol Rhinol Laryngol*. 1967;76:975–987
5. Medina JE. A rational classification of neck dissections. *Otolaryngol Head Neck Surg*. 1989;100:169–176,
6. Byers, RM, Clayman GL, Guillamondegui OM, Peters LJ, Goepfert H. Resection of advanced cervical metastasis prior to definitive radiotherapy for primary squamous carcinomas of the upper aerodigestive tract. *Head Neck*. 1992;14(2):133–138
7. Medina JR, Byers RM. Supraomohyoid neck dissection: rationale, indications, and surgical technique. *Head Neck*. 1989;11(2):111–122

CHAPTER 5

Surgical Approaches to the Nasopharynx

William Ignace Wei, MS, FRCSE, DLO, FACS, and Po Wing Yuen, MS, DLO, FRCSE

The nasopharynx is located in the center of the head. It is difficult to perform a thorough examination of the region with conventional methods. It is even more difficult to expose the region adequately for a surgical procedure to be carried out to remove pathologies in the region satisfactorily, particularly when an oncological resection has to be undertaken.

Anatomically, the nasopharynx and the paranasopharyngeal space are anterior to the brain stem and the upper cervical spine, thus it is not practical to approach the region from posteriorly. Superior approaches to the area have been reported and lesions in the nasopharynx have been removed with the trans-skull base technique.[1] Under these circumstances, the subarachnoid space is exposed and contamination by pathogens of the nasal cavity is unavoidable. The associated morbidity is also not negligible. Complications such as meningitis, development of encephalocele, and diabetes insipidus have all been reported.[2]

THE LATERAL APPROACH

Pathologies in the nasopharynx and the paranasopharyngeal region can be removed via the lateral approach.[3] With this operation, a radical mastoidectomy has to be carried out first and some other structures have to be mobilized or divided. These include the zygomatic arch and the bony component of the floor of the middle cranial fossa with the middle meningeal artery and the mandibular branch of the fifth cranial nerve (Figure 5–1). The internal carotid artery also has to be exposed and isolated from the middle ear to the skull base to gain adequate mobility so that it can be displaced to allow entrance into the nasopharynx.

This approach is suitable for pathologies of limited extent with the main bulk located in the paranasopharyngeal region, lateral to the nasopharynx. It has the advantage of gaining control of the internal carotid artery, but the exposure of the nasopharynx itself is not adequate to allow an oncological procedure to be carried out for tumors located mainly in the nasopharynx. This is particularly so when the tumor crosses the midline of the nasopharynx, as with this approach it is difficult to control the resection margin at the opposite pharyngeal recess.

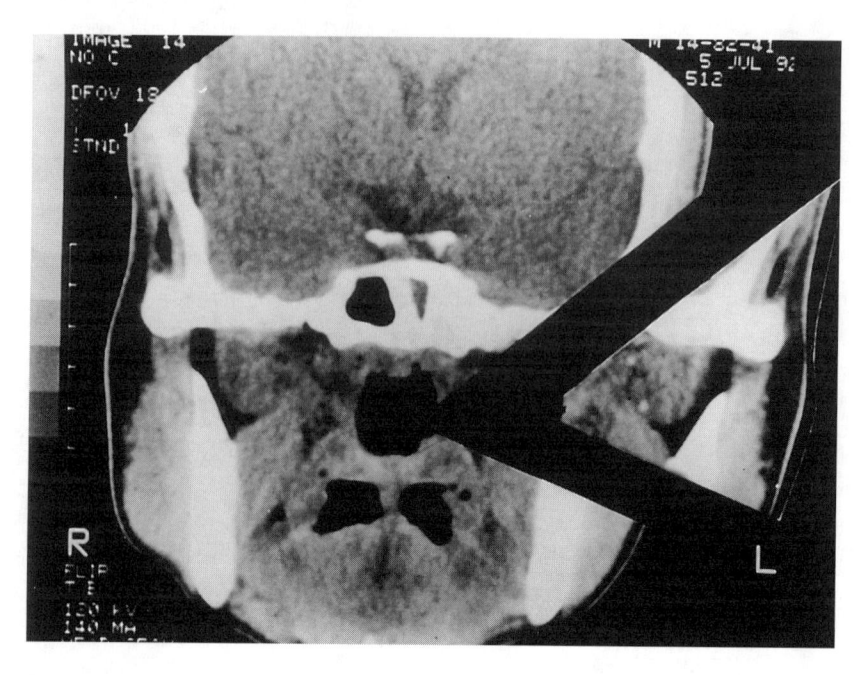

FIG 5–1. Schematic computed tomography showing the lateral approach to the nasopharynx.

THE INFERIOR APPROACH

Transpalatal

The nasopharynx can be approached inferiorly via the transpalatal route or transcervically. For a patient with a wide nasopharynx, the soft palate can be retracted with two catheters inserted through the nostrils and the nasopharynx can then be exposed. Successful removal of a chordoma in the region by this method has been reported.[4] More extensive exposure is possible when the palate is incised and retracted. A transverse incision placed at the junction of the soft and hard palates detaches the soft palate, which can then be retracted posteriorly to improve the exposure of the nasopharynx.[5] The palatal incision can also be placed along the inner margin of the upper alveolus, and the mucoperiosteum of the hard palate is lifted as a flap (Figure 5–2). Posterior retraction of this flap as well as removal of the posterior part of the hard palate contribute significantly toward better exposure of the nasopharynx.[6] The palate can also be incised in the midline extending from the uvula to the lingual margin of the upper incisor. The split soft palate together with the mucoperiosteum over the hard palate can be retracted laterally to expose the nasopharynx (Figure 5–3). A transverse limb at the anterior end of the longitudinal incision over the palate can be added. This allows retraction of the palatal flap laterally to improve exposure of the nasopharynx.[7]

The advantages of approaching the nasopharynx from the inferior aspect are that the operative procedures, both exposure and reconstruction, are less difficult. The associated morbidity is also minimal and adequate exposure can be achieved for lesions located in the central posterior wall of the nasopharynx. Although tumors in the nasopharynx have been successfully removed using the transpalatal approach,[8] the lateral aspect of the nasopharynx cannot be adequately exposed. Although tumors in the nasopharynx can be exposed with this approach (Figure 5–4) and radioactive gold grains can be inserted as a brachytherapy source under direct vision[9], it is difficult to carry out an oncological resection. However, with this approach alone, exposure of the paranasopha-

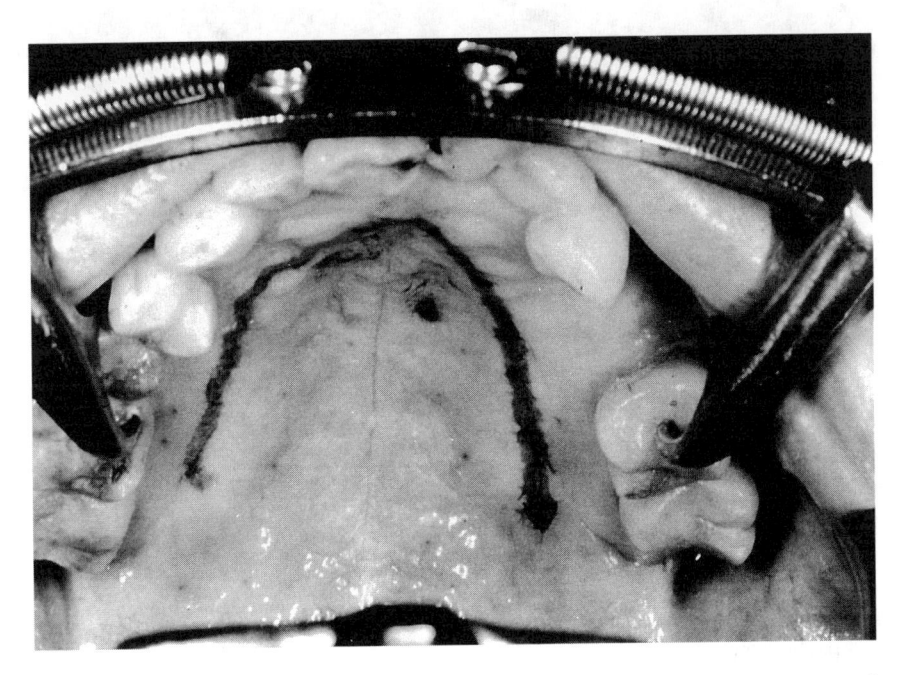

FIG 5–2. Incision placed along the inner border of the upper alveolus to allow elevation of mucoperiosteum off the hard palate.

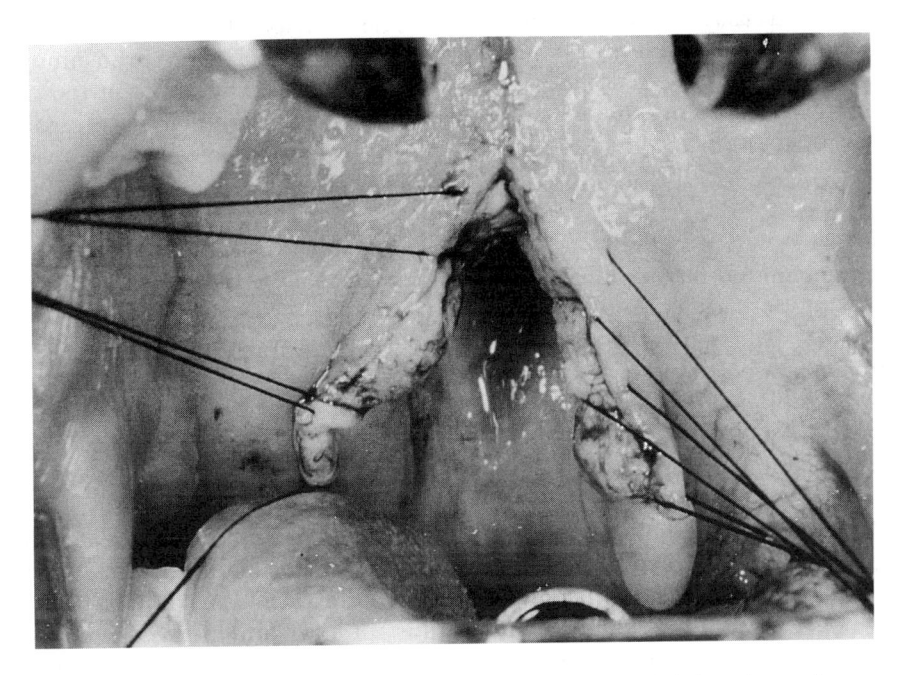

FIG 5–3. Midline incision over the hard and soft palates to allow their lateral retraction to expose the nasopharynx.

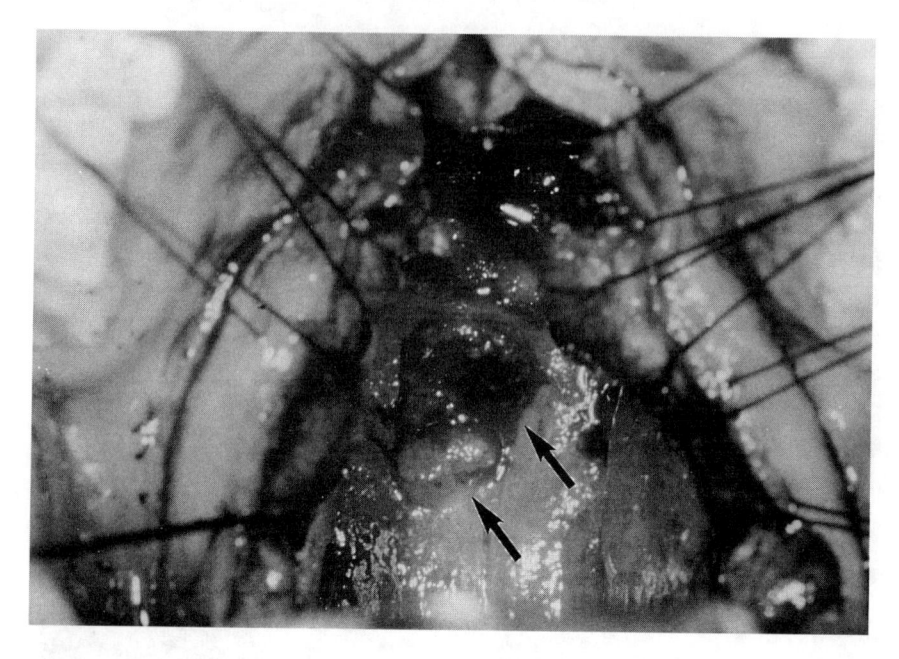

FIG 5–4. Exposure of the tumor (*arrows*) in the posterior wall of the nasopharynx with the split palate approach.

ryngeal space is limited and lesions that have extended to areas lateral to the nasopharynx cannot be removed easily under direct vision. Control of the internal carotid artery is also not easy with this approach. In addition, patients with trismus are not suitable candidates for this operation.

Transcervical

Lesions located around the nasopharyngeal area can also be approached through a transcervical route.[10] The paranasopharyngeal region can be exposed through a neck incision, medial to the mandible, employing a deep retractor. The use of the operating microscope also contributes to better visualization. For proper resection of pathologies in the region, the lip and the mandibular symphysis can be temporarily divided to facilitate retraction and enhance exposure.[11,12] Krepsi and Sisson[13] removed part of the mandible and the posterior part of the maxilla to achieve a wider exposure of the pathologies and adequate removal with less morbidity. The internal carotid artery could be identified and traced cephalically through the neck incision and protected during the removal of the pathology.[13]

The transpalatal and the transcervical approaches can be employed simultaneously to remove pathologies in the nasopharynx. Recurrent nasopharyngeal carcinoma has been removed successfully employing the combined approaches.[14]

ANTERIOR APPROACHES

The various anterior approaches to the nasopharynx via the transnasal or the transantral route just described[15] did not expose the region adequately for an oncological procedure to be carried out. Increased exposure of the nasopharynx could be gained with down fracture of the entire hard palate following a transverse maxillary osteotomy.[16] Lesions in the central skull base could be removed with this approach and the exposure was claimed to be adequate.[17] Exposure could be further improved with subtotal maxillectomy or extended maxillotomy,[18] although the coronoid process needs to be mobilized and the partial maxillectomy defect requires further reconstruction. En bloc resection of the tumor of the nasopharyngeal carcinomas that extend to the lateral wall of the nasopharynx and into paranasopharyngeal space could not be easily achieved with these anterior approaches.

THE ANTEROLATERAL APPROACH

The nasopharynx and the paranasopharyngeal region are usually widely exposed, at the completion of total maxillectomy, when a patient undergoes total maxillectomy for one reason or another. The whole maxilla bone has been removed to provide access for removal of tumor in the region and, after the resection, it is possible to reinsert the maxilla bone as a free graft.[19] Although there is no bone resorption at 15 months, its application in patients who have had previous radiotherapy requires further consideration.

The retromaxillary area can be accessed with the transfacial approach. All four walls of the maxillary antrum can be detached from the roof and the hard palate and moved laterally. The hard palate, however, was left intact.[20] With this method, the superiolateral wall of the nasopharynx is not widely exposed.

The whole maxillary antrum with the hard palate attached to the anterior cheek flap is turned laterally as an osteocutaneous flap (Figure 5–5). The nasopharynx and the paranasopharyngeal space is widely exposed with this approach.[21] Pathologies located in the region can be confidently removed under direct vision.[22]

Surgical Technique

Before the operation, a dental plate is made to fit the patient's hard palate. This will be used to fix the maxilla after it is returned to its original location.

The operation is done under general anesthesia with the patient in a supine position. Endotracheal intubation is performed through the nostril opposite to the side of the operation. An extended Weber Ferguson Longmire incision is made over the face, as in a maxillectomy. The incision over the lip is continued between the central incisors in the midline over the hard palate until it reaches the junction between the hard and soft palates, and it then turns laterally behind the maxillary tuberosity on the side of the swing (Figure 5–6).

The soft tissue over the anterior wall of the maxilla is incised and lifted off just enough to expose a strip of bone for osteotomy. When the osteotomy site is determined, miniplates are positioned at the zygomatic-malar bone region and across the midline. Holes for the screws for these plates are drilled before the osteotomy as this greatly aids the accurate positioning of the maxilla bone on its return. A thin blade oscillating saw is then employed to divide the anterior wall of the maxilla just below the roof of the orbit. The osteo-

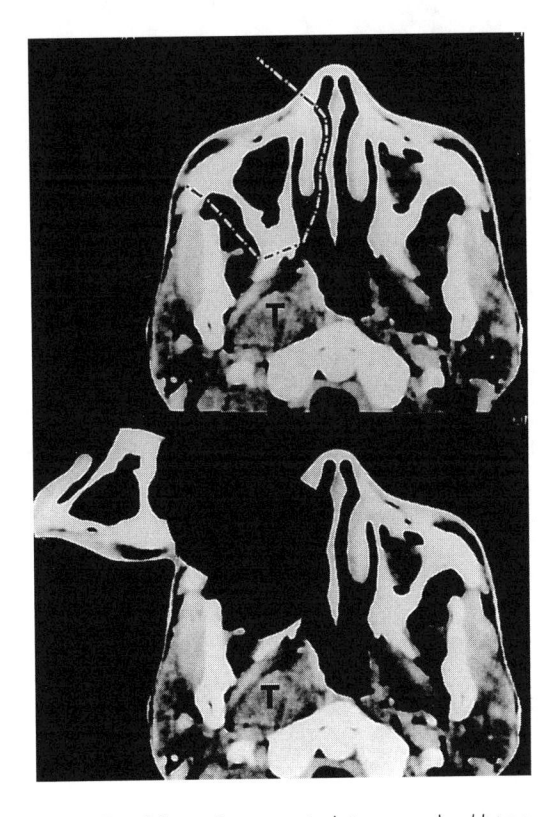

FIG 5–5. Schematic computed tomography. *Upper:* osteotomy sites marked with dotted line. *Lower:* the osteocutaneous complex is swung laterally while remaining attached to the overlying cheek flap. Tumor (T) in nasopharynx and paranasopharyngeal space is exposed.

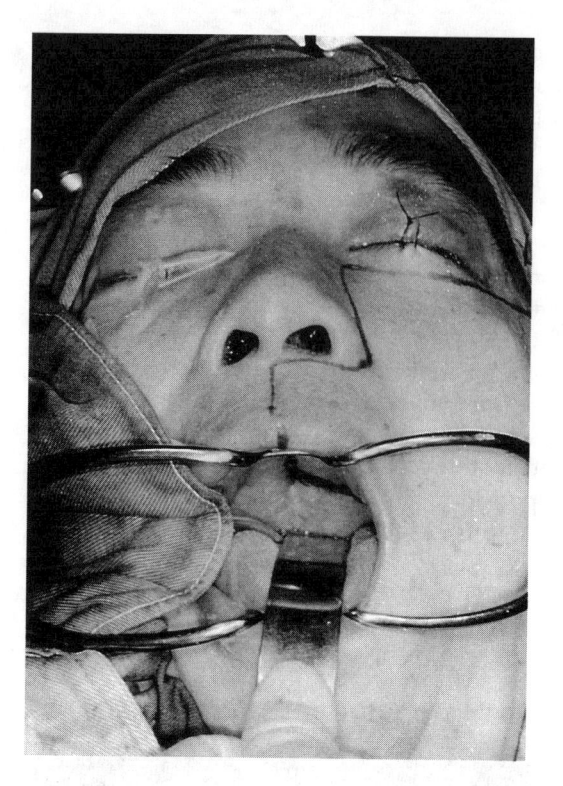

FIG 5–6. Facial incision that continues onto the hard palate and turned laterally to behind the maxillary tuberosity.

tomy is continued onto the zygomatic arch and divides it at its lower border (Figure 5–7). The medial wall of the nose is divided just below the middle turbinate and an osteotomy is also made over the midline of the hard palate. A curved osteotome is then used to separate the pterygoid plates from the maxillary tuberosity.

After severing the bony connections, the whole maxillary antrum is dropped inferiorly, but still remains attached to the anterior cheek flap from which it receives its blood supply. The whole osteocutaneous complex can then be swung laterally to expose the nasopharynx and the paranasopharyngeal area (Figure 5–8).

The tumor in nasopharynx and the parapharyngeal region can be removed en bloc. The posterior part of the nasal septum and the anterior wall of the sphenoid sinus can be removed to gain additional margin (Figure 5–9). After complete removal of pathology in the region, inferior turbinectomy is performed on the side of the swing and an antrostomy is done to allow better drainage of the antrum. The mucosa of the inferior turbinate can be removed and laid onto the raw area in the nasopharyngeal area as a free graft to facilitate healing. Nasal packing is carried out to hold the graft in position and for hemostasis. The maxilla can then be returned to its original position and the dental plate is placed in position temporarily to facilitate accurate apposition before the bony fixation is completed with screws and miniplates. The dental plate is then removed to allow suturing of the mucoperiosteum over the hard palate and reattaching the soft palate to the hard palate on the side of the swing. The facial wound is then closed in layers. The dental plate is then fixed to the hard palate by wiring onto the teeth on both sides. This gives additional stability and is left in situ for 6 weeks.

Clinical Application and Results

Patients

The anterolateral approach has been employed for the removal of lesions in and around the nasopharyngeal region.[22] Between February 1989 and January 1996, we have employed the anterolateral (maxillary swing) approach in 37 patients in our department. Twenty-nine patients were suffering from recurrent primary nasopharyngeal carcinomas after radiotherapy; the remaining eight had pathologies in the central skull base or infratemporal fossa. These included adenocarcinoma of the nasopharynx, neurofibroma, chordoma, and recurrent deep lobe parotid tumors. The efficacy of treatment of these lesions depends on the extent and pathologic nature of the tumor.[22]

In the 29 patients with recurrent primary nasopharyngeal carcinoma, the resection margins were subjected to frozen section examination during operation to ensure tumor clearance. Only when all the margins were negative was the resection considered to be curative. This was achieved in 26 patients.

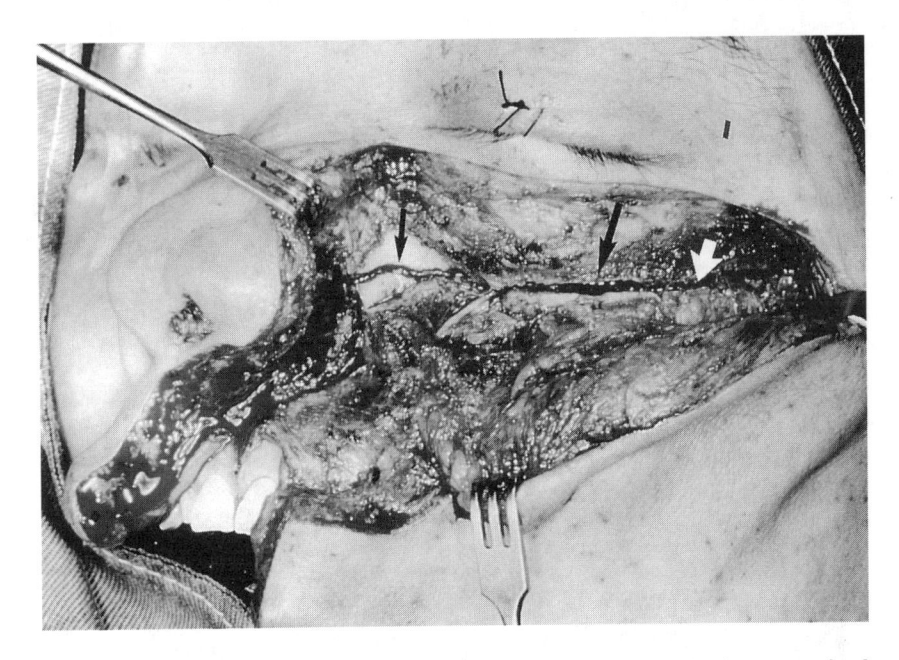

FIG 5–7. Osteotomy over the anterior wall of the maxilla. Only a limited amount of soft tissue is lifted to allow osteotomy to be carried out. Anterior wall osteotomy (*arrows*).

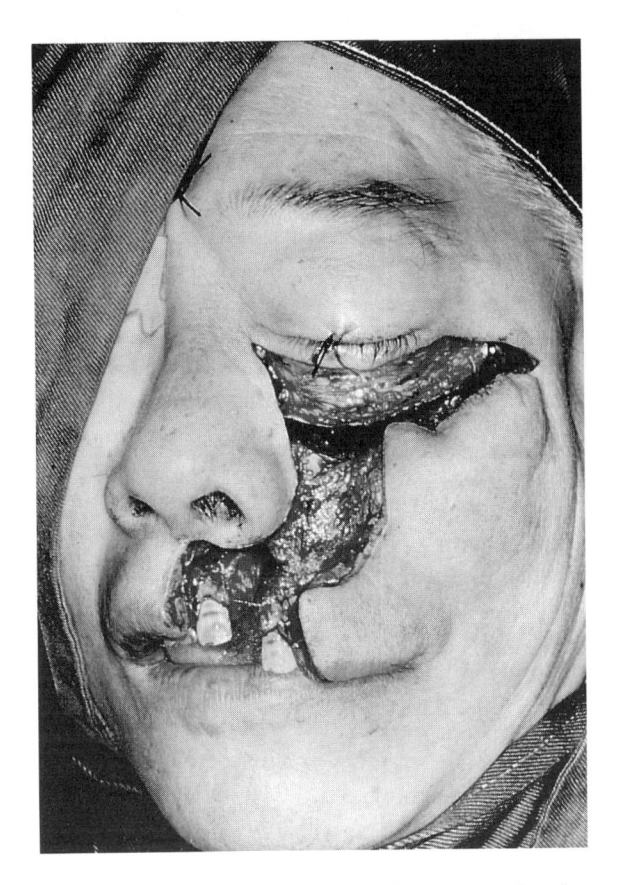

FIG 5–8. After completion of all the osteotomies, the whole osteocutaneous complex moves inferiorly.

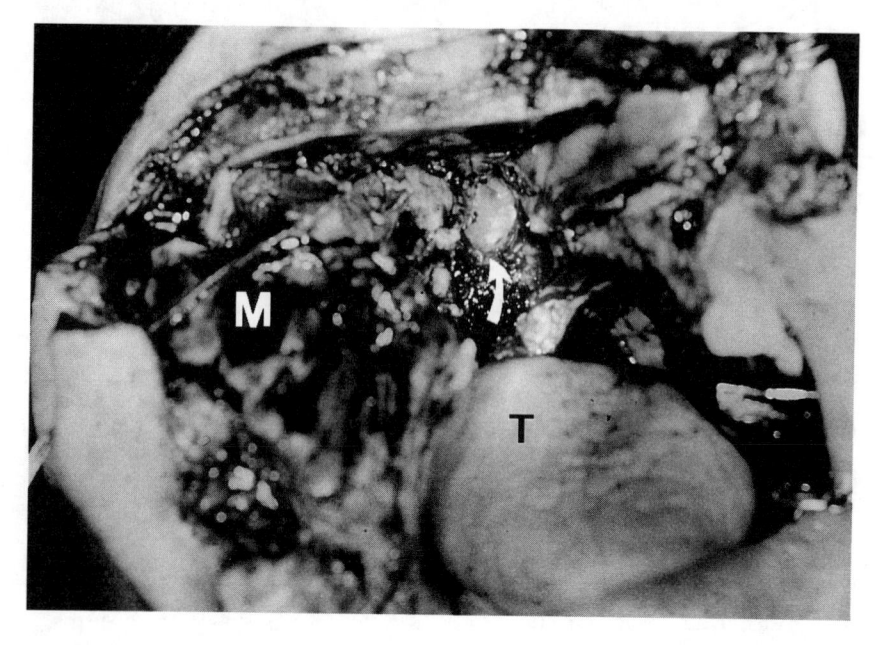

FIG 5–9. After resection of tumor, the posterior part of the nasal septum and the anterior wall of the sphenoid sinus were removed with wide exposure of the sphenoid sinus (*arrow*). Swinged maxilla (*M*), Tongue (*T*)

These included 25 men and 1 woman, ranging in age from 33 to 74 years (median, 54 years). All patients had received radical external radiotherapy before operation with dosages ranging from 59.9 to 120 Gy (median 63.5 Gy). Prior to surgery, computed tomography was performed for all 26 patients. In 16, the recurrent tumor was shown to be localized in the nasopharynx; in the other 10 patients, it had extended to the paranasopharyngeal space. In 3 of the 26 patients, the local recurrence detected after external radiotherapy was initially treated with brachytherapy. Two patients had cesium intubation and one patient had split palate insertion of gold grain (Au[198]) as the brachytherapy source. However, the tumor recurred in all three patients and salvage nasopharyngectomy was then carried out. The disease-free interval between the last radiation treatment and the present recurrence in these 26 patients ranged from 2 to 70 months (median, 12 months).

Biopsy of the recurrent tumor in the nasopharynx revealed anaplastic carcinoma in 25 and nonkeratinizing squamous cell carcinoma in the remaining patient. The follow-up period of the group ranged from 6 to 76 months (median, 24 months).

Nasopharyngectomy via the anterolateral (maxillary swing) approach as outlined above was performed for the 26 patients. Most of the recurrent nasopharyngeal carcinomas were located in the lateral wall of the nasopharynx and ranged in size from 1 to 3 cm in diameter. Macroscopic tumor was removed with at least 1 cm margin. The extent of resection usually involved the posterior wall, roof, and the lateral wall of the nasopharynx, including the Eustachian tube on the side of the tumor. The posterior part of the septum extending across the midline to the fossa of Rosenmüller on the opposite side was also resected when indicated, as was the anterior wall of the sphenoid sinus as additional margins of resection. Thus the sphenoid sinus was usually exposed at the end of the resection (Figure 5–9). In patients whose preoperative imaging studies showed tumor involvement of the paranasopharyngeal area, tissue in the region was removed en bloc with the nasopharyngectomy.

Results

All of the 26 patients survived the operation and were discharged from hospital. Their facial wounds healed primarily and they were able to tolerate oral diet on the third postoperative day. On removing the dental plate 6 weeks after the operation, a palatal fistula was detected in seven patients (27%). There was no necrosis of the maxilla.

At the time of assessment, four patients had developed local recurrent tumor. Two patients had died of regional disease and one from distant metastasis. Two patients died of causes unrelated to the tumor. The remaining 17 patients were alive and free of disease. The 5-year actuarial control of tumor in the nasopharynx was 42.4% and the 5-year actuarial survival of this group of patients was 36.8%, with a median survival of 53 months.

On histologic examination, these tumors showed a tendency to infiltrate beyond the mucosa despite the macroscopic appearance of localized tumor in the nasopharynx (Figure 5–10). The recurrent tumors were also noticed to extend into the submucosal region and were in close proximity to the cartilage of the Eustachian tube crura (Figure 5–11).

Complications and Their Management

All patients survived the operation and were discharged from the hospital. No necrosis of the maxilla bone was detected. One patient developed a granuloma over the lateral aspect of the facial wound related to a small sequestrum lying close to the upper lateral miniplate (Figure 5–12). The sequestrum and the plate were removed under local anesthesia and the wound healed subsequently. The facial wounds in all the other patients healed primarily.

Seven patients who had a radical dose of radiation for the primary nasopharyngeal carcinoma developed a palatal fistula. Four of the fistulas were behind the maxillary tuberosity; the other three were in the midline, at the junction of the hard and soft palates. In two patients, a palatal flap was used successfully to close the central fistula

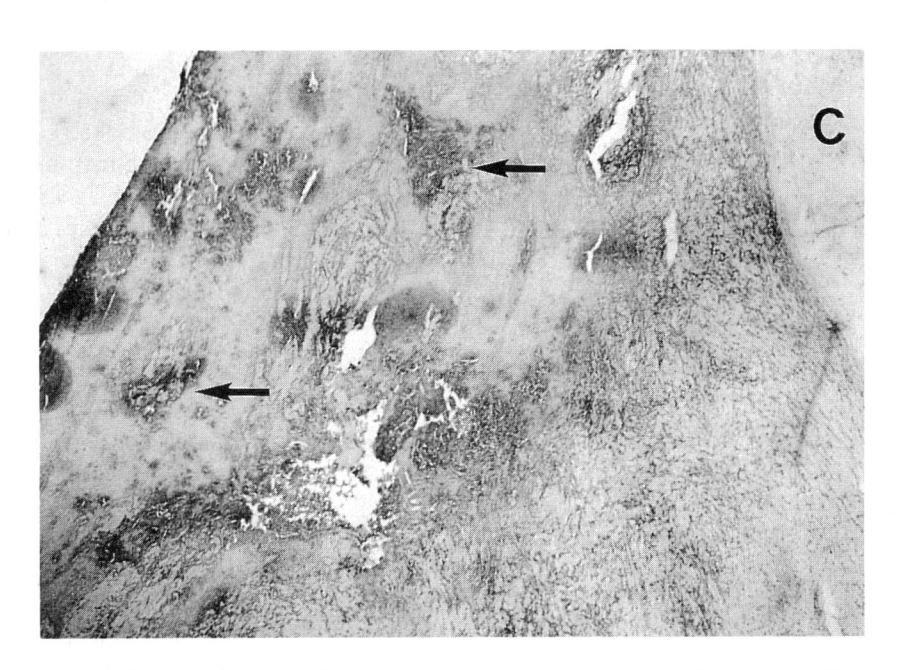

FIG 5–10. Tumor cells were frequently seen in the submucosa (*arrows*) close to the Eustachian tube crura (C) (Hematoxylin and eosin ÷ 100).

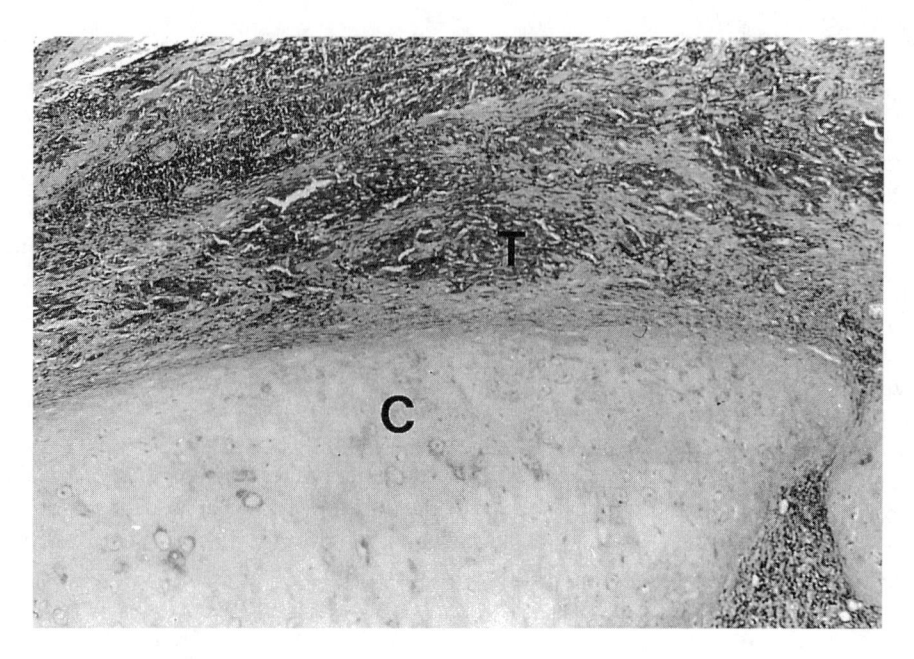

FIG 5–11. Sheets of tumor (T) were located in close proximity to the Eustachian tube crura (C) (Hematoxylin and eosin ÷ 150).

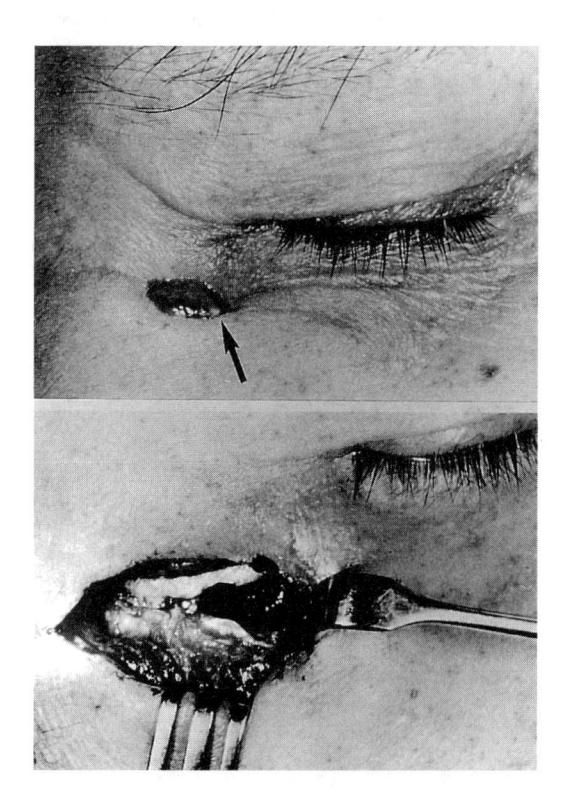

FIG 5–12. *Upper*: Granuloma situated over the lateral aspect of the facial wound (*arrow*). *Lower*: Underlying sequestrum identified and subsequently removed.

(Figure 5–13). The other patients were managed successfully with dental plates.

Contraction of the wound under the eyelid resulted in ectropion in two patients. Both were corrected with full thickness skin graft taken from behind the pinna.

After the operation, all patients suffered from trismus of varying degrees. This was worse in patients who had further radiation after surgery. This could be prevented by early mobilization of the muscles of mastication. If trismus still develops, active conservative management with stretching is usually effective in achieving a functionally adequate interalveolar distance.

COMMENTS

The options for salvage treatment of recurrent nasopharyngeal carcinoma are limited. The inferior approach to the nasopharynx, by splitting the palate, allows the implantation of radioactive gold grains. When the tumor volume is small, this form of brachytherapy is effective in the control of disease in the nasopharynx and the associated mor-

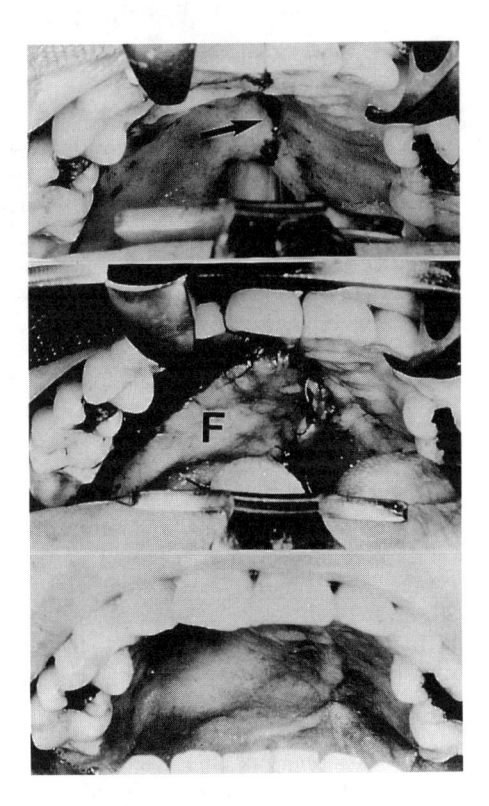

FIG 5–13. *Upper:* Palatal fistula (*arrow*). *Middle:* Palatal flap raised (*F*). *Lower:* Fistula closed despite the significant trismus.

bidity is low.[9] The limitation of this form of therapy is that the effective radiation range of gold grain is short. It is not effective in treating large recurrent tumors or tumors that have extended to the paranasopharyngeal space. It is also difficult to position the gold grains into the cartilaginous crura to treat tumors situated on, or in close proximity to, the tubal opening. Under these circumstances, surgical resection is an alternative salvage option for salvage treatment.

Among the different approaches employed for resection of lesions in the nasopharynx and its vicinity, the anterolateral route to the nasopharynx with the maxillary swing approach provides wide exposure of the whole nasopharynx and the paranasopharyngeal space. Adequate exposure is mandatory for an oncologic resection of the recurrent nasopharyngeal tumor after radiotherapy.

Although macroscopically recurrent tumors often seem to be localized, histologically, there may be extensive submucosal infiltration. Wide exposure of the nasopharynx is necessary to remove the tumor with an adequate margin to effect a curative resection. As the recurrence may be in close proximity to the crura of the nasal opening of the auditory tube, the cartilaginous portion of the Eustachian tube must be included in the resection for complete tumor extirpation. Surgical dissection in this region and in the paranasopharyngeal space may damage the internal carotid artery, which lies in the vicinity. The extensive exposure provided by the anterolateral approach allows digital palpation of pulsation of the internal carotid artery, thus helping to prevent its injury during surgical resection. Whenever tumor presence in the paranasopharyngeal tissue is suspected, soft tissue in the area should be removed en bloc with the nasopharyngectomy. The anterolateral route with the maxillary swing approach to the nasopharynx offers a wide exposure for oncological resection and is associated with a low morbidity.

REFERENCES

1. Derome PJ. The transbasal approach to tumors invading the base of the skull. In: Schmidek HH, Sweet WH, eds. *Operative Neurosurgical Techniques.* New York: Grune & Stratton; 1982; 1:357–359.
2. Van Buren JM, Ommaya AK, Ketcham AS. Ten years' experience with radical combined craniofacial resection of malignant tumors of the paranasal sinuses. *J Neurosurg.* 1968;28: 341–350.
3. Fisch U, Pillsbury HC. Infratemporal fossa approach to lesions in the temporal bone and base of the skull. *Arch Otolaryngol Head Neck Surg.* 1979;105:99–107.
4. Mullan S, Naunton R, Hekmat-Panah J, Vailati G. The use of an anterior approach to ventrally placed tumors in the foramen magnum and vertebral column. *J Neurosurg.* 1966; 24:536–543.
5. Ruddy LW. A transpalatine operation for congenital atresia of the choanae in the small child or the infant. *Arch Otolaryngol Head Neck Surg.* 1945;41:432–438.
6. Wilson CP. The approach to the nasopharynx. *Proc R Soc Med.* 1951;44:353–358.

7. Crumley RL, Gutin PH. Surgical access for clivus chordoma: the University of California, San Francisco experience. *Arch Otolaryngol Head Neck Surg.* 1989;115:295–300.
8. Tu GY, Hu YH, Xu GZ, Ye M. Salvage surgery for nasopharyngeal carcinoma. *Arch Otolaryngol Head Neck Surg.* 1988;114:328–329.
9. Wei WI, Sham JST, Choy D, Ho CM, Lam KH. Split-palate approach for gold grain implantation in nasopharyngeal carcinoma. *Arch Otolaryngol Head Neck Surg.* 1990;116:578–582.
10. Stevenson GC, Stoney RJ, Perkins RK, Adams JE. A transcervical transclival approach to the ventral surface of the brain stem for removal of a clivus chordoma. *J Neurosurg.* 1966;24:544–551.
11. Wood BG, Sadar ES, Levine HL, Dohn DF, Turcker HM. Surgical problems of the base of the skull. An interdisciplinary approach. *Arch Otolaryngol.* 1980;106:1–5.
12. Biller HF, Shugar JMA, Krepsi YP. A new technique for wide-field exposure of the base of the skull. *Arch Otolaryngol.* 1981;107:698–702.
13. Krepsi YP, Sisson GA. Skull base surgery in composite resection. *Arch Otolaryngol.* 1982;108:681–684.
14. Fee WE Jr, Roberson JB Jr, Goffinet DR. Long-term survival after surgical resection for recurrent nasopharyngeal cancer after radiotherapy failure. *Arch Otolaryngol Head Neck Surg.* 1991;117:1233–1236.
15. Wilson CP. Observations on the surgery of the nasopharynx. *Ann Otol Rhinol Laryngol.* 1957;66:5–40.
16. Belmont JR. The Le Fort I osteotomy approach for nasopharyngeal and nasal fossa tumors. *Arch Otolaryngol Head Neck Surg.* 1988;114:751–754.
17. Uttley D, Moore A, Archer DJ. Surgical management of midline skull-base tumors: a new approach. *Neurosurg.* 1989;71:705–710.
18. Cocke EW Jr., Robertson JH, Robertson JT, Crook JP Jr. The extended maxillotomy and subtotal maxillectomy for excision of skull base tumors. *Arch Otolaryngol Head Neck Surg.* 1990;116:92–104.
19. Schuller DE, Goodman JH, Brown BL, Frank JE, Ervin-Miller KJ. Maxillary removal and reinsertion for improved access to anterior cranial base tumors. *Laryngoscope.* 1992;102:203–212.
20. Hernandez AF. Transfacial access to the retromaxillary area. *J Maxillofac Surg.* 1986;14:165–170.
21. Wei WI, Lam KH, Sham JST. New approach to the nasopharynx: the maxillary swing approach. *Head Neck.* 1991;13:200–207.
22. Wei WI, Ho CM, Yuen PW, Fung CF, Sham JST, Lam KH. Maxillary swing approach for resection of tumors in and around the nasopharynx. *Arch Otolaryngol Head Neck Surg.* 1995;121:638–642.

CHAPTER 6

Targeted Cisplatin Chemotherapy for Advanced Head and Neck Cancer

K. Thomas Robbins, MD

Combination chemotherapy, particularly cisplatin-based, has been shown to be highly active for head and neck cancer. Unfortunately, when used alone or in the neoadjuvant setting, studies have repeatedly failed to demonstrate any associated survival advantage. There is evidence to suggest that treatment failure in patients receiving chemotherapy is related to rapidly acquired drug resistance following exposure to the agents. In the case of cisplatin, it is possible that this resistance could be circumvented through the delivery of higher doses of cisplatin. A novel, targeted cisplatin drug delivery technique was developed for this purpose.[1] It involves rapid, superselective intra-arterial infusions combined with intravenous sodium thiosulfate for systemic cisplatin neutralization. Dose intensities of cisplatin equivalent to tenfold standard intravenous cisplatin regimens are possible using this strategy. Intratumor platinum levels are 2- to 20-fold greater than measurements obtained after intravenous infusions, confirming that it is possible to obtain high concentrations of the agent into the tumor bed.[2]

LABORATORY EVIDENCE FOR CISPLATIN RESISTANCE

Using in vitro models, there is evidence that acquired cisplatin resistance by tumors is mild to moderate and can be overcome with drug concentrations 5- to 10-fold greater than the therapeutic equivalent.[3,4,5] Teicher et al demonstrated a linear dose response relationship for a head and neck carcinoma cell line which indicated that an additional log 10 ÷ 2 of cell kill occurred by doubling the cisplatin dose.[3]

Using a sponge-gel supported histoculture, 43 tumor specimens from patients with squamous cell carcinoma (SCC) of the upper aerodigestive tract (UADT) were grown and exposed to cisplatin.[6] Growth inhibition by the drug, in concentrations equivalent to peak therapeutic doses (1.5 µg/ml) and concentrations 10- and 25-fold greater (15 and 37.5 µg/ml), were measured in specimens from patients with previously untreated and recurrent lesions. In vitro, the overall rate of sensitivity of the tumor samples to cisplatin concentrations of 1.5, 15, and 37.5 µg/ml were 22%, 62%, and 83%, respectively. In patients with previously untreated disease, the respective rates were 25.9%, 63.3%, and 79.3% compared to 10.0%, 55.6%, and 85.6% for patients with recurrent disease. The response difference between cisplatin concentrations of 1.5 and 15 µg/ml was statistically significant. The decadose effect of cisplatin on growth inhibition was 2.44-fold for untreated lesions and 5.56-fold for recurrent tumors. The results indicate that resistance to standard doses of cisplatin by squamous cell carcinoma (SCC) of the UADT can be substantially overcome with a decadose (10 ÷) increase and is more pronounced in tumors from patients with recurrent disease. Progress toward improving survival of patients may be possible by incorporating decadose cisplatin therapy into a multimodality treatment plan.

Since the development of several new and effective methods to circumvent dose-limiting toxicity, high dose chemotherapy has recently become an important focus of clinical research. The premise for high dose chemotherapy is based on the well known principle that cumulative response of a biologic system to an inciting agent can be mathematically described by a sigmoidal curve. For drugs, this is referred to as the dose response curve comprising a lag phase, a linear phase, and a plateau phase. Cisplatin dose response curves have been determined for a variety of cell lines from different organ sites, including the head and neck.[3,7] In general, the curve is relatively steep and a 10-fold increase of drug concentration produces several logarithmic powers of additional cell kill. Even for cell lines that have been selectively made resistant to cisplatin, this resistance is relative and can usually be overcome by increasing the concentration of the cisplatin. It is significant to note that it is difficult to render resistance to cisplatin in cell lines greater than 10-fold, whereas the magnitude of resistance to other drugs such as methotrexate is substantially higher. Thus, with in vitro systems, cisplatin resistance to various cancers is usually mild to moderate and can be overcome with a 10-fold increment in concentration.

A practical limitation to the strategy of overcoming drug resistance by increasing the dose is toxicity to normal cells. Prior to the use of hydration and diuresis, cisplatin doses exceeding 50 mg/m^2 frequently caused nephrotoxicity. Thus the results of early clincal trials with cisplatin using relatively low doses showed only modest response rates. After hydration was instituted, subsequent studies employing cisplatin in doses ranging between 80–120 mg/m^2 q 3–4 weeks were then possible.[8-10] However, even with this "high dose" cisplatin exposure, the average overall response rates (CR and PR) in 267 patients with recurrent head and neck cancer collected from eight studies was only 28% (range: 14–41%).[11]

The major dose-limiting toxicity beyond this amount continued to be renal and gastrointestinal (severe nausea and vomiting). More recently, the use of seratonin uptake inhibitors have abrogated much of the gastrointestinal toxicty for cisplatin at conventional doses. Nevertheless, clinical trials using cisplatin in doses above this level have not been practical because of excessive toxicity.

TARGETED SUPRADOSE CISPLATIN TECHNIQUE

Developed at the University of California, San Diego, the use of this drug delivery technique makes it possible to saturate the tumor bed with cisplatin in concentrations that are much greater than the intravenous drug delivery route.[1,12] It also permits the administration of repeated cisplatin infusions at dose intensities equivalent to 10-fold higher than standard methods. Cisplatin is rapidly infused over 3–5 minutes through a microcatheter placed angiographically to selectively encompass only the dominant blood supply of the targeted tumor. Simultaneous with starting the IA infusion of cisplatin, sodium thiosulfate (9 gm/m^2 over 30 minutes, followed by 12 gm/m^2 over 6 hours) was given intravenously. This allows the tumor bed to initially receive the full dose of cisplatin prior to the neutralizing agent and the systemic organs to receive the neutralizing agent prior to the cisplatin (Fig 6–1). Patients receive pretreatment IV hydration over 2 hours consisting of 2 liters of normal saline containing 20 mEq KCl and 2 gm magnesium sulfate. Cisplatin is dissolved in 400 ml normal saline. Post-treatment hydration consists of 1 liter of normal saline containing 20 mEq KCl and 2 gm magnesium sulfate over 6 hours. Decadron is also administered IV or PO, 4 mg every 6 hours until the following morning.

Patients are admitted to the hospital and hydrated overnight. The catheterization is done by interventional radiologists under local anaesthesia in the interventional radiology suite. Transfemoral carotid arteriography is first done to assess the vascular anatomy and any pathology.[13] The appropiate vessels supplying the region of primary disease are then infused with cisplatin. This is usually achieved by placing a microcatheter, introduced transaxially through a tracker catheter, into the external carotid artery at the level of the orifice of the dominant branching artery to the tumor. Thus, on its initial exposure cisplatin can be rapidly infused to selectively encompass only the territory of the targeted tumor. In selected patients with excessively bulky disease crossing the midline, bilateral transfemoral catheterizations are performed to permit simultaneous infusions of the contralateral disease. In each patient, the goal is to infuse the component of the disease considered to be bulky and/or infiltrative and likely to fail radiotherapy alone. No specific attempt is made to infuse the regional lymph nodes. Instead, this disease component is treated with radiotherapy in appropiate doses. Simultaneous with starting the IA infusion of cisplatin, sodium thiosulfate is infused IV. This allows the tumor bed to receive the full dose of cisplatin prior to the neutralizing agent and the systemic organs to receive the neutralizing agent prior to the cisplatin.

In a phase I study, it was determined that the maximum tolerated dose of cisplatin that could be administered is 150 mg/m^2/week ÷ 4.[1] Cohorts of patients received dose intensity

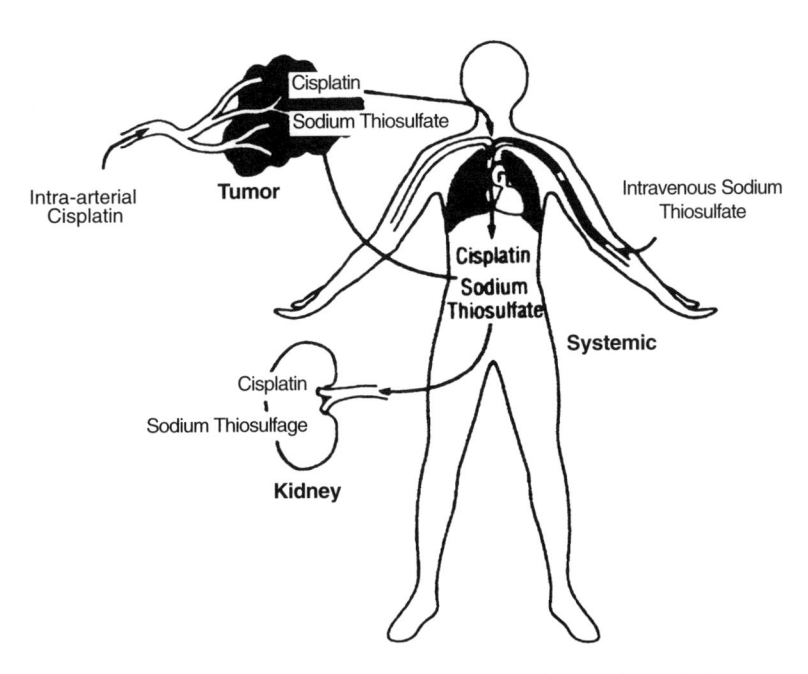

FIG 6–1. Schematic representation of targeted supradose cisplatin infusion technique with systemic sodium thiosulfate neutralization.

schedules of 50, 100, 150, and 200 mg/m²/week. Dose limiting toxicity was found to be a severe leakage of electrolytes from the kidney, which could be alleviated by intravenous replacement therapy until there was recovery. None of the patients had irreversible nephrotoxicity. Other grade III–IV toxicities noted during this trial were gastrointestinal (4 events) and neutropenia (1 event).

The response of tumor to this treatment among 22 patients with previously untreated disease was: 9 complete responses (CR) (41%) and 10 partial responses (PR) (45%) for a major response rate of 86%. Among the 16 patients with recurrent disease, 4 had a CR (25%) and 6 had a PR (38%) for a major response rate of 63%. Because this was a dose escalating study in which the dose intensity schedule ranged between 32.5 and 200 mg/m²/week, a more detailed analysis of the response effects of cisplatin at specific dose intensities was done.[14] The overall response rate (CR and PR) to cisplatin therapy at dose intensity intervals of 0–74, 75–149, and 150–200 mg/m²/week were 45.5%, 72.7%, and 100%, respectively. The average received dose intensity for nonresponders (NR) versus responders (CR and PR) was 57.8 and 120.7 mg/m²/week respectively ($p = 0.031$). For patients with previously untreated disease, the average planned dose intensity for nonresponders was 85.5 mg/m²/week compared to 106.3 mg/m²/week for responders ($p = 0.1403$). For patients with recurrent disease, the average planned dose intensity for nonresponders was 56.2 mg/m²/week compared to 159.3 mg/m²/week for responders ($p = 0.0073$). These data indicate that high-dose cisplatin exposure increases the rate of tumor response in SCC of the UADT and supports the hypothesis that acquired cisplatin resistance by these tumors is usually mild to moderate and can be circumvented by 10-fold concentrations of the drug. The decadose effect was achieved by increasing the dose and condensing the overall treatment time. Calculated as the dose intensity value, this increased cisplatin exposure reaches an equivalent 10-fold greater than standard cisplatin protocols.

Intra-arterial chemotherapy for head and neck cancer has been investigated for over the past three decades. Trials have been conducted with cisplatin alone or in combination with other agents. In patients with previously untreated disease, the average overall and complete response rates in 85 patients treated with cisplatin alone from three collected studies was 76.5% (range 70.8–82%) and 29.9% (range 24.2–32%), respectively.[14-17] The average overall and complete response from IA cisplatin combined with one or more other drugs was 78.5% (range 46–94%) and 21.6% (range 7.7–43%), respectively, in 167 patients with previously untreated disease collected from 6 studies.[18-22] The results from the IA trials are variable but several studies, particularly those using cisplatin-based regimens, indicate that a high response rate can be achieved. Others have argued that the best results of IA chemotherapy do not surpass the best response rates from IV chemotherapy, and when combined with the increased risk of local toxicity, there is no advantage to this approach. Most of the technical complications have been related to catheter placements, including thrombosis, dislodgement, and hemorrhage. However, newer and safer angiographic techniques as used in the targeted chemotherapy program now permit highly selective placements of microcatheters into small arteries under direct vision using fluoroscopy.[23] These advances in interventional vascular radiology make it possible to selectively and repeatedly infuse chemotherapeutic agents into head and neck tumors with minimal side effects.[21]

The theoretical advantage of IA chemotherapy over standard intravenous (IV) chemotherapy is that a higher concentration of the drug can be delivered directly to the tumor bed than to other organs. Depending on the amount of drug uptake by the tumor during this first pass, it is also possible to infuse a higher concentration of cytotoxic agent through this route than would be tolerated by the IV route. It is important to remember that the entire advantage of IA delivery must be achieved during this first pass. After the drug leaves its target and enters the systemic circulation, it behaves as if it were injected IV. The pharmacokinetics of IA therapy were described by Eckman et al.[24] The relative advantage of IA infusion is directly proportional to the plasma clearance of the drug and inversely proportional to the plasma flow to the tumor. Thus, the faster the drug is excreted, and the slower the tumor plasma flow, the larger the relative advantage for infusing by the IA route. In the case of head and neck lesions, Wheeler et al reported the mean tumor blood flow estimated by radionuclide washout techniques was 13.6 ± 6.7 ml/100g/ml compared to 4.2 ± 2.1 ml/100g/min for normal tissue (scalp).[25] This provided a mean tumor: normal tissue blood flow ratio of 3.9 ± 2.7 ml/100g/min, thus favoring drug delivery to the tumor contained within the infused region.

Although the IA route for drug delivery provides a theoretical advantage for higher concentrations of the drug to reach the tumor, only conventional doses have been administered in almost all of the previous trials. Very few trials have been conducted with high-dose cisplatin in patients with UADT tumors. In a study using high dose cisplatin (200 mg/m^2 q 4 weeks), a high response rate (72%) was achieved in a group of 22 patients, 16 of whom had recurrent disease.[26] Haines et al treated 51 patients (Stage III–IV disease) with 187.5–200 mg/m^2 of cisplatin and 60 U/m^2 of bleomycin q 4 weeks resulting in an overall response of 69% (CR 24%, PR 45%.[27] Kish et al reported a 90% response rate (CR 45%) in 11 patients treated with cisplatin 150–200 mg/m^2 and 5-FU 1000 mg/m^2 q 3 weeks.[28] Both authors concluded that the higher dose schedule showed no added benefit for response whereas toxicity was greater. When evaluating these studies, it is important to underscore the difference between *high dose* and *high dose intensity*. In all of these previous head and neck studies, the maximum dose intensity of the cisplatin schedule was 66.7 mg/m^2/week, equivalent to two- or three-fold the standard dose.

Prior to the targeted chemotherapy program, a decadose cisplatin effect had not previously been tested, primarily because such doses are highly toxic when given by conventional methods. The exploitation of the chelating reaction of sodium thiosulfate with cisplatin and the new technology of selective vascular catheterization has permitted the use of a drug delivery technique that involves the preferential supersaturation of the tumor bed with cisplatin. Thus the major barrier precluding the use of extremely high dose intensity cisplatin in humans, nephrotoxicity, has been substantially pushed back.

Thiosulfate reacts covalently with cisplatin to produce a complex that is still soluble but is totally devoid of either toxicity or antitumor activity.[29] When this neutralization occurs in the plasma it effectively increases the plasma "clearance" of cisplatin. The extent of reaction is a function of the concentration of both agents. Thiosulfate is not a very potent neutralization agent and molar thiosulfate/cisplatin ratios in excess of 10 are required before the reaction is fast enough to contribute significantly to the clearance of cisplatin.[30] Thiosulfate itself is very nontoxic and doses in excess of 72 gm can be given acutely, which is well above that needed to provide effective cisplatin neutralization. Pharmacokinetic studies have demonstrated an important additional feature of thiosulfate: it is extensively concentrated (>25-fold) in the urine, and this provides excellent protection against cisplatin-induced nephrotoxicity.

Subsequently, emphasis has been given to the use of concomitant therapy in which chemotherapy is given simultaneously with radiation therapy or sandwiched between courses of radiation therapy. There are many interactions between radiation and chemotherapeutic agents that theoretically could make concurrent use more effective than sequential use. The mechanisms are based on differential activity of drug and radiation against specific tumor cell subpopulations such as hypoxic cells,[31] pH differences in tumor cells,[32] cell cycle phase distribution patterns,[33] or mechanical factors such as reduced tumor bulk leading to improved drug delivery and reoxygenation of hypoxic cells. Other mechanisms may require direct interactions between the drug and radiotherapy and include inhibition of repair of radiation damage, cell cycle synchronization, or the elimination of inherent resistance to the drug or radiation as single agents.[34-36]

Cisplatin has been well studied as a radiation sensitizer. Zak and Drobnik first described enhanced radiation cytotoxicity in the presence of cisplatin in a murine tumor.[37] It was later demonstrated that radiation cytotoxicity could be enhanced with cisplatin in mammalian cells.[34] Other chemotherapy agents including 5-FU, mitomycin, and hydroxyurea are also capable of enhancing the cytotoxic effects of radiation.[35]

Clinical trials using concomitant chemoradiation have provided some evidence that this approach is better than radiation alone for patients with unresectable disease. Trials have been conducted using cisplatin alone[38-41]; cisplatin and 5-FU[40,42,43]; and other combinations[44,45] for patients with previously untreated head and neck cancer. The highest response rate was 84% reported in 27 patients with nasopharyngeal carcinoma.[41] Very few randomized chemoradiation studies have compared cisplatin/XRT to XRT alone. Using a low dose cisplatin regimen, Haselow et al[39] found no difference in response rate (CR: 30 % vs 34 %) and survival.[39] However, Merlano et al[42] reported improved survival using rapidly alternating cisplatin/5 FU chemotherapy and radiation therapy compared to radiation alone. Paccagnella et al[46] recently reported better overall survival among patients with unresectable disease treated with induction cisplatin/5 FU followed by radiation versus radiotherapy only. However, there was no demonstrable survival advantage for patients with resectable disease, a result in keeping with numerous other randomized studies testing similar induction chemotherapy regimens. Chemoradiation may also have potential benefits when used in the postoperative setting.[47]

Chemotherapy and radiotherapy also have the potential to avoid major loss of organ function, particularly as this relates to the larynx. The initial thrust of the organ preservation approach was to preserve the larynx in patients with laryngeal cancer using induction chemotherapy followed by radiation. Several trials for preserving the larynx[48,49] or other organs have been done.[50-52] The benchmark study was a randomized trial for advanced laryngeal cancer conducted by the Veterans Administration Intergroup.[51] In this, approximately two thirds of the patients receiving induction chemotherapy (cisplatin /5-FU) were spared total laryngectomy. Survival was nearly the same as the group receiving standard care (total laryngectomy/XRT). However, others have argued that organ preservation can be be achieved with primary radiotherapy alone,[53] particularly if hyperfractionation schedules are employed.[54-56] The results of a randomized study conducted by the EORT for patients with intermediate oropharyngeal cancer showed an improved survival for the group treated with hyperfractionated radiation therapy.[56] Further support for this approach may be forthcoming on completion of an RTOG study in which induction chemotherapy is being compared to standard versus hyperfractionated radiotherapy.

Subsequent studies using the targeted drug delivery concept have focused on investigations combining cisplatin infusions with radiation therapy. The preliminary reports indicated an extremely high, complete pathological response rate, a very high organ preservation rate, sustained disease control above the clavicles, and a relatively low rate of toxicity.[57-59] The most recent analysis included 83 patients treated between 1991–1994 for whom the follow-up ranged between 17–61 months (median 24 months).[60] All patients had tumors arising in the oral cavity, oropharynx, hypopharynx, or larynx. Distribution by specific subsite was as follows: base of tongue (11 patients), oropharyngeal wall (10 patients), piriform sinus (8 patients), glottic larynx (4 patients), and supraglottic larynx (9 patients). One third of the lesions were massive and anatomically unresectable; two thirds were potentially resectable by technical (anatomical) criteria but removal would have caused the loss of one or more organs necessary for speech and swallowing. Forty-seven patients (56%) had T4 disease; 30

(36%) had T3 disease; and only 6 (8%) had T2 disease. The distribution of disease by N stage was: 20 (24%) had N0 disease; 12 (14%) had N1; 44 (52%) had N2; and 7 (10%) had N3. Thus, only 24% of patients had stage III disease. The remaining 76% had stage IV disease.

Conventional external beam irradiation was used in daily fractions (180–200 cGy/fraction) to a total dose of 68.5–74.0 Gy given over 7–8 weeks. All patients received intra-arterial (IA) cisplatin and IV sodium thiosulfate infusions concurrently on days 1, 8, 15, and 22 of radiotherapy. Planned neck dissection was done 2 months post-treatment on patients whose original nodal disease was considered to be N2 or N3. Salvage surgery was done on patients who developed recurrent disease that was considered to be resectable.

Of the 78 patients evaluable for response to treatment in the *primary site*, 70 (92%) had a complete response; 5 (6%) had a partial response; and 1 (1%) had no response. Five patients were unevaluable for response assessment. Planned neck dissection was performed on 30 of the 52 patients with bulky (N2–N3) nodal disease. For this subset of patients, staging of response to treatment in the neck was based on the pathological findings of the neck dissection specimen. For the remaining patients with bulky nodal disease, and the patients who had class N0–N1 disease, staging was based on clinical and radiological criteria. Of the 78 patients evaluable for response to treatment in the *regional lymph nodes*, there was a complete response in 64 patients (84%), and a partial response in 11 patients (14%). The only patient who had no response in the primary site also had no response in the neck.

The overall rate of severe toxicity to chemotherapy was 5% as determined by the 18 grade III–IV events among the 83 patients undergoing a cumulative total of 323 cycles. This included 9 gastrointestinal, 7 hematologic, 1 neurologic, and 1 death during therapy secondary to a pulmonary embolus. There were no events of grade III–IV ototoxicity or renal damage. Seventy-two patients (87%) received all four cycles of cisplatin, 9 (11%) received three cycles, and 2 (2%) received less than three cycles.

An inherent problem with treatment protocols combining concomitant radiation with chemotherapy is toxicity, particularly mucositis.[45,61] Although this is more commonly associated with the use of 5-FU, toxicity of the mucosa and other organs have been prevalent side effects of cisplatin-based protocols. Thus treatment delays and dose reductions are common. In contrast, there were 25 patients (30%) who developed grade III–IV mucositis, all but 2 of whom were categorized as grade III. Only one patient required a delay in radiotherapy because of mucositis. Only one patient in the series required an interruption of radiotherapy, a lower incidence than one would expect from radiotherapy alone. The 30% rate of confluent mucositis is lower than one would expect from radiation therapy alone. This raises the possibility that sodium thiosulfate may exert a radioprotective effect on the surrounding normal mucosa.

Among the total number of 323 transfemoral, super-selective IA infusions performed, 6 patients had postinfusion central nervous system dysfunction, 3 of whom had a cerebrovascular accident and 3 had a transient ischemic attack. None of these patients developed any severe impairment as a consequence of these complications. This low rate of technical complications appears to justify the invasive approach chosen because of its ability to deliver high concentrations of cisplatin directly into the tumor bed. Three patients developed a pulmonary embolus, one of whom died after successfully completing 4 weekly infusions. Two additional patients died immediately after the treatment regimen was completed, one from acute coronary ischemia and one from suspected aspiration pneumonia. Another patient developed femoral vein thrombosis without any adverse sequelae.

At a median follow-up of 30 months, the overall and disease-related survival was 58% and 74% respectively. The projected Kaplan Meier 5-year overall and disease-related survival rates were 40% and 58%, respectively.

The rate of disease control above the clavicle for all patients was 76/83 (90%) (Fig 6–2). Twenty-one patients developed recurrent disease: 4 within the primary site, 3 within the regional lymph nodes, and 14 in distant sites (lung-8 patients, bone-5 patients, brain-1 patient). One of the patients with lung metastases also had liver and brain lesions. Successful surgical salvage was possible for three of the four patients who developed recurrent disease in the primary site, and all three of the patients who developed recurrent disease in the regional lymph nodes.

The data indicate that high-dose intensity intra-arterial cisplatin infusions combined with radiation therapy administered to patients with advanced head and neck cancer has an antitumor effect that is sufficiently powerful and sustained to render almost every patient disease free.

The overall rate of grade III–IV chemotoxicity was only 5% and 87% of patients were able to receive all four cycles of DDP. The low rate of toxicity and high rate for delivering all of the prescribed chemotherapy regimen was attributed to the systemic cisplatin-neutralizing effects of sodium thiosulfate.[62] There were no events of grade III–IV renal toxicity, presumably because sodium thiosulfate is concentrated in the kidneys and thereby has an added protective effect. It was also observed that ototoxicity was much reduced relative to experiences using intravenous cisplatin without systemic neutralization.[63]

A major goal of this research was to identify a new strategy that could offer patients an improved survival outcome while avoiding major loss of organ function. Towards improving survival, the data strongly suggest that subjects are remaining alive at a rate that

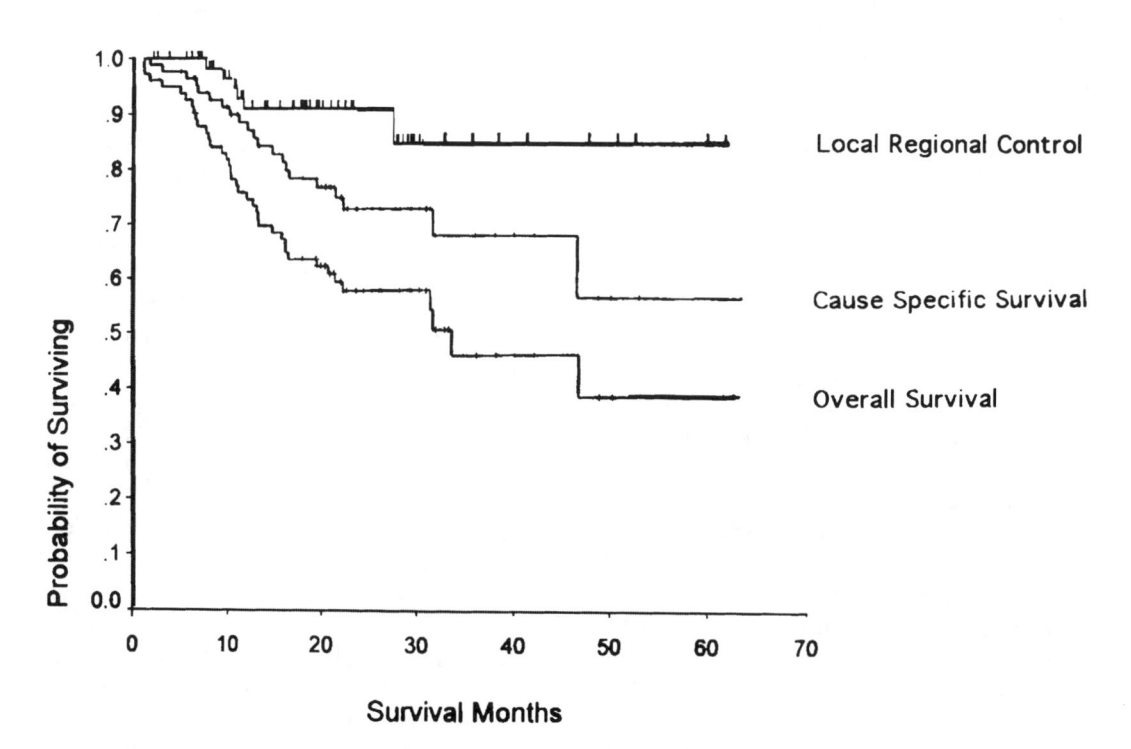

FIG 6–2. Projected Kaplan-Meier survival plots for 83 patients with Stage III–IV upper aerodigestive tract squamous cell carcinoma treated with targeted supradose cisplatin and concomitant radiation therapy.

is significantly higher than expected. Previous survival results reported for patients with stage IV disease vary from 10–40%. The higher figures reflect the results among surgical patients with resectable lesions; whereas the very low figures are typical of patients with unresectable lesions treated with radiation alone.

Death from persistent or recurrent disease within the primary site or the neck is often associated with catastrophic suffering related to marked alterations of important bodily functions, severe pain, and disfigurement. Only three patients in the study succumbed to persistent disease following initial therapy and only two patients died of recurrent disease above the clavicle. The majority of patients who died of disease did so because of recurrent tumor at distant sites, most commonly the lungs. This pattern of cancer death is different from most head and neck cancer trials in which death from locoregional disease is by far more common. It is likely that distant metastatic disease among patients with head and neck cancer is usually masked by locoregional disease. With improved methods to control disease above the clavicle, one can expect an unmasking of clinical distant disease among patients who had occult metastatic disease prior to therapy. The emerging problem of death from distant disease will require designing subsequent studies to include a systemic treatment component, particularly for patients who are at greatest risk.

Although the organ preservation therapeutic approach used in this study potentially has highly significant advantages over standard surgical treatment protocols, one must temper this enthusiasm because organ preservation does not necessarily imply preserving function. For example, one would not expect to see return of normal laryngeal function in a patient whose advanced tumor had effaced a large part of the organ. Instead, one might expect to see some degree of dysphonia and possibly compromised respiration and/or aspiration with associated dysphagia.

Detailed analyses of functional impairment are currently being done on our patients to better assess this problem. This includes the development and validation of objective measures of phonation[64] and application of swallowing assessment and quality of life questionnaires applicable to head and neck cancer patients.[65] The latter also reflects the patient's ability to tolerate the therapy, which is particularly important to monitor among patients undergoing aggressive treatment with chemotherapy and radiation.

In an attempt to improve the dismal prognosis for patients with advanced cancer involving the temporal bone, the targeted cisplatin chemotherapy technique was piloted as part of a multimodality treatment approach for patients presenting with this challenging problem.[66,67] Rapid supradose cisplatin infusions selectively delivered to the lesion and concurrent systemic cisplatin neutralization were given to 14 patients with carcinoma involving the temporal bone. Four patients received chemotherapy alone, four had concomitant irradiation, and six had subsequent irradiation and/or temporal bone surgery. All of the patients tolerated the chemotherapy without any significant complications or toxicity. All three of the patients with previously untreated disease responded to chemotherapy (2 CRs, 1 PR); three of the seven patients with recurrent disease responded to chemotherapy; and all four patients treated with chemoradiation had a complete responses (including one patient with recurrent disease). At a median follow-up of 19 months (range 5–63 months), 9 of the 14 patients were alive, including the 4 who were treated with targeted chemoradiation. The data support further investigations using targeted high-dose chemotherapy, particularly when it is given simultaneously with radiation, for patients with malignant skull base lesions and potentially improve the outcome

CONCLUSION

Despite the earlier failures to demonstrate an effective role for chemotherapy in head and neck cancer, there remains the promise for successfully incorporating this approach into the multimodality therapy for this disease. The targeted supradose cisplatin program is one strategy that appears to provide a lasting state of disease control without having to sacrifice the function of major organs. Further work is needed to demonstrate the ability to safely use this technique in multiple centers and to duplicate its effectiveness. Ultimately, randomized trials may be indicated to determine whether this approach can increase survival, maintain organ function, and improve the quality of life.

REFERENCES

1. Robbins KT, Storniolo AMS, Kerber C, Vicario D, Seagren S, Shea M, Hanchett C, Los G, Howell SB. Phase I study of highly selective supradose cisplatin infusions for advanced head and neck cancer. *J Clin Oncol.* 1994;12:2113–2120.
2. Los G, Barton R, Heath DD, Blommaert FA, den Engelse L, Hanchett C, Vicario D, Weisman R, Robbins KT, Howell SB. Selective intra-arterial infusion of high dose cisplatin in advanced head and neck cancer patients resulting in high tumor platinum concentrations and cisplatin-DNA adduct formation. *Cancer Chemotherapy Pharmacology.* 1995;37(1–2):15–154.
3. Teicher BA, Holden SA, Kelley MJ, Shea TC, Cucchi CA, Rosowsky A, Henner WD, Frei E III. Characterization of a human squamous carcinoma cell line resistant to cis-diamminedichloroplatinum (11). *Cancer Res.* 1987;47:388–393.
4. Waud W. Differential uptake of cis-diamminedichloroplatinum (11) by sensitive and resistant murine L1210 leukemia cells. *Cancer Res.* 1987;47:6549–6555.
5. Van Hoff DD, Clark GM, Weiss GR, Marshall MH, Buchok JB, Knight WA, LeMaistre CF. Use of in vitro dose response effects to select antineoplastics for high-dose or regional administration regimens. *J Clin Oncol.* 1986;4(12):1827–1834.
6. Robbins KT, Hoffman R. Decadose effects of cisplatin on squamous cell carcinoma of the upper aerodigestive tract: part I, histoculture experiments. *Laryngoscope.* 106,1996;37–42.
7. Andrews PA, Murphy MP, Howell SB. Characterization of cisplatin-resistant COLO 316 human ovarian carcinoma cells. *Eur J Cancer Clin Oncol.* 1989;25(4):619–625.
8. Randolph VL, Vallejo A, Spiro RH, Shah J, Strong EW, Huvos AG, Wittes RE. Combination therapy of advanced head and neck cancer induction of remissions with diamminedichloroplatinum (II), bleomycin and radiotherapy. *Cancer.* 1978;41:460–467.
9. Hayat M, Bayssas M, Brule G, Cappelaere P, Cattan A, Chauvergne J, Clavel B, Gouveia J, Guerrin J, Laufer J, Pommatau E, Szpirglas H, Muggia F, Mathe G. Cis-platinum-diammino-dichlor (CPID) in chemotherapy of cancers. Phase II therapeutic trial. *Biochimi.* 1978;60:935–940.
10. Wittes R, Heller K, Randolph V, Howard J, Vallejo A, Farr H, Harrold C, Gerold F, Shah J, Spiro R, and Strong E. cis-Dichlorodiammineplatinum (II)-based chemotherapy as inital treatment of advanced head and neck cancer. *Cancer Treat Rep.* 1979;63:1533–1538.
11. Al-Sarraf M. Chemotherapy strategies in squamous cell carcinoma of the head and neck. *CRC Crit Rev Oncol/Hematol.* 1989;1(4):323–355.
12. Robbins KT, Storniolo AM, Kerber C, Seagren S, Berson A, Howell SB. Rapid superselective high dose cisplatin infusion for advanced head and neck malignancies. *Head Neck.* 1992;14:364–371.
13. Kerber CW, Wong WHM, Robbins KT. Treatment of head and neck cancers with a new intraarterial infusion strategy. In: Conner B, ed. *Neurointerventional technique.* (In press)
14. Robbins KT, Storniolo AMS, Hryniuk WH, Howell SB. Decadose effects of cisplatin on squamous cell carcinoma of the upper aerodigestive tract: part II, clinical studies. *Laryngoscope.* 1996;106:37–42.
15. Frustaci S, Barzan L, Carusco G, Ghirado R, Foladore S, Carbone A, Conoretto R, Serafini I, Monfardini S. Induction intra-arterial cisplatin and bleomycin in head and neck cancer. *Head Neck.* 1991;13:291–297.
16. Mortimer JE, Taylor ME, Schulmans, Cummings C, Weymuller E, Laramore G. Feasibility and efficacy of weekly intraarterial cisplatin in locally advanced (stage III and IV) head and neck cancers. *J Clin Oncol.* 1988;6:969–975.
17. Galmarini FC, Yoel H, Abulafia J, Nakasone J, Temperley G. Intra-arterial cisplatinum in head and neck cancer—controlled clinical trial in phases I and II. *Head Neck Surg.* 1981 (Jan/Feb):257.

18. Cheung DK, Regan J, Savin M, Gibberman V, Soessner W. A pilot study of intraarterial chemotherapy with cisplatin in locally advanced head and neck cancers. *Cancer*. 1988; 61:903–908.
19. Claudio F, Rotondi M, Bonassi S, Cacacer F, Comella G, Coucourde F, Claudia PP, Bevilacqua AM, Ionna F, Toma S. Factors affecting response and survival in advanced head and neck cancers treated with intraarterial chemotherapy. *Reg Cancer*. 1992:4:180–187.
20. Forastiere AA, Baker SR, Wheeler R, Medvec BR. Intra-arterial cisplatin and FUDR in advanced malignancies confined to the head and neck. *J Clin Oncol*. 1987;5:1601–1606.
21. Lee YY, Dimery I, Van Tassel P, De Pena C, Blacklock B, Goepfert H. Superselective intra-arterial chemotherapy of advanced paranasal sinus tumors. *Arch Otolaryngol Head Neck Surg*. 1989;115:503–511.
22. Molinari R. Preliminary intra-arterial chemotherapy in cancer of the oral cavity: long-term results of combined treatments with surgery and radiotherapy. In Cretian PB, Johns ME, Shedd DP, et al, eds. *Head and Neck Cancer*. Philadelphia, Pa: Decker; 1985:456–461.
23. Wolpert SM, Kwan ES, Heros D, Kasdon DL, Hedges TR. Selective delivery of chemotherapeutic agents with a new catheter system. *Radiology*. 1988;166:547–549.
24. Eckman WW, Patlak CS, Fenstermacher JD. A critical evaluation of the principles governing the advantages of intra-arterial infusions. *J Pharmacokinet Biopharm*. 1974;2:257–285.
25. Wheeler RH, Ziessman HA, Medvec BR, et al. Tumor blood flow and systemic shunting in patients receiving intraarterial chemotherapy for head and neck cancer. *Cancer Res*. 1986;46:4200–4204.
26. Forastiere AA, Takasuri BJ, Baker SR, Wolf, Kudla-Hatch V. High-dose cisplatin in advanced head and neck cancer. *Cancer Chemother Pharmacol*. 1987;19:155–158.
27. Haines I, Bosl G, Pfister D, Spiro R, Gerold F, Sessions R, Shah J, Strong E, Vikram B, Harrison L. Very-high-dose cisplatin with bleomycin infusion as initial treatment of advanced head and neck cancer. *J Clin Oncol*. 1987;5:1594–1600.
28. Kish JA, Ensley JF, Jacobs JR, Binns P, Al-Sarraf M. Evaluation of high-dose cisplatin and 5-FU infusion as initial therapy in advanced head and neck cancer. *Am J Clin Oncol*. 1988;II(5):553–557.
29. Elferink WJF, van der Vijah IK, Pinedo HM. Interaction of cisplatin and carboplatin with sodium thiosulfate: reaction rates and protein binding. *Clin Chem*. 1986;32:642–645.
30. Shea M, Koziol JA, Howell SB. Kinetics of sodium thiosulfate, a cisplatin neutralizer. *Clin Pharmacol Ther*. 1984;35(3):419–425.
31. Sartorelli AC. Therapeutic attack of hypoxic cells of solid tumors: presidential address. *Cancer Res*. 1988;48:775–778.
32. Tannock IF, Rotin D. Acid pH in tumors and its potential for therapeutic exploitation. *Cancer Res*. 1989;49:4373–4384.
33. Sinclair WK. Hydroxyurea: effects on Chinese hamster cells grown in culture. *Cancer Res*. 1967;27:297–308.
34. Douple EB, Richmond RC. Platinum complexes as radiosensitizers of hypoxic mammalian cells. *Br J Cancer*. 1978;37:98–102.
35. Muggia FM, Glatstein E. Summary of investigations on platinum compounds and radiation reactions. *Int J Radiol Oncol Biol Phys*. 1979;5:1407–1409.
36. Alvarez MV, Cobreros G, Heras A, Zumel Ma CL. Studies on cisdichlorodiammineplatinum (II) as a radiosensitizer. *Br J Cancer*. 1978;37: 68–72.
37. Zak M, Dobnik J. Effects of cis-dichlorodiammineplatinum (II) on the post-irradiation lethality in mice after irradiation with X-rays. *Strahlentherapie*. 1971;142:112–115.
38. Marcial VA, Pajak TF, Mohiuddin M, Cooper JS, Al-Arraf M, Mowry PA, Curran W, Crissman J, Rodriguez M, Velez-Garcia E. Concomitant cisplatin chemotherapy and radiotherapy in advanced mucosal squamous cell carcinoma of the head and neck. *Cancer*. 1990;66:1861–1868.
39. Haselow RE, Warshaw MG, Oken MM, et al. Radiation alone versus radiation with weekly low dose cis-platinum in unresectable cancer of the head and neck. In: Fee WE Jr, Goepfert H, Johns ME, et al, eds. *Head Neck Cancer*, Philadelphia, Penna: BC Decker; 1990;2: 279–281.
40. Slotman GJ, Cummings FJ, Glicksman AR, Doolittle CL, Leone LA. Preoperative simultaneously administered cis-platinum plus radiation therapy for advanced squamous cell carcinoma of the head and neck. *Head Neck Surg*. 1986:159–164.
41. Al-Sarraf M, Pajak TF, Cooper JS, Mohiuddin M, Herskovic A, Ager PJ. Chemo-radiotherapy in patients with locally advanced naso-

pharyngeal carcinoma: a radiation therapy oncology group study. *J Clin Oncol.* 1990; 8(8):1342–1351.
42. Merlano M, Grimaldi A, Benasso M, Bacigalupo A, Toma S, Scarpati D, Corvo R, Santelli A, Garaventa G, Rosso R. Alternating cisplatin-5-fluorouracil and radiotherapy in head and neck cancer. *Am J Clin Oncol (CCT).* 1988;11(5):538–542.
43. Taylor SG IV, Murthy AK, Caldarelli DD, Showel JL, Kiel K, Griem KL, Mittal BB, Kies M, Hutchinson JC Jr, Holinger LD, Campanella R, Witt TR, Hoover S. Combined simultaneous cisplatin/fluorouracil chemotherapy and split course radiation in head and neck cancer. *J Clin Oncol.* 1989;7(7): 846–856.
44. Wendt TG, Hartenstein RC, Wustrow TPU, Lissner. Cisplatin, fluorouracil with Leucovorin calcium enhancement, and synchronous accelerated radiotherapy in the management of locally advanced head and neck cancer: a phase II study. *J Clin Oncol.* 1989;7(4):471–476.
45. Vokes EE, Weichselbaum RR. Concomitant chemoradiotherapy: rationale and clinical experience in patients with solid tumors. *J Clin Oncol.* 1990;8(5):911–934.
46. Paccagnella A, Orlando A, Marchiori C, et al. Phase III trial of initial chemotherapy in stage III or IV head and neck cancers: a study by the Gruppo di Studio sui Tumori della Testa e del Collo. *J Nat Cancer Inst.* 1994;86:265–272.
47. Larramore GE, Scott CB, Al-Sarraf M, et al. Adjuvant chemotherapy for resectable squamous cell carcinomas of the head and neck: report on Intergroup Study 0034. *Int J Radiat Oncol Biol Phys.* 1992;23:705–713.
48. Demard F, Chauvel P, Santini J, et al. Response to chemotherapy as a justification for modification of the therapeutic straegy for pharyngolaryngeal carcinomas. *Head Neck Surg.* 1990;12:225–231.
49. Pfister DG, Harrison LB, Strong EW, Bosl GJ. Current status of larynx preservation with multimodality therapy. *Oncology.* 1992;6(3): 33–38.
50. Jacobs C, Goffinet DR, Goffinet L, Kohler M, Fee WE. Chemotherapy as a substitute for surgery in the treatment of advanced resectable head and neck cancer. *Cancer.* 1987; 60:1178–1183.
51. Wolf GT, Hong WK, Fisher SG, Urba S, Endicott JW, Close L, Fisher SR, Toohill RJ, Karp D, Miller DM, Cheung NK, Weaver A, Hillel AD, Spaulding M, Chang BK, Dougherty B, DeConti R, Garwal H, Fry C. Induction chemotherapy plus radiation compared with surgery plus radiation in patients with advanced laryngeal cancer. The Department of Veterans Affairs Laryngeal Study Group. *N Engl J Med.* 1991;324:1685–1690.
52. Lefebvre JL, Chevalier D, Luboinski B, Kirkpatrick L, Collette L, Sahmoud T. Larynx preservation in pyriform sinus cancer: preliminary results of a European organization for research and treatment of cancer phase III trial. *JNCI.* 1996;88(13):890–898.
53. Harwood AR, Hawkins NV, Beale FA, et al: Management of advanced glottic cancer: a 10 year review of the Toronto experience. *Int J Radiat Oncol Biol Phys.* 1979;5:899–904.
54. Peters LJ, Ang KK. The role of altered fractionation in head and neck cancers. *Sem Radiat Oncol.* 1992;2(3):180–194.
55. Wendt CD, Peters LJ, Ang K, et al. Hyperfractionated radiotherapy in the treatment of squamous cell carcinomas of the supraglottic larynx. *Int J Radiat Oncol Biol Phys.* 1989;17: 1057–1062.
56. Horiot JC. The EORTC radiotherapy group experience: phase III trials in hyprefractionation (HF) and accelerated fractionation (AF) in head and neck cancers. In: *Proceedings of the American Society for Therapeutic Radiology and Oncology 33 Annual Meeting*, Washington DC, November 4–8, 1991. *Int J Radiat Oncology Biol Phys.* 1991;21 (Suppl II):108. [Abstract]
57. Robbins KT, Vicario D, Seagren S, Weisman R, Orloff L, Pelliteri P, Kerber C, Los G, Howell SB. A targeted supradose cisplatin chemoradiation protocol for advanced head and neck cancer. *Am. J. Surg.* 1994;168:419–421.
58. Robbins KT, Fontanesi J, Wong FSH, Vicario D, Seagren S, Kumar P, Weisman R, Pelliteri P, Thomas R, Gold R, Palmer R, Weir A, Kerber C, Murry T, Ferguson R, Los G, Howel S B. A novel organ preservation protocol for advanced carcinoma of the larynx and pharynx. *Arch Otolaryngol.* 1996;122:853–857.
59. Robbins KT, Kumar P, Regine WF, Kun LE, Hanchett C, Palmer R, Fontanesi J, Paig CU, Harrington V, Flick PA, Ferguson R, Murry T, Wong FSH, Weir AB III , Niell HB. Efficacy of supradose intra-arterial targeted (SIT) cisplatin (P) and concurrent radiation therapy (RT) in the treatment of unresectable stage III–IV head and neck carcinoma: The Memphis experience. *Int J Radiat Oncol Biol Phys.* 1997;38(2):263–271.

60. Robbins KT, Kumar P, Weisman RA, Wong FSH, Hartsell W, Weir AB, Niell B, Los G, Christen R, Palmer R, Seagren SL, Fergusen R, Flick P, Kerber CW, Howell SB. Phase II trial of targeted supradose cisplatin (DDP) and concomitant radiation therapy (RT) for patients with stage III–IV head and neck cancer. *Proceedings of ASCO*. 1996;15:323.
61. Al-Sarraf M, Pajak TF, Marcial V, Mowry P, Cooper J, Stetz J, Ensley JF, Velez-Garcia E. Concurrent radiotherapy and chemotherapy with cisplatin in inoperable squamous cell carcinoma of the head and neck: a RTOG study. *Cancer*. 1987;59:259–265.
62. Howell SB, Pfeifle CE, Wung WE, Ohshen RA, Lucas WE, Yon JL, Green M. Intraperitoneal cisplatin with systemic thiosulfate protection. *Ann Int Med*. 1982;97:845–851.
63. Madasu R, Ruckenstein M, Robbins KT. Ototoxic effects of targeted supradose cisplatin chemoradiation and systemic sodium thiosulfate neutralization for advanced head and neck cancer. *Arch Otolaryngol*. (In press).
64. Woodson G, Rose C, Murry T, Madasu R, Wong F, Hengesteg A, Robbins KT. Assessing vocal function after chemoradiation for advanced larngeal carcinoma. *Arch Otol-HNS*. 1996;122: 858–864.
65. Murry T, Martin A, Robbins KT, Madasu R. Acute and chronic changes in swallowing and quality of life (QOL) following intra-arterial chemoradiation for organ preservation in patients with advanced head and neck cancer. *Head Neck J.* (In press).
66. Robbins KT, Pellitteri P, Harris J, Hanchett C, Kerber C, Vicario D, Highly selective infusions of supradose cisplatin for cranial base malignancies. *Skull Base Surgery*. 1994;4:3.
67. Robbins KT, Pellitteri P, Vicario D, Kerber C, Robertson J, Hanchett C, Howell S. Targeted infusions of supradose cisplatin with systemic neutralization for carcinomas invading the temporal bone. *Skull Base Surg*. 1996;6(1):53-60.

CHAPTER 7

Endoscopic Resection of Laryngeal Cancer

R. Kim Davis, MD

DEVELOPMENT OF ENDOSCOPIC LASER RESECTION

Primary endoscopic surgical management of early glottic cancer was first reported in 1920 by Lynch but gained little acceptance.[1] In 1973 Lillie and DeSanto reported excellent results with patients treated by endoscopic transoral cordectomy using nonlaser techniques.[2]

Transoral CO_2 laser excision of carcinoma *in situ* and early T1 glottic cancer was introduced in America by Strong, Jako, and Vaughan in the 1970s.[3,4] Resections were limited to the anterior true vocal cord, including the vocal process of the arytenoid cartilage when necessary to gain clear margins. Complete arytenoid cartilage resection was not done to avoid the presumed complication of severe aspiration. Additionally, there was significant concern that, when cancer extended to the body of the arytenoid cartilage, paraglottic spread of cancer beyond the safe limits of laser cordectomy could often be present, as suggested by the studies of Kirchner, thereby rendering endoscopic resection oncologically unsound.[5]

Supraglottic resection with the CO_2 laser was initially described by Vaughan at Boston University in 1979.[6] Davis et al reported on transoral CO_2 laser epiglottectomy in several benign conditions and as a definitive therapeutic option for T1 suprahyoid epiglottic cancer in 1983.[7] These resections were done through a large-bore tubed laryngoscope and basically accomplished by transecting the epiglottis from pharyngoepiglottic fold to pharyngoepiglottic fold. Patients undergoing transoral epiglottectomy had minimal postoperative problems with aspiration or swallowing. Additionally, postoperative bleeding was not seen.

Additional experience in supraglottic cancer resection was gained by attempting to stabilize the airway of patients undergoing staging endoscopy for far advanced supraglottic cancer in whom extubation was not possible due to tumor swelling and bleeding after biopsy.[8] It became evident that the airway could be secured through vigorous CO_2 laser excision of supraglottic cancer as a biopsy procedure. In these patients, epiglottectomy, resection of one aryepiglottic fold, and in some cases further resection to include the ventricular fold stabilized the airway and was extremely well tolerated. In this group of patients, no significant postoperative aspiration or hemorrhage was seen. Airway stabilization allowed these patients to be worked up in an orderly way without tracheotomy and then treated by standard total laryngectomy with postoperative irradiation or to participate in clinical trials utilizing induction chemotherapy followed by surgery and irradiation.

In light of how well patients tolerated transoral supraglottic resection, the question naturally arose as to whether transoral partial supraglottic resection could be done with curative intent as a definitive primary therapy. As is true in most new tumor therapies, patients initially treated for curative or even palliative intent by transoral CO_2 laser supraglottic resection were patients who were not candidates for standard open supraglottic laryngectomy or patients who adamantly refused any type of open procedure. Initial patients underwent supraglottic resections with the intent of gaining complete tumor excision before definitive radiation therapy.[9] The rationale of this approach was that removal of all known cancer would increase the effectiveness of later definitive irradiation. Additionally, some of the problems seen with radiation therapy, like significant epiglottic, aryepiglottic fold, or arytenoid area edema were decreased due to the prior removal of these tissues by the laser. The initial patient workup, therapeutic approach, surgical approach, and contraindications to supraglottis CO_2 laser resection will be presented. The further evolution and current state of both glottic and supraglottic endoscopic resection of cancer is the focus of this chapter.

ENDOSCOPIC RESECTION OF STAGE I AND STAGE II GLOTTIC CANCER

Endoscopic resection of glottic cancer started with the premise that the arytenoid cartilage could not be resected without inducing life-threatening aspiration. With this limitation in mind, Davis and Jako described the anatomical limitations of endoscopic glottic cancer resection in 1982.[10] This cadaver study concluded that excision could be accomplished at a right angle across the vocal process of the arytenoid cartilage through the paraglottic space to the thyroid cartilage. This incision line was determined to be the posterolateral extent to which safe laser excision could be accomplished. Anteriorly, it was determined that the thyroid cartilage could be easily approached. The anterior inferior limitation to resection was felt to be the cricothyroid membrane through which tumor could escape to the soft tissues of the neck, thereby contraindicating any conservation operation. These limitations to transoral CO_2 laser resection of glottic cancer have largely remained in place in the United States.

The successful application of this approach was reported by the Boston University group in 1984.[11] Patients underwent excisional biopsy of T1 glottic cancers at the time of their definitive staging endoscopy. In this study, 50 patients with clear margins after excisional biopsy underwent laser excision alone and had a 3-year no evidence of disease (NED) rate of 92%. Thirty-eight were found to have residual cancer in the vocalis muscle after laser excision. Thirty-four of these patients were treated by radiation therapy with a 3-year NED rate of 85%. Four patients underwent vertical partial laryngectomy and obtained 100% control at 3 years. For the total group, 90% of patients had local control by the above mentioned methods. It is important to note that the reported local control in this study was obtained from the primary therapies and did not include later salvage surgery.

Similar results were reported by the University of Utah where 70 patients were selected for laser excision or definitive irradiation therapy.[12] Patients with T1a carcinoma of the true vocal cord were selected to undergo laser excision according to the Boston regimen. None of these patients had positive margins, and the 5-year NED rate was 93%. Several other papers in the

American literature have reported results of laser excision in stage I glottic cancer with 3-year NED rates ranging from 80 to 92%.[13,14]

In the Utah series, stage Ib glottic cancer patients did not undergo laser resection and were treated by irradiation alone. Only 67% were rendered free of cancer at the 3-year follow-up period. Although stage Ib glottic cancer is obviously more threatening than stage Ia cancer, the poor survival with irradiation alone is clearly unacceptable. Further, the reported series of patients with stage II glottic cancer treated by conventional irradiation alone is also troubling.

At the University of Virginia, the 3-year disease-free survival for irradiated patients with stage II glottic cancer was 75.5%.[15] Failure was most commonly seen in patients with persistent hoarseness after radiotherapy and in patients with impaired true vocal cord mobility before cancer therapy. In a large series of 114 patients with stage II glottic cancer from the MD Anderson Hospital in Houston, Texas, the local control rate following definitive radiotherapy was 68%.[16] In a series from the Geisinger Medical Center, 48 patients with T2 glottic cancer underwent definitive irradiation with a 3-year local control rate of 73%.[17] Patients with impaired true vocal cord mobility or anterior commissure cancer were identified as being at increased risk of recurrence after primary radiation therapy.

In light of the decreased efficacy of radiotherapy in T2 cancers with extension of disease either to the anterior commissure or to the arytenoid cartilage area, the vast majority of American head and neck surgeons favor conventional open vertical partial laryngectomy in these patients. With this approach, cancer can be widely resected with excellent local control. However, standard open vertical partial laryngectomy has attendant morbidity, including perioperative tracheotomy and feeding tube placement as well as generally poor voice. Both of these observations, the excellent local control and the resultant morbidity, have raised the question of whether extended endoscopic resection could replace open surgery in treating these cancers. Success in accomplishing exactly this challenge has been reported by Steiner et al in Germany.[18]

In the Steiner series, stage II glottic cancer patients were treated if the true vocal cord could be fully visualized endoscopically from the anterior commissure through and including the arytenoid area. Following intubation, moistened neurosurgical cottonoids were placed through the glottis to protect the underlying cuff of the endotracheal tube. Laser excision was started by cutting tangentially through the posterior one third of the cancer, with this incision line carried laterally until normal tissue could be visualized in the paraglottic space (see Fig 7-1). Cutting vertically through tumor in this manner was determined to best allow the depth of tumor extension to be ascertained. Once this was accomplished, the posterior aspect of the cancer was excised with posterior margins first obtained. Similar excision was then carried anteriorly until the complete tumor was excised, usually as one or two additional specimens. Where necessary, the vocal process of the arytenoid cartilage was fully transected and excision carried out immediately adjacent to the arytenoid body. Cancer present posterolateral to the body of the arytenoid and in the upper portion of the arytenoid body was also excised. If cancer extended posteriorly to the arytenoid, the full arytenoid cartilage was removed.

Where cancer extended to the anterior commissure, the anterior commissure was fully exposed. Laser resection was carried to the anterior perichondrium, which was raised by microsurgical instruments and resected if needed to encompass the cancer. If cancer extended to involve the perichondrium, part of the thyroid cartilage was also excised. In Steiner's series, all stage II glottic cancer patients without impaired true vocal cord mobility were resected in this manner and did not receive postoperative irradiation.

Thirty-four patients had stage IIa (full vocal cord mobility) glottic cancer and underwent laser resection alone. Local con-

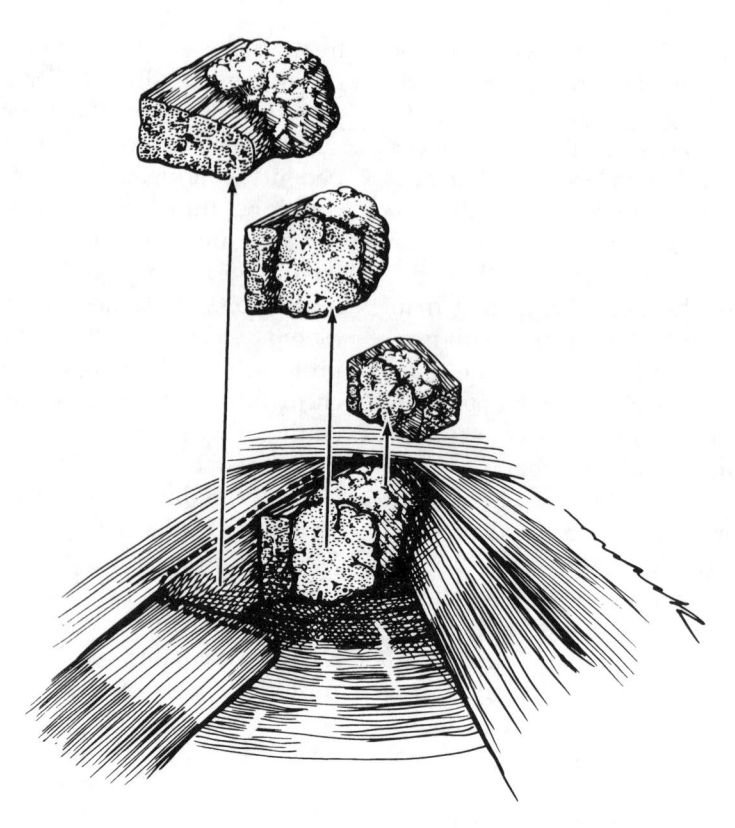

FIG 7–1. Vertical partial laryngectomy is first accomplished by making a laser incision tangential to the vocal process of the arytenoid or membranous posterior vocal cord and carrying this incision to a depth that goes beyond the deepest extent of tumor. The posterior aspect is removed as illustrated. The operation then involves moving anteriorly and taking further resections until the tumor is completely cleared.

trol was obtained in 32 of 34 patients (94%). Two-year survival was 94% and 5-year survival was 78%. All deaths in these patients came from either second primary cancers or intercurrent disease. No T2a patient died because of local failure.

Twenty-five patients with T2b glottic cancer underwent laser excision alone. Local control was obtained in 17 of 25 patients, or 68%. Late regional metastases were seen in 20% of these patients and distant metastases in 8%. Second primary cancer was seen in 12% of patients. Two patients were salvaged by total laryngectomy. The survival at 5 years in this group was 80%.

Transoral CO_2 laser excision of selected stage IIb glottic cancer patients has also been accomplished at the University of Utah Health Sciences Center. In contrast to the German series, all Utah patients underwent initial resection of the ipsilateral hemiepiglottis and aryepiglottic fold before glottic resection. Initial supraglottic resection uncaps the paraglottic space from above, allowing full visualization of this space, which is much more difficult to obtain by starting the excision at the false or true vocal cord level.

In the Utah series, 91% local control was obtained by transoral vertical partial laryngectomy and postoperative irradiation. The patient who failed locally was salvaged by total laryngectomy. No stage II patient required tracheotomy, either at the time of cancer excision or subsequently during follow-up. Seventeen percent of patients required postoperative feeding tubes, for times varying between 2 and 4 weeks.

Endoscopic laser excision of stage I squamous cell carcinoma of the glottis limited to the anterior true vocal cord is a well established, successful treatment option for this cancer. This is well illustrated by the papers already cited. Certainly radiation therapy remains the other viable alternative treatment for early glottic cancer. In practice, most patients are treated either due to the biases of the diagnosing physicians or by the treatment plan that best suits their individual needs. In the setting of a regional medical center like the University of Utah, many patients live in outlying communities in which radiation therapy facilities are not available. Limited endoscopic excision of their cancers clearly has major advantages in their lifestyles as they do not need to leave home and work for extended periods of time to undergo irradiation. As reported cure rates are at least as high as those seen in patients treated with radiation therapy, endoscopic surgery is simply better for these patients.

If the initial endoscopic staging procedure is coupled with the definitive surgical resection, the cost of endoscopic resection of stage I glottic cancer is significantly less than the cost of treating these patients by full course irradiation therapy. Additionally, the lifelong morbidity of irradiation is eliminated, and the ability to use irradiation for more threatening lesions yet remains.

The argument used in favor of definitive irradiation over surgery in early glottic cancer is that vocal quality is better in the irradiated group. Most evidence either for or against this statement comes from anecdotal experiences of the treating physicians. The few studies done to document vocal quality postirradiation or postsurgery suggest there is very little difference in outcome between the two modalities. Although surgery certainly results in scarring to the vocal cord and altered true vocal cord vibrational mechanics on the operated side, the contralateral cord remains normal. Conversely, as both cords are treated in irradiated patients, scarring and edema in Reinke's space can be present on both sides.

Endoscopic laser excision of stage IIa glottic cancer has generally not been done in America. These patients have either been irradiated or treated by open vertical partial laryngectomy. Because of the poor results in stage IIb glottic cancer patients treated by radiation alone, the University of Utah study cited earlier was done to determine if endoscopic excision used as an adjuvant therapy to full course irradiation could improve the otherwise poor treatment results in these patients when irradiated alone. This, in fact, did occur in a limited number of treated patients for whom the 3-year NED rates were greater than 90%.

Professor Steiner's work in Germany suggests that endoscopic resection alone of stage IIb cancers will confer local control rates at least comparable to those seen in patients treated by irradiation alone. Very importantly, Dr. Steiner's work with more limited T2a cancers treated by endoscopic resection shows local control rates greater than 90%. Our experience at the University of Utah confirms Steiner's reported results and suggests that these cancers can readily be treated endoscopically with the expectation of gaining clear margins and excellent local control. In light of this, the earlier stated anatomical limitations to transoral laser resection certainly are too restrictive.[10] Additionally, treating T2a by standard open technique is very likely excessive therapy and unnecessarily morbid.

ENDOSCOPIC RESECTION OF SUPRAGLOTTIC CANCER

All patients with supraglottic cancer, except those having T1 suprahyoid epiglottic cancer, undergo preoperative computed tomographic scanning (CT) or magnetic resonance imaging (MRI). This is done to determine the presence or absence of pre-epiglottic space invasion. T1 suprahyoid epiglottic lesions, by definition, do not have pre-epiglottic space invasion. On the other hand, as Zeitels and his associates have clearly shown, even T1 infrahyoid epiglottic lesions can have occult pre-epiglottic space invasion in 30% to 40% of cases.[19] Where preoperative scans show no apparent pre-epiglottic space invasion, transoral supraglottic resection can proceed. Where preoperative scanning shows gross invasion of the pre-epiglottic space, endoscopic resection should not be attempted.

Following intubation with a laser protected endotracheal tube, an adjustable laryngoscope is placed. One blade of the laryngoscope is placed in the vallecula and the other blade placed over the endotracheal tube. As the scope is opened, it should be possible to visualize the epiglottis from pharyngoepiglottic fold to pharyngoepiglottic fold. A large neurosurgical cottonoid is then moistened with saline and placed over the endotracheal tube to further protect it from laser impact.

Prior to the initiation of resection, a microlaryngeal suction is placed in the side port of the laryngoscope and attached to a smoke evacuator. If the laryngoscope does not have a specific portal for placement of the suction, it may be necessary for an assistant to hold the suction between the open leaves of the laryngoscope to the side out of the field of vision. Additionally, a standard microsurgical suction is attached to a conventional canister to help with any evacuation of secretions or blood.

The procedure is started by retracting the epiglottis inferiorly to expose the lingual surface. Using a small cups forceps or a specially designed microcautery, the pharyngoepiglottic fold area on each side is cauterized to prophylactically control vessels that enter the epiglottis through this area. With a CO_2 laser that provides a microspot of approximately 1 mm a power setting of 4 to 8 watts is selected with the laser on continuous mode. The initial incision is carried from one pharyngoepiglottic fold to the midline. A similar incision is then made with the laser from the opposite side. The level of transection is demonstrated in Fig 7–2. It is typically best to carry this incision down to epiglottic cartilage along the full length of the incision. When cartilage is encountered, there is a typical fluorescent glow that clearly identifies the cartilage. Once the incision reaches the cartilage, the epiglottis is grasped near one lateral edge and the incision carried through and through the epiglottis from side to side and the suprahyoid epiglottis delivered.

Depending on the nature of the cancer present, the actual tumor may or may not be transected in this first resection of the epiglottis. With the suprahyoid epiglottis removed from the field, visualization is significantly enhanced. Usually, at this point in time, it is possible to see the underlying true vocal cords in the posterior aspect. Attention is taken to redirect placement of the neurosurgical cottonoid to ensure that the endotracheal tube and true vocal cords are protected. Often it is reasonable to replace the cottonoid with a new moist cottonoid or to simply instill saline to an already well positioned neurosurgical cottonoid.

Using a velvet-tipped suction (ie, a suction with portals on the side but not on the end) and/or a cups forceps, the residual epiglottis is manipulated to fully visualize the extent of tumor. The cups or velvet-tipped suction is then used to push the residual epiglottis posteriorly, which allows further resection over the top of transected epiglottis into the tissue overlying the pre-epiglottic space. An incision is then made parallel to and approximately 4 or 5 mm in front of the lingual edge of the transected epiglottis. This incision is carried inferiorly into pre-epiglottic fat. Typically in the center of this area, few blood vessels are found and the incision can be readily conducted. Not only is this area easy to visualize, but the crackling sound of vaporizing fat gives a very distinct identifying characteristic to laser resection in this area. This incision is then carried laterally toward the aryepiglottic fold and superior paraglottic aspect of one false vocal cord.

With careful visualization of the tumor, an incision is made in the aryepiglottic fold at a level below the inferior extent of the cancer. Determination of the exact area to start

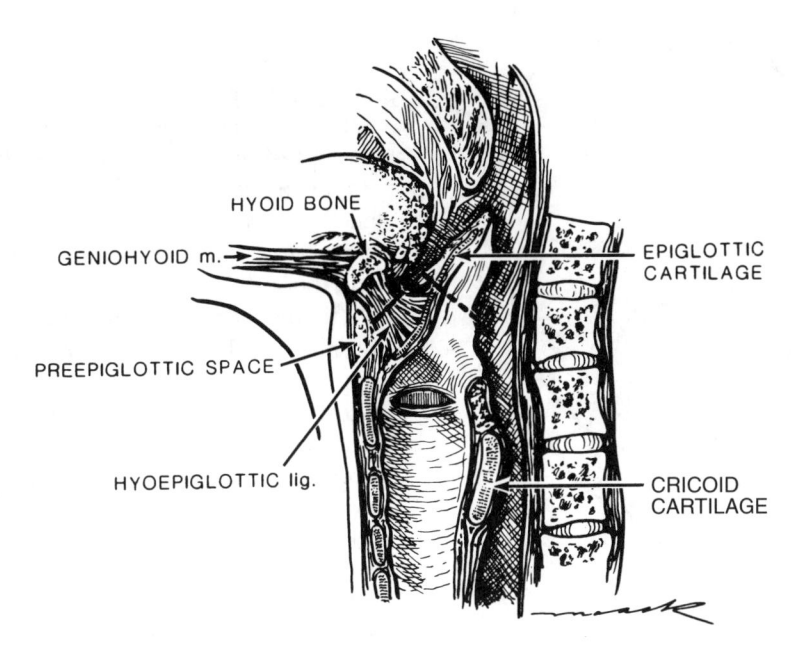

FIG 7–2. This cross sectional view of the larynx depicts well the relationship between the epiglottic cartilage, hyoepiglottic ligament, and pre-epiglottic space. The dotted line across the epiglottis represents the first excision line. With the suprahyoid epiglottis resected, the area of the hyoepiglottic ligament is readily seen and laser dissection through this opens the pre-epiglottic space. Where possible, the full pre-epiglottic space from hyoid bone to the superior aspect of the thyroid cartilage can be transected.

requires some experience and it is best helped by manipulating the residual epiglottis and tumor to see the exact level of the false and true vocal cords. This incision is best made at a level that does not violate the arytenoid body and allows the incision to be carried forward into the false vocal cord. Using very careful laser excisional technique, the anterior or pre-epiglottic incision is connected to the lateral or aryepiglottic fold–false vocal cord incision.

After transection of the suprahyoid epiglottis, the residual epiglottis can be manipulated to show the extent of the laryngeal surface that is involved. If the tumor is in the midline, a vertical incision is made through the epiglottis from the transected superior edge through and through the epiglottis, joining the incision placed earlier in the pre-epiglottic space (see Fig 7–3). This incision is carried inferiorly to the full extent needed to go beyond the inferior most extent of tumor involvement. This incision, of course, should not extend beyond the anterior commissure area of the endolarynx. Typically, the incision will come to the area of the petiole of the epiglottis. This incision then is joined to the previously placed incisions in the pre-epiglottic space and through the aryepiglottic fold–false vocal cord. Full completion of this step allows the residual hemiepiglottis (AE fold–false vocal cord specimen) to be removed.

In cases of extensive involvement of the laryngeal aspect of the epiglottis by cancer, a similar procedure is accomplished on the opposite side. After removal of both hemiepiglottic specimens, in most cases the full supraglottic tumor will have been removed. If residual cancer still exists, it will usually be possible to identify under the microscope. Further excision is then taken in the areas needed to gain full tumor resection.

When the full tumor has been resected, final margins are taken from the patient. The aryepiglottic fold is further resected approx-

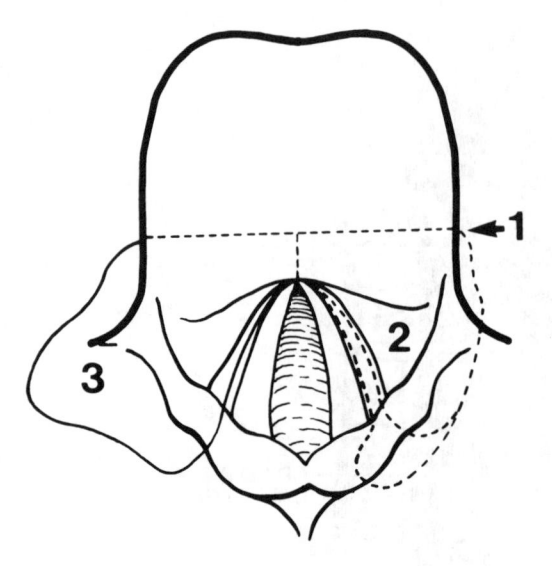

FIG 7–3. The major steps in supraglottic resection are illustrated. Step 1 involves the transection of the epiglottis at approximately the level of the hyoid bone. The two illustrated incision lines in area 2 show laser resection through and through the epiglottis into the pre-epiglottic space as well as the division of the aryepiglottic fold and the false vocal cord. Area 3 shows the contralateral supraglottis which is removed to accomplish a full supraglottic laryngectomy.

imately 4 or 5 mm below the edge of the earlier excision line. If the cancer was very extensive, this margin may come across the upper part of the body of the arytenoid cartilage. If this partial arytenoid resection is needed, the main part of the body of the arytenoid must be spared. The upper aspect of the arytenoid body can be excised as part of the aryepiglottic fold margin. It should be noted that such resection often results in unilateral true vocal cord fixation. The petiole area of the epiglottis is again resected as a final anterior margin. Resection of residual false vocal cord can be readily accomplished as a final lateral margin.

As the initial resection passes through the aryepiglottic fold into the false vocal cord, it is very easy to carry this incision to the upper aspect of the thyroid cartilage. Cartilage again is readily identified by first blackening of the perichondrium from laser impact and then by the fluorescent glow of the cartilage when it is impacted by the CO_2 laser. When the thyroid cartilage is encountered, the perichondrium can be raised using microsurgical instruments. If there is any question of tumor extension below the upper aspect of the thyroid cartilage, it is necessary to raise the thyroid cartilage perichondrium for 3 or 4 mm. Perichondrium and the soft tissue adjacent to it can be resected to the needed inferior extent. Exposed thyroid cartilage is then partially vaporized to promote later granulation and healing. Interestingly, experience has shown that such exposure and vaporization of a part of the upper aspect of the thyroid cartilage has not led to later chondronecrosis. In fact, healing seems to be stimulated and helped by this procedure.

When all of the above excision has been accomplished for aryepiglottic fold lesions, the contralateral infrahyoid epiglottis and aryepiglottic fold as well as the contralateral false vocal cord will remain. Where a full endoscopic supraglottic laryngectomy is needed, the upper aspect of both true vocal cords will be readily visualized. If there is the unexpected finding of tumor extension into the lateral paraglottic space, now totally uncapped by the previous excision, biopsies should be taken. Patients with extensive involvement into the lateral pre-epiglottic space which was not appreciated preoperatively have T3 cancers. In this case, the endoscopic approach is not oncologically sound, and open surgical therapy is needed. Where careful preoperative staging by CT scan has been done, this circumstance can be avoided.

T1 suprahyoid epiglottic cancers are widely resected transorally using microsurgical laser technique. Neck dissection or postoperative irradiation is not indicated in this group.

T1 carcinomas of the infrahyoid epiglottis, aryepiglottic fold, or false vocal cord are also treated by transoral laser microsurgery. In these cases, even with N0 necks by preoperative CT scanning, neck therapy is indicated. Patients may be treated either by postoperative irradiation or bilateral functional neck dissection removing lymph node regions II, III, and IV. In America, neck dissections typically are done at the time of transoral laser resection, but in Europe they are often done 1 to 2 weeks following definitive laser resection.

Patients with T2 supraglottic primaries are readily treated by transoral CO_2 laser resection with the extent of surgery tailored to the specific area defined by tumor invasion.

SUMMARY AND FUTURE DIRECTIONS

Endoscopic laser excision of stage I and II glottic and supraglottic cancers has evolved to a point of being a highly successful, reproducible technique. This approach to cancer resection does not change any time-honored oncological principles related to the treatment of these cancers. Endoscopic resection represents a less morbid technique of accomplishing the same operation done through open techniques without the attendant morbidity. Tracheotomy and feeding tubes are far less frequently needed with endoscopic laser surgery as normal structures do not need to be taken apart for tumor access and then repaired after tumor excision. Margins obtained endoscopically are similar to those obtained through external approaches. Clearly cancers that extend beyond the limits defined for classical open conservation laryngeal surgery should not be treated endoscopically.

Protocols that will allow the study of a large number of patients being treated endoscopically are currently being developed to allow needed prospective evaluation of these newer techniques.

REFERENCES

1. Lynch RC. Intrinsic carcinoma of the larynx, with a second report of the cases operated on by suspension and dissection. Trans Am Laryngol Assoc. 1920;42:119–126.
2. Lillie JC, DeSanto LW. Transoral surgery of early cordal carcinoma. Trans Am Acad Ophthalmol Otolaryngol. 1973;77:92–96.
3. Strong MS. Laser excision of carcinoma of the larynx. Laryngoscope. 1975;85:1286–1289.
4. Vaughan DW, Strong MS, Jako GJ. Laryngeal carcinoma. Transoral treatment utilizing the CO_2 laser. Am J Surg. 1978;136:490–493.
5. Kirchner JA, Cornog JL, Holmes RE. Transglottic cancer: its growth and spread within the larynx. Arch Otolaryngol 1974;99:247–251.
6. Vaughan CW. Transoral laryngeal surgery using the CO_2 laser. Laboratory experiments and clinical experience. Laryngoscope. 1978;88:1399–1420.
7. Davis RK, Shapshay SM, Strong SM, Hyams V. Transoral partial supraglottic resection using the CO_2 laser. Laryngoscope. 1983;93:429–432.
8. Davis RK, Shapshay SM, Vaughan CW, Strong MS. Pretreatment airway management in obstructing carcinoma of the larynx, Otolaryngology Head Neck Surg. 1981;89(2):209-214.
9. Davis RK, Kelly SM, Hayes J. Endoscopic CO_2 Laser excisional biopsy of early supraglottic cancer. Laryngoscope, 1991;100:680–683.
10. Davis RK, Jako GJ, Hyams VJ, Shapshay SM. The anatomical limitations of CO_2 laser cordectomy. Laryngoscope 1992;92:980–984.
11. Blakeslee D, Vaughan CW, Shapshay SM, et al. Excisional biopsy in the selected management of T1 glottic cancer: a 3-year follow-up study. Laryngoscope. 1984;94:488–494.
12. Davis RK, Kelly SM, Parkin JL, Stevens MH, Johnson LP. Selective management of early glottic cancer. Laryngoscope. 1990;100:1306–1309.
13. McGuirt WF, Koufman JA. Encoscopic laser surgery. Arch Otolaryngol Head Neck Surg. 1987;113:501–505.
14. Wetmore SJ, Key M, Suen JY. Laser therapy for T1 glottic carcinoma of the larynx. Arch Otolaryngol Head Neck Surg. 1986;112:853–855.
15. Kelly MD, Hahn SS, Spaulding CA, Kersh CR, Constable WC, Cantrell RW. Definitive radiotherapy in the management of stage I and II carcinomas of the glottis. Ann Otol Rhinol Laryngol. 1989;98(3):235–239.
16. Howell-Burke D, Peters LJ, Goepfert H, Oswald MJ. T2 glottic cancer. Recurrence, salvage and survival after definitive radiotherapy. Arch Otolaryngol Head Neck Surg. 1990;116(7):830–835.
17. Pellitteri PK, Kennedy TL, Vrabec DP, Beiler D, Hellstrom M. Radiotherapy in the mainstay in the treatment of early glottic carcinoma. Arch Otolaryngol Head Neck Surg. 1991;117(3):297–301.

18. Steiner W. Results of curative laser microsurgery of laryngeal carcinoma. *Am J Otolaryngol.* 1993;14(2):116–121.

19. Zeitels SM, Vaughan CW. Pre-epiglottic space invasion in "early" epiglottic cancer. *Ann Otol Rhinol Laryngol.* 1991;100:789–792.

CHAPTER 8

Supracricoid Partial Laryngectomy

Gregory S. Weinstein, MD, and Ollivier Laccourreye, MD

In 1959, approximately ten years after Alonso's[1] first description of the supraglottic laryngectomy, Majer and Reider[2] published the first description of a partial laryngectomy in which the reconstruction was performed by suturing the hyoid to the cricoid. A number of other authors including Labayle and Bistmuth and Piquet et al in the 1970s further refined these techniques. A plethora of names have been used to describe these techniques, including subtotal laryngectomy and reconstructive laryngectomy. Nonetheless, the term supracricoid partial laryngectomy (SCPL) best describes the extent of resection (Fig 8–1) and the term cricohyoidopexy (CHP) or cricohyoidoepiglottopexy (CHEP) best describes the mode of reconstruction. The SCPLs are conservation laryngeal surgeries in which the functional goal is speech and swallowing without a permanent tracheostomy.

One concept that is not always clearly expressed in the literature is that there are two types of SCPL which are utilized for distinct indications. In addition, it cannot be overemphasized that these techniques are utilized only for cancers that remain endolaryngeal without extension to the pharynx. The first technique, which is utilized for selected supraglottic and transglottic carci-

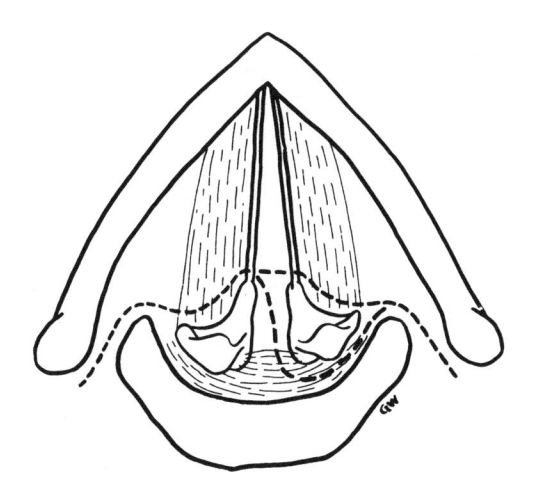

SUPRACRICOID LARYNGECTOMY

FIG 8–1. Axial view of the larynx at the level of the glottis showing the resected tissue following SCPL (tissue posterior to the dotted lines is preserved).

nomas, results in the resection of the whole epiglottis, pre-epiglottic space, the whole thyroid cartilage, bilateral paraglottic spaces, true and false folds. The cricoid, hyoid, and at least one arytenoid must be spared. The closure is performed by creating a pexy between the remaining cricoid and the hyoid and tongue base and hence the name cricohyoidopexy (CHP). The second technique is utilized for selected glottic carcinomas, and in this procedure the resection includes the whole thyroid cartilage, the petiole of the epiglottis, the bilateral paraglottic spaces, and the true and false folds. In this technique, the upper portion of the epiglottis, the cricoid, hyoid, and at least one arytenoid is spared.

The literature indicates that these techniques have been utilize during the last two decades throughout Europe and Asia. The Practice Guidelines of the American Society of Head and Neck Surgery and The Society of Head and Neck Surgeons recommend the use of SCPL in selected cases of laryngeal carcinoma.[3] The question arises as to where these techniques fit within the spectrum of "organ preserving surgical techniques" for laryngeal carcinoma such as the vertical partial laryngectomies (VPLs), supraglottic laryngectomies (SGLs), or endoscopic excision with and without the laser. The focus of this chapter is to outline not only the technique itself but to detail the oncologic rationale and role of these techniques within the spectrum of surgical alternatives for laryngeal carcinoma. Finally, in our opinion, there are preoperative, intraoperative, and postoperative techniques that optimize functional outcome. The final section in this chapter discusses these perioperative techniques and our management recommendations.

SURGICAL TECHNIQUE

Suprcricoid Partial Laryngectomy with Cricohyoidopexy

Exposure

The skin incision can be made either as a wide apron flap to incorporate a unilateral or bilateral neck dissection or as a smaller incision if no neck dissection is to be done. In either case, the skin incision is routinely created to include the tracheostomy site. This superiorly based subplatysmal flap should always be elevated to at least 1 cm above the hyoid bone or skin retraction will result after closure. The next step is to identify the midline raphe of the strap muscles in the midline. The raphe is divided from the sternal notch to the level of the hyoid. The sternohyoid is transected bilaterally at the upper border of the thyroid cartilage. Following this, the thyrohyoid muscle is transected, again at the upper border of the thyroid cartilage (Fig 8–2). The thyrohyoid muscle is then elevated laterally and inferiorly, exposing the oblique line of the thyroid cartilage and the insertion of the sternothyroid muscle on the larynx. This muscle is now transected at the inferior border of the thyroid cartilage, taking care not to create bleeding around the thyroid gland or the vessels underlying the muscles in this area. The next step in the exposure is the transection of the inferior constrictor muscles at their attachment to the posterior lateral edge of the thyroid cartilage (Fig 8–3). The external thyroid perichondrium is also cut in a superior to inferior fashion and then the internal thyroid perichondrium is elevated with the pyriform sinuses bilaterally, to preserve these structures. Two or three 3-0 vicryl sutures are passed through the cut edge of the constrictor muscles, bilaterally, approximately a centimeter apart. The needles are removed and hemostats are attached to the sutures. These sutures will be utilized later in the case to reapproximate the pyriform sinus during the closure. The cricothyroid joints are disarticulated bilaterally taking special care to avoid damaging the recurrent laryngeal nerves (Fig 8–4). At this point, the thyroid isthmus is transected and ligated in the midline.

The final step of the exposure is a finger dissection of the cervicomediastinal trachea. Prior to this, the surgeon should transect and ligate any anterior thyroid veins extending inferiorly from the isthmus so that these do not tear, and bleed, during the final clo-

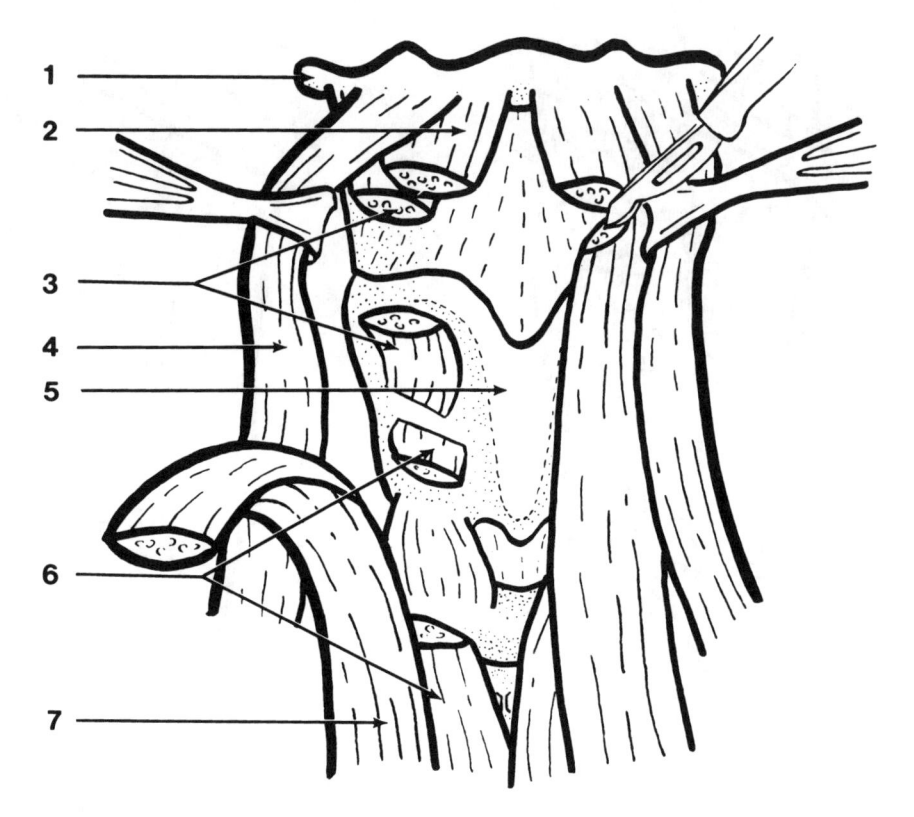

FIG 8–2. Anterior exposure—transection of the strap musculature. 1. Hyoid bone, Sternohyoid muscle. 3. Sternothyroid muscle. 4. Omohyoid muscle. 5. Thyroid cartilage. 6. Sternothyroid muscle. 7. Sternohyoid muscle.

sure. The tracheal rings are identified just below the level of the thyroid isthmus and a plane is developed inferiorly towards the mediastinum. Care is taken to keep the finger right on the trachea. A slow gentle rocking lateral motion with the finger allows for a slow progression into the mediastinum to the carina. Care is taken not to devascularize the trachea laterally. This will allow the trachea and the cricoid to be pulled superiorly to the hyoid at the time of closure.

Resection

A horizontal cricothyrotomy is made just above the level of the cricoid. A flexible armored tube is placed and the orotracheal tube is removed. At this point, the larynx is entered just inferior to the hyoid bone. This is accomplished by first elevating the portions of the strap musculature that were preserved above the thyroid cartilage. These straps are elevated off the thyrohyoid membrane to the level of the inferior aspect of the hyoid bone. The pre-epiglottic space is separated from the inferior aspect of the hyoid bone. This is only done centrally, between the lesser cornua of the hyoid bone using an elevator. Once the bluish discoloration of the submucosa of the vallecula is noted, the pharynx is opened through the vallecula. The superior aspect of the epiglottis is grasped and pulled anteriorly through the mucosal opening. A curved Mayo scissors is then utilized to make a superior to inferior transection just lateral to the epiglottis bilaterally. Once the top of the thyroid cartilage is reached, one scissors blade is placed between the thyroid cartilage and the previously elevated internal thyroid cartilage perichondrium and the other blade is placed into the lumen of the larynx (Fig 8–5). The

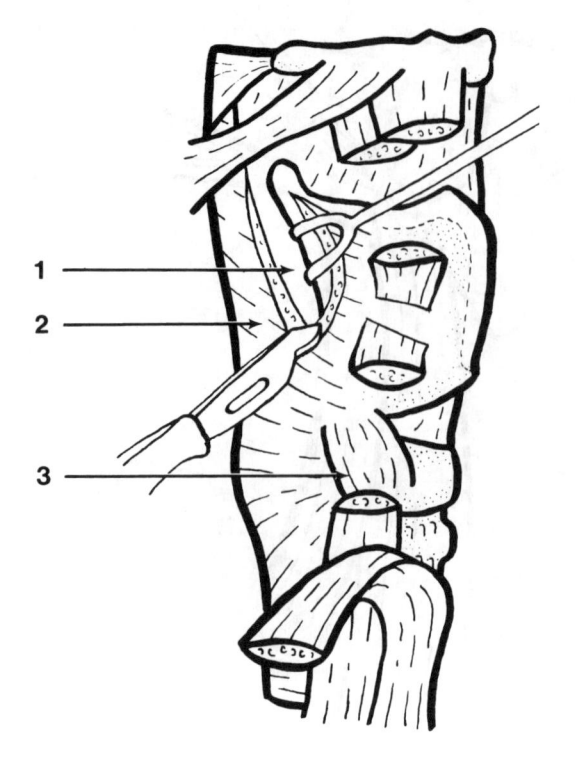

FIG 8–3. Lateral Exposure—transection of the constrictor muscles. 1. Internal thyroid perichondrium. 2. Constrictor muscles. 3. Cricothyroid muscle.

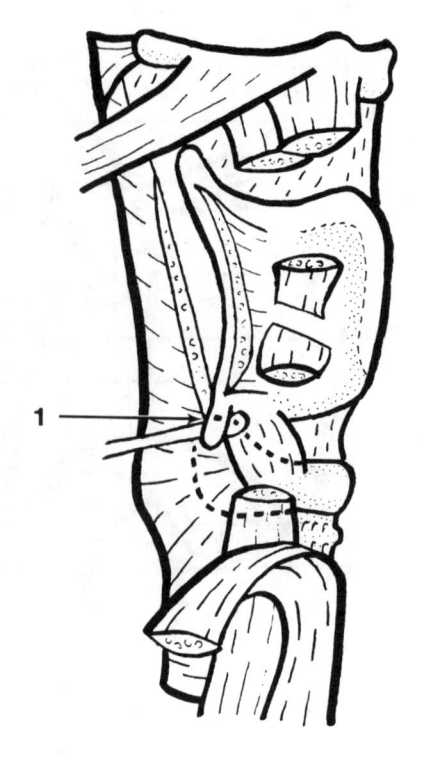

FIG 8–4. Lateral Exposure—disarticulation of the cricothyroid joint. 1. Cricothyroid joint.

superior to inferior transection is continued on the side of the larynx with the least tumor burden. The transection is made just anterior to the top of the arytenoid, resecting the whole false vocal fold and then continued just posterior to the ventricle. At this point the anterior aspect of the vocal process is transected, and the entire vocal fold is resected. Care must be taken to orient the axis of the scissors blades in the coronal plane of the larynx to avoid cutting posteriorly and entering the cricoarytenoid joint. Once the cricoid is reached, with the scissors, the transection is brought anteriorly through the cricothyroid musculature and the subglottic mucosa to connect anteriorly with the previously made horizontal cricothyrotomy.

Now the larynx is opened like a book on the anterior spine. The resection is continued on the tumor-bearing side from inferior to superior under direct vision. The entire arytenoid cartilage may be resected on the involved side; however, it is critical to save all of the posterior arytenoid mucosa for the closure. The resection on the tumor-bearing side may be accomplished with a curved Mayo scissors or a fifteen blade.

Closure

The first step in the closure is to pull the arytenoids anteriorly by placing one or two 4-0 vicryl sutures just above the vocal process and suturing it to the ipsilateral anterolateral cricoid cartilage. This suture serves as as an "air-knot" that keeps the arytenoid from prolapsing posteriorly. When one arytenoid cartilage is resected, the preserved posterior arytenoid mucosa is sutured anteriorly with a submucosal "air-knot" to the ipsilateral cricoid cartilage. At this point, three 1 vicryls, with large (45–65 mm) needles are utilized to perform the cricohyoidopexy (CHP) sutures. The first stitch is placed in the midline, submucosally around the cricoid cartilage. The suture is then passed in the midline sub-

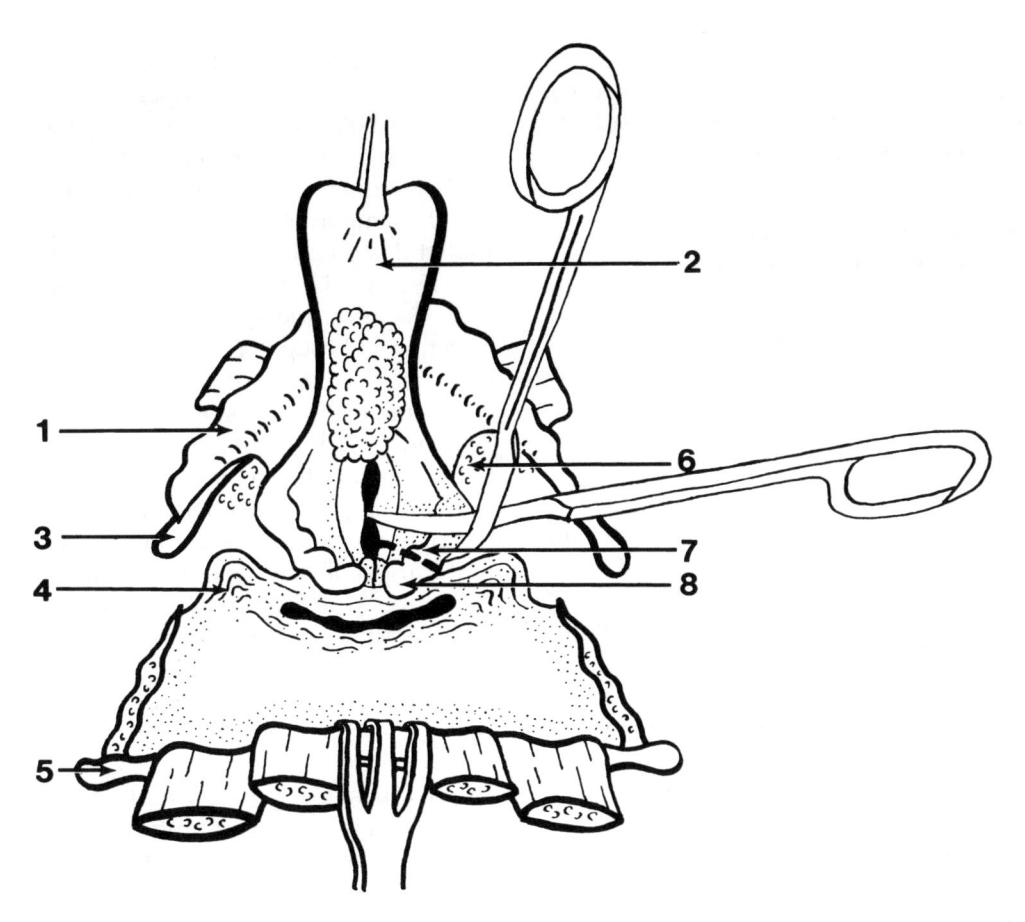

FIG 8–5. Superior exposure showing resection SCPL with CHP. 1. Vallecular mucosa. 2. Epiglottis. 3. Thryoid cartilage. 4. Pyriform sinus. 5. Hyoid bone. 6. Paraglottic space. 7. Prearytenoid incision. 8. Arytenoid cartilage.

mucosally around the hyoid bone deep into the tongue base and then back out through the suprahyoid musculature. The sutures are not tied until all three have been placed. The next two sutures are placed in the same fashion, precisely 1 cm from the midline submucosally around the cricoid cartilage and 1 cm from the midline suture around the hyoid bone and deep into the tongue base. After passing these sutures out of the tongue base through the suprahyoid musculature, they are passed back through the remaining portions of the sternothyroid and sternohyoid muscles. It is important not to place the two lateral CHP sutures too far laterally to avoid compression of the hypoglossal nerves or the lingual arteries, either of which will result in poor function of the tongue. At this point the previously placed 3-0 vicryl sutures, which were placed in the constrictor muscles, are tied gently over the CHP closure. This reapproximates the pyriform sinuses. Once all three CHP sutures have been placed, the endotracheal tube is removed, and the two lateral sutures are tightened, which pulls up the trachea and cricoid. A tracheostomy is then performed in line with the skin incision. After tightening the two lateral CHP sutures, the central suture is tied. It is critically important that the cricoid be aligned properly with the hyoid and that they be approximated closely. After the central suture is tied, the two lateral ones are tied.

The strap musculature is then closed in the midline and superiorly in the form of a

"T." Following the placement of closed suction drains, the skin is closed, with particular attention to separating the tracheostomy site from the remainder of the wound.

Supracricoid Partial Laryngectomy with Cricohyoidoepiglottopexy

Exposure

The exposure is precisely the same as outlined above for the SCPL with CHP.

Resection

The difference in the resection between the SCPL with cricohyoidoepiglottopexy (CHEP) and the SCPL with CHP is that the upper portion of the epiglottis and pre-epiglottic space is spared in the former. Following a horizontal cricothyrotomy a flexible armored tube is put into place and the oroendotracheal tube is removed. The larynx is entered just above the superior aspect of the thyroid cartilage. A curved Mayo scissors is placed just above the thryoid notch and pointed inferiorly towards the anterior commissure. The entry into the larynx is done only in the midline, just above the notch. Once the larynx is entered, the petiole is grasped with a clamp and pulled anteriorly, out of the lumen of the larynx. Curved Mayo scissors are then utilized to make a superior to inferior transection just lateral to the remainder of the epiglottis bilaterally. One blade of the scissors is placed between the thyroid cartilage and the previously elevated internal thyroid cartilage perichondrium and the other blade is placed into the lumen of the larynx (Fig 8–6). As in the CHP, the superior to inferior transection is continued on the side of the larynx with the least tumor burden. Again the transection is carried out just anterior to the top of the arytenoid, resecting the whole false vocal fold and then continued just posterior to the ventricle. At this point the anterior aspect of the vocal process is transected, and the entire vocal fold is resected. During this resection it is important to refrain from sparing some or all of a noninvolved true vocal fold because this soft tissue will impair the mobility of the arytenoid postoperatively. Care must be taken to avoid entering the cricoarytenoid joint by orienting the blades of the scissors in the coronal plane of the larynx. It is important to resect the entire vocal fold at this point and continue the resection inferiorly to the cricoid. At this point, the scissors are reoriented anteriorly and the resection is brought forward to the previously made cricothyrotomy.

The tumor-bearing side of the larynx is now exposed by cracking the larynx open like a book on the anterior spine of the thyroid cartilage. The tumor-bearing side is resected under direct vision, taking as much of the arytenoid cartilage as is oncologically necessary. As in SCPL with CHP, it is necessary to spare the posterior arytenoid mucosa for the reconstruction.

Closure

To avoid posterior prolapse of the arytenoid cartilages it is necessary to suture them anteriorly. This is accomplished by placing one or two 3-0 vicryl sutures above the level of the vocal process of each arytenoid and suturing it anteriorly with an "air-knot" to the anterolateral aspect of the ipsilateral cricoid cartilage. In the event that all or a portion of an arytenoid is resected, the preserved posterior arytenoid mucosa is sutured anteriorly in a similar fashion.

As in the CHP, three number 1 vicryls, with large (45–65 mm) needles are utilized to perform the cricohyoidopexy. The first suture is placed in the midline, submucosally around the cricoid cartilage. It is then used to attach the inferior transected edge of the epiglottis at the midline. This suture passes submucosally through a small amount of the epiglottic cartilage. The needle is then regrasped and passed through the thyrohyoid membrane and pre-epiglottic space and then passed in the midline submucosally around the hyoid bone deep into the tongue base and then back out through the suprahyoid musculature. To avoid misplacement and asymmetry the sutures are left untied until all three are placed. The next two

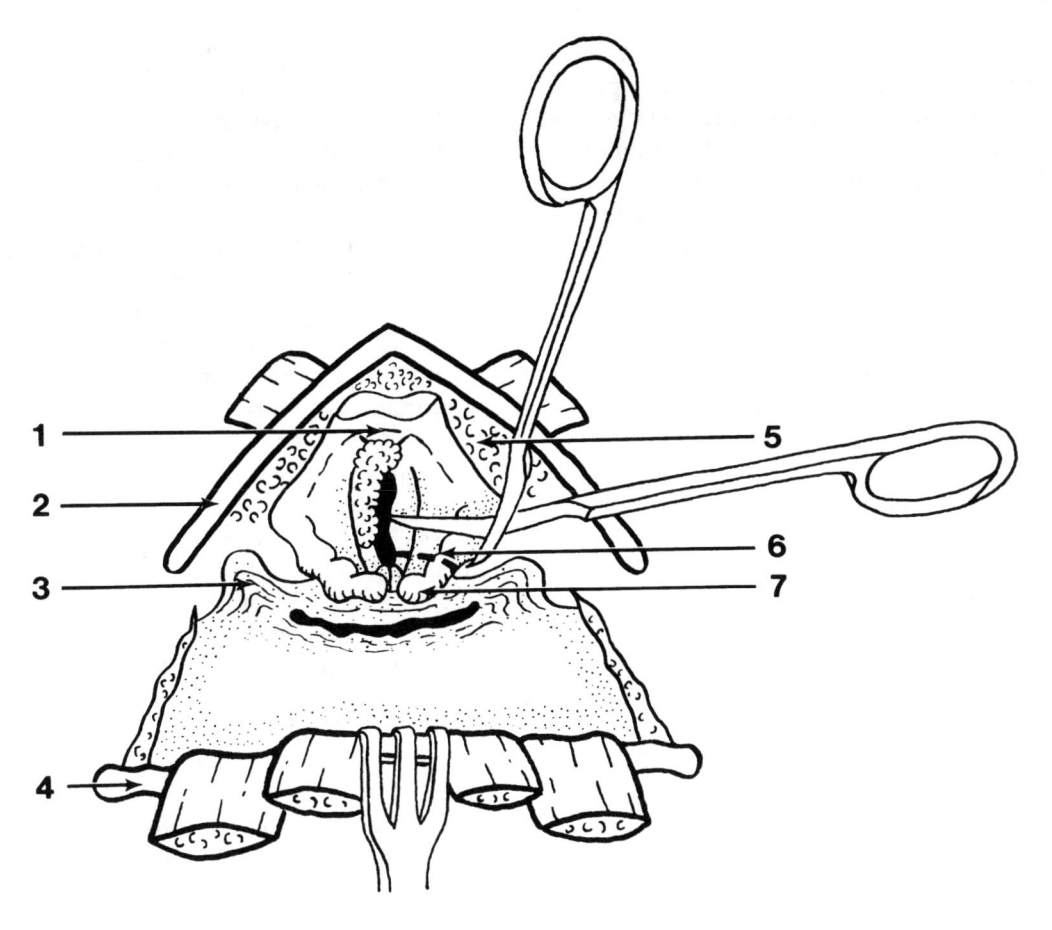

FIG 8–6. Superior exposure showing resection SCPL with CHEP. 1. Epiglottis. 2. Thyroid cartilage. 3. Pyriform sinus. 4. Hyoid bone. 5. Paraglottic space. 6. Prearytenoid incision. 7. Arytenoid cartilage.

sutures are placed in the same fashion, precisely 1 cm from the midline submucosally around the cricoid cartilage and 1 cm from the midline suture, through the inferior aspect of the epiglottis, back into the pre-epiglottic space and around the hyoid bone and deep into the tongue base. After passing these out of the tongue base through the suprahyoid musculature, the sutures are passed back through the remaining portions of the sternothyroid and sternohyoid muscles. As in the CHP, it is important to avoid too lateral a placement to avoid damaging the hypoglossal nerves and the lingual artery. Damage to these structures may result in poor functional outcome.

The tracheostomy is performed prior to tying the CHEP stitches. This allows the surgeon to properly place the tracheostomy site in line with the skin incision. To do this, the endotracheal tube is removed, and the two lateral sutures are tightened, thus pulling the trachea up to its final postoperative position. The tracheotomy is then performed in line with the skin incision. With the lateral sutures still under tension, the central suture is tied, and then the two lateral ones are tied. Special care must be made to approximate the cricoid and the hyoid, taking care to avoid an assymetrical closure. Although the three CHEP sutures may seem to be a minimal closure for this wound, these represent only the internal mucosal and submucosal sutures; additional sutures are also utilized for the closure of the strap muscles, as an additional layer.

After the CHEP stitches are tied down, two more closure steps are taken: reapproximation of the pyriform sinuses and closure of the strap muscles. The previously placed inferior constrictor sutures are tied over the CHEP closure to gently hold them forward. The strap muscles are closed in a "T," and the skin is closed, taking special care to separate the tracheostomy site from the remainder of the wound.

ONCOLOGIC RATIONALE, INDICATIONS, AND CONTRAINDICATIONS

The two main advantages of the SCPLs are (1) the avoidance of total laryngectomy for intermediate size lesions and (2) substitution for the standard conservation procedures (ie, VPL and SGL) to improve local control. Examples of lesions amenable to SCPL that otherwise would require a total laryngectomy (or near-total laryngectomy) include selected (a) transglottic carcinomas, (b) supraglottic carcinomas not amenable to supraglottic laryngectomy, (c) T4 laryngeal carcinomas, (d) T3 glottic carcinomas, and (e) recurrent laryngeal carcinomas following radiation therapy. The second role for the SCPL is to improve local control over traditional conservation surgeries for lesions such as selected (a) T2 glottic carcinomas and (b) T3 supraglottic carcinomas. The Europeans advocate these procedures for selected early as well as advanced cancers. However, the concepts and discussion in this section are limited to medium and advanced staged tumors.

Oncologic Rationale of the SCPL with CHP

The SCPL with CHP is utilized for selected cases of supraglottic and transglottic carcinoma. A number of retrospective series have noted excellent local control in these patients. In 1990, Laccourreye et al reported no local failures among 68 patients who underwent SCPL with CHP (T1 = 1, T2 = 40, T3 = 26, T4 = 1).[4] In another series specifically evaluating the role of SCPL with CHP for supraglottic lesions with pre-epiglottic space invasion, Laccourreye et al[5] noted a 5.6%(1/19) local failure rate with a minimum of 5 years follow-up. Chevalier et al[6] noted comparable results, of 3.3% (2/61) local failure rates, in their 1994 report of SCPL with CHP for selected supraglottic carcinomas. In 1996, Vincentiis et al[7] reported a series of supraglottic and transglottic carcinomas with a local failure rate of 7.1% (5/70) following SCPL with CHP.

The management of supraglottic carcinoma in the United States utilizes an eclectic approach, the planning of which takes into account patient factors and "institutional opinion." All options are presented to the patient in the context of the opinion of the clinician. Patient factors include, among other things, the patient's preconceived notions concerning surgery or other treatment modalities, overall constitution, pulmonary status, age, and expectations concerning functional outcome. "Institutional opinion" is a mixture of the opinion of the clinician and, many times, the institution's tumor board, which is based on a thorough understanding of the literature interpreted in the context of the collective experience of the involved clinicians. A review of the literature focusing on the management of supraglottic carcinoma in the United States reveals that some institutions strongly favor primary surgical approaches, others favor nonsurgical approaches, and still others utilize a mixture of both surgical and nonsurgical approaches. A review of the major series reported from institutions in the United States reveals that 47% to 90% of patients underwent primary surgical management for supraglottic carcinoma.[8-11] Among the major series published in the United States between 1976 and 1990 that included data concerning the numbers of patients undergoing partial or total laryngectomy for supraglottic carcinoma, the local failure rate for patients undergoing primary surgical management was consistently less than 3%.[8,9,11] Although the local control following primary surgical management is consistently excellent, the percentage of patients undergoing conservation laryngectomy, most of which were SGL, was reported as 45%,[8] 25%,[9] 34%,[10] and 36%.[11] So, although primary surgical management of supraglottic carcinoma yields excellent local control rates, when the option for conservation surgery is limited to SGL many patients will undergo total laryngectomy.

A number of factors may contribute to the limited number of supraglottic carcinomas amenable to SGL. Standard SGL is useful for endolaryngeal carcinomas, without extension below the false vocal fold, with normal true vocal cord mobility.[12] There are a number of extensions of the standard SGL including tongue base resection, pyriform sinus resection, and arytenoid resection.[13] Nonetheless, some series in the United States performed only standard SGL,[11] which therefore limited the number of partial laryngectomies in those series. Another factor that limits the utility of SGL is the significant number of supraglottic carcinomas that extend to the glottic level, a contraindication to SGL. Although in the past it was suggested that supraglottic cancer rarely extends to the glottis,[14] a recent whole organ section analysis as well as a review of other reports on whole organ sectioning indicates that the incidence of spread of supraglottic carcinoma to the glottis is in fact between 20% and 54%.

SGL is very useful for selected T1 and T2 supraglottic carcinomas;[16,17] however, it must be used with great caution to avoid local failure or functional problems in selected cases of T3 and T4 carcinomas of the supraglottis.[18,19] The addition of SCPL with CHP to the spectrum of conservation surgeries for selected cases of T2, T3, and T4 supraglottic carcinoma is of value for avoiding total laryngectomy and improving local control.

Indications and Contraindications for SCPL with CHP[4]

The indications include (1) supraglottic carcinomas with glottic extension, (2) supraglottic carcinomas with pre-epiglottic space invasion, (3) transglottic carcinomas, and (4) selected supraglottic carcinoma with limited thyroid cartilage invasion.

The contraindications include (1) massive invasion of the pre-epiglottic space, because involvement of the hyoid bone would preclude preservation of this structure; (2) involvement of the pharynx or interarytenoid area; (3) cricoid cartilage invasion and infraglottic extension of the tumor reaching the cricoid; (4) arytenoid cartilage fixation; and (5) respiratory impairment.

The presence of arytenoid fixation deserves special comment. Brasnu et al[20] have shown, with serially sectioned larynges, that different pathologic patterns of spread account for true fold versus arytenoid fixation. Although tumor bulk from supraglottic carcinoma can result in decreased motion of the arytenoid, fixation of this cartilage is typically caused by cancer invasion of the cricoarytenoid joint or the cricoarytenoid musculature. Hence, when these structures are involved, it is not possible to save the cricoid, and SCPL with CHP is contraindicated.

Oncologic Rationale of the SCPL with CHEP

The SCPL with CHEP is utilized for selected glottic carcinomas. Several reports have indicated excellent local control rates following SCPL with CHEP for selected glottic carcinomas. Laccourreye et al[21] reported a 5-year actuarial local control of 94.4% (3/67) patients with T2 glottic carcinoma. In another series, Laccourreye et al[22] reported a 10% (2/20) local failure rate for selected T3 glottic carcinomas managed with SCPL with CHEP. Piquet et al[23] reported a local failure rate of 5% among 104 patients who underwent SCPL with CHEP (T1 = 12, T2 = 77, T3 = 15).

When series of T2 glottic carcinoma with more than 100 patients followed for a minimum of 3 years are considered, a 22–24% local failure rate following VPL and a 22–43.5% local failure rate following radiation therapy is noted.[21] When the series of T2 glottic carcinoma in the English literature (not limited to >100 patients) treated by VPL and reporting results by T stage are reviewed, the local failure ranges from 4–24%.[24-28] Even greater variability in local control is noted when the series of VPL for T3 glottic carcinomas are reviewed. When two series from the English literature with five patients or less are excluded, the local failure rates reported for VPL for T3 glottic carcinoma are 11% (3/27),[29] 17% (3/18),[30] 36% (4/11),[31] 41% (9/22),[32] 42% (11/26),[26] and 46% (6/13).[33]

There are a number of advantages for the utilization of the SCPL with CHEP for lesions at high risk for local recurrence following VPL. As noted above, a number of series have consistently reported more than 90% local control following SCPL with CHEP for selected T2 and T3 glottic carcinoma.[21-23,34] A second issue relates to the surgical techniques. One of the challenges that has faced surgeons utilizing extended VPL for T2 and T3 glottic carcinomas has been to devise a reconstruction that would result in consistently adequate functional outcome. When the literature is reviewed it is noted that there is a plethora of reported reconstructions after extended VPL.[35-38] It is our opinion that VPL is most useful for selected T1 glottic carcinomas[39] and that the large number of reconstructions reported following extended VPL may be a reflection of the difficulty in performing a functionally reproducible outcome following these procedures. So another advantage of the SCPL with CHEP is that only one reconstructive technique, the CHEP, is utilized for a wide range of lesions, with the one variation being the resection of one arytenoid. The application of one technique for a wider range of lesions has advantages from the teaching perspective, as well. The addition of SCPL with CHEP for selected cases of T2, T3, and T4 glottic carcinoma is of value in terms of avoiding the need for a permanent stoma from total laryngectomy, improving local control, and providing the surgeon with a single technique for the management of a wide range of lesions with a reproducible reconstruction.

Indications and Contraindications for the SCPL with CHEP

The indications[34] include selected lesions with: (1) bilateral cord involvement (ie, horseshoe lesions), (2) impaired true vocal cord mobility with limited subglottic (less than 1 cm) and ventricular extension, or (3) true vocal cord fixation without arytenoid fixation.

The contraindications include: (1) pre-epiglottic space invasion (utilize SCPL with CHP in this case), (2) cricoid cartilage invasion or infraglottic invasion reaching the cricoid cartilage, (3) arytenoid cartilage fixation, or (4) respiratory impairment.

When evaluating glottic carcinoma prior to performing SCPL with CHEP, it is important to evaluate vocal cord mobility separately from arytenoid mobility. Whole organ section studies have revealed that fixation of the true vocal fold is due to thyroarytenoid muscle invasion,[32] which is not a contraindication to SCPL with CHEP. Arytenoid fixation, on the other hand, is related to cricoarytenoid joint or musculature invasion, which is a contraindication to SCPL with CHEP. In our opinion, in all cases of T3 glottic carcinoma, the arytenoid cartilage on the tumor-bearing side should be resection to ensure a thorough resection of the posterior paraglottic space and the entire thyroarytenoid muscle.

OPTIMIZING FUNCTIONAL OUTCOME FOLLOWING SUPRACRICOID PARTIAL LARYNGECTOMY

The expected functional outcome following SCPL is temporary dysphagia, temporary interruption of laryngeal respiration (temporary tracheostomy), and permanent hoarseness. A review of the world literature reveals that range of days to ending tube feeding ranges from 9 to 50 days for the SCPL with CHEP[23,34,40-44] and from 13 to 365 days for the SCPL with CHP.[4,5,42,44-49]

Obtaining successful functional results following supracricoid partial laryngectomy requires proper patient selection and preoperative evaluation beginning with a thorough medical history. Severe chronic obstructive pulmonary disease is a contraindication to the procedures. We utilize the same pulmonary criteria for SCPL as have been recommended for SGL, which is the patient's ability to ascend two flights of stairs without becoming short of breath. Gastroesophageal reflux should be treated aggressively preoperatively. This avoids irritation of the remaining supraglottic and epilaryngeal mucosa, which may lead to edema and interfere with postoperative deglutition. A history of rheumatoid arthritis necessitates the evaluation of arytenoid mobility by both direct and indirect laryngoscopy.

The surgeon should be cognizant of the location of the superior laryngeal nerves (SLN) during the resection of the primary and the regional lymph nodes. Some of the peripheral branches of the SLN will be cut during the SCPL with CHEP. More branches of the SLN will be cut when performing the SCPL with CHP due to the more extensive supraglottic resection. Care must be taken, both at the time of neck dissection and resection of the primary tumor, to avoid injury to the main trunk of the SLN. Loss of the SLN results in a sensation deficit to the ipsilateral hypopharynx and remaining supraglottic larynx that interferes with the patient's ability to sense secretions and food in those areas.[50] The only indication for the sacrifice of the main trunk of the SLN is direct cancer invasion of the nerve.

The lymphatic drainage from the supraglottis is via the lymphatic trunks, which pass through the thyrohyoid membrane and parallel the SLN and vessels.[51] These high-risk lymph nodes can be removed at the time of radical or modified neck dissection. This dissection results in the identification of the SLN and thereby avoids injury to the main nerve trunk during the primary resection. The limits of the "superior laryngeal node dissection" are the hypoglossal nerve superiorly, the superior thyroid artery inferiorly, the pharyngeal constrictor muscles and the thyrohyoid membrane anteriorly, the carotid artery posteriorly, and the superior laryngeal nerve deep and medially (Fig 8–7).

One of the goals of the reconstruction is to allow for proper positioning of the arytenoids postoperatively. It is important to preserve at least one "cricoarytenoid unit" to allow for function postoperatively. The cricoarytenoid unit includes the cricoarytenoid joint, the cricoarytenoid musculature, the recurrent laryngeal nerve, and the superior laryngeal nerve. During phonation and swallowing, the lateral cricoarytenoid and interarytenoid musculature contract, closing the neoglottis. These muscles relax and the lateral cricoarytenoid muscles contract during respiration, opening the neoglottis.[52] The absence of the vocal ligament appears to

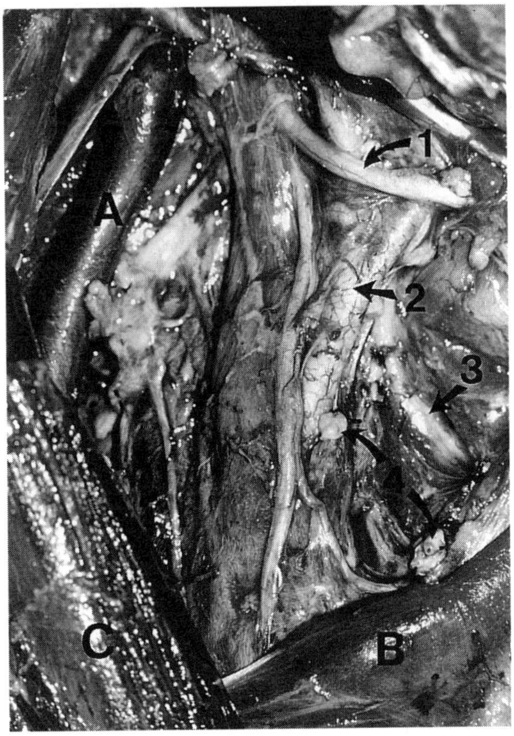

FIG 8–7. Anatomy following superior laryngeal lymph node dissection. A. Internal jugular vein, B. Omohyoid muscle, C. Sternocleidomastoid muscle. 1. Hypoglossal nerve. 2. Carotid bulb. 3. Internal branch of the superior laryngeal nerve. 4. Ligated ends of the superior thyroid artery.

allow the arytenoid cartilage to prolapse anteriorly to abut against the tongue base following CHP or the epiglottis following CHEP.

A number of technical maneuvers during closure have been found to improve functional rehabilitation. It is important to place one or two 3-0 vicryl stitches between the antero-superior aspect of the arytenoid and the anterolateral aspect of the ipsilateral cricoid cartilage. These stitches compensate for the resection of the thyroarytenoid muscles and lift the arytenoids from the posterior pharyngeal mucosa. This may facilitate swallowing by placing the arytenoids under the tongue during deglutition. When one arytenoid is preserved the posterior arytenoid mucosa on the involved side is preserved and also sutured to the anterolateral aspect of the ipsilateral cricoid arch. This provides a cushion against which the preserved arytenoid will abut during phonation and swallowing.

The proper placement of the CHP sutures is important for the timely recovery of deglutition. When passing the sutures around the hyoid it is necessary to arc the suture at least 2–3 cm from the hyoid bone (Fig 8–8, top) The three deep sutures, which are located 1 cm on either side of the midline, gather the bulk of the tongue base medially and rotate it posteriorly, both covering the neoglottis and allowing for diversion of the food bolus into the pyriform sinuses bilaterally.

The closure of the CHEP is modified by the presence of the residual epiglottis. Following the placement of the sutures submucosally around the cricoid cartilage, the sutures are then passed submucosally through the epiglottis (Fig 8–8, bottom). The stitch is then passed out of the pre-epiglottic space close to the inferior border of the hyoid bone prior to being passed back into the tongue base and arched around the hyoid bone as in the CHP. The inclusion of the epiglottis in the stitch prevents it from becoming horizontally oriented, which might compromise the airway postoperatively. This is similar to the epiglottic stitch that ensures proper placement of the epiglottis during the closure of the VPL.[53] A key point in the closure of the CHEP or CHP is that the mucosa of the epiglottis or base of tongue, respectively, abuts the mucosa of the anterior internal surface of the cricoid facilitating primary healing.

The reapproximation of the pyriform sinuses, bilaterally, is accomplished after the CHP or CHEP stitches are tied. This is done by passing two sutures through the transected edge of the constrictor muscles. These are placed just after these muscles are cut from the posterior lateral edge of the thyroid cartilage. These stitches should be tied gently over the anterior aspect of the larynx. A recent study revealed that pyriform repositioning was the only variable that statistically reduced the risk of aspiration.[54]

The functional rehabilitation at the University of Pennsylvania Medical Center has undergone an evolution. Presently, our ap-

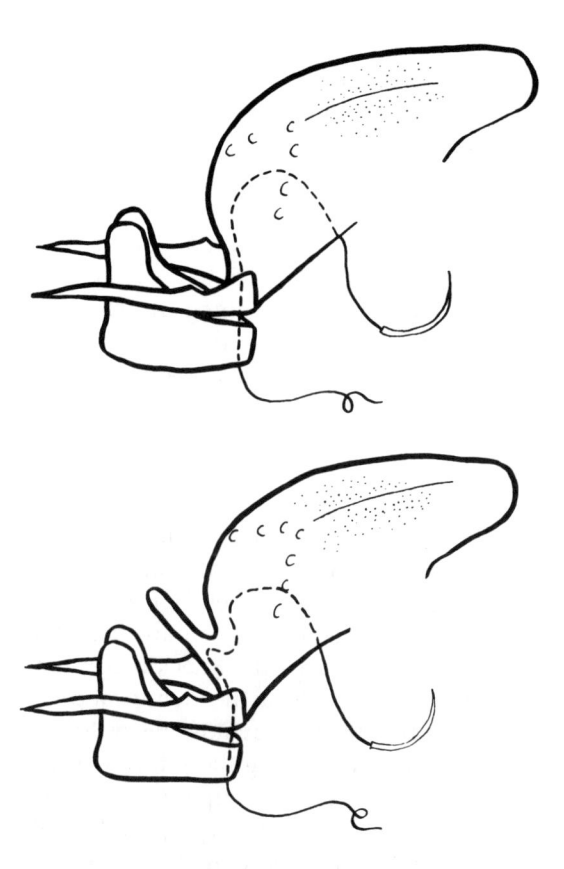

FIG 8–8. *Top,* lateral view of schematic of cricohyoidopexy suture. *Bottom,* lateral view of schematic of cricohyoidoepiglottopexy stitch.

proach includes a modification of the Laennec Hospital rehabilitation program. Rehabilitation is predicated on the principle that active mobilization of the oropharyngeal musculature during the early postoperative period will facilitate early resumption of deglutition. From postoperative day 1, the patient is encouraged to expectorate all secretions into a container without the aid of suction devices. Expectoration both clears the secretions from the pharynx and oral cavity and is an active process that mobilizes the oropharyngeal musculature, compared to suctioning of oral secretions which is a passive process.

The tracheostomy is changed to a cuffless tube on postoperative day 5. Once the swelling has decreased, the tracheostomy is corked. Presently, at the University of Pennsylvania Medical Center, our goal is to discharge patients within the first postoperative week with their tracheostomy in place and corked as tolerated. They are not encouraged to swallow their own secretions during the first postoperative week. Tube feedings are continued on an outpatient basis.

Swallowing rehabilitation is managed on an outpatient basis. During the second posoperative week, the patient is taught the "safe swallow" technique, which is adopted from the technique utilized at Laennec Hospital. This technique consists of having the patient flex the neck and raise the shoulders in an attempt to touch the chin to the chest. The patient then thrusts the tongue base against the posterior pharyngeal wall and swallows forcefully. This is begun first with saliva only, then followed in a few days by pureed foods and, finally, by liquids. Once full nutrition is taken by mouth, tube feedings are stopped. At the University of Pennsylvania Medical Center and Laennec Hospital, clinical assessment is utilized in lieu of modified barium swallow during swallowing rehabilitation.

The tracheostomy is removed once a stable airway is observed without evidence of significant edema or granulation tissue. Decannulation is typically delayed if the patient has had previous laryngeal radiation therapy.[55]

Initially the voice is breathy. As the mobility of the arytenoids improves, voice quality also improves. The vocal quality following SCPL has been studied prospectively and by the sixth postoperative month the speech parameters of phrase groupings and the number of words per minute were similar to normal speakers.[56] Of note, the mean fundamental frequency was lower and wider than normal indicating postoperative voice instability, and the degree of voicelessness parameters was increased, suggesting problems with neoglottic closure during speech.[56] Piquet et al noted that the voice tends to be deep with a fundamental frequency of 80 Hz and an intensity between 60–70 dB following SCPL with CHEP.[57] Similar results were noted by Vincentiis et al[7] following SCPL with CHEP in which the fundamental frequency ranged from 49 to 131 Hz to a maximum of 98 to 220 Hz, with an intensity range of 55 to 95 dB. Although the expected voice quality is similar to chronic laryngitis, the quality of the postoperative voice allows normal social interaction.[34]

SUMMARY

The role of the SCPLs in the management of selected laryngeal carcinomas has been reviewed. The operative technique, oncologic rationale, and techniques for optimizing functional outcome were presented. The tradeoff when performing these procedures appears to be permanent hoarseness in exchange for improved local control and avoidance of a permanent stoma. In conclusion, the SCPLs are useful techniques for both avoiding total laryngectomy and improving local control in selected cases of laryngeal carcinoma.

REFERENCES

1. Alonso JM. Conservative surgery of the larynx. *Trans Am Acad Opthalmol Oto-laryngol.* 1947;51:633–642.
2. Majer HaR, W. Technique de laryngectomie permetant de conserver la permeabilité respi-

ratoire la cricohyoido-pexie. *Ann Otolaryngol Chir Cervicofac.* 1959;76:677–683.
3. Medina JE. *Clinical Practice Guidlines for the Diagnosis and Management of Cancer of the Head and Neck.* Arlington, Va: The American Society for Head and Neck Surgery and The Society of Head and Neck Surgeons; 1996:32.
4. Laccourreye H, Laccourreye O, Weinstein, G, Menard, M, Brasnu, D. Supracricoid laryngectomy with cricohyoidopexy: a partial laryngeal procedure for selected supraglottic and transglottic carcinomas. *Laryngoscope.* 1990;100:735–741.
5. Laccourreye O, Brasnu, D, Merite-Drancy A, Cauchois R, Chabardes E, Menard M, Laccourreye H. Cricohyoidopexy in selected infrahyoid epiglottic carcinomas presenting with pathological preepiglottic space invasion. *Arch Otolaryngol Head Neck Surg.* 1993; 119:881–886.
6. Chevalier D, Piquet JJ. Subtotal laryngectomy with cricohyoidopexy for supraglottic carcinoma: review of 61 cases. *The Am J Surg.* 1994;168:472–473.
7. Vincentiis M, Minni, A, Gallo A. Supracricoid laryngectomy with cricohyoidopexy (CHP) in the treatment of laryngeal cancer: a functional and oncologic experience. *Laryngoscope.* 1996;106:1108–1114.
8. DeSanto LW. Cancer of the supraglottic larynx: a review of 260 patients. *Otolaryngol Head Neck Surg.* 1985;93:705–711.
9. Coates HL, DeSanto LW, Devine KD, Elveback LR. Carcinoma of the supraglottic larynx: a review of 221 cases. *Arch Otolaryngol.* 1976;102:686-9.
10. Lee NK, Goepfert H, Wendt CD. Supraglottic laryngectomy for intermediate-stage cancer: UT MD Anderson Cancer Center experience with combined therapy. *Laryngoscope.* 1990; 100:831–836.
11. Lutz CK, Johnson JT, Wagner RL, Myers EN. Supraglottic carcinoma: patterns of recurrence. *Ann Otol Rhinol Laryngol.* 1990;99: 12–17.
12. Montgomery W. *Surgery of the Upper Respiratory System.* Philadelphia: Lea and Febiger; 1989.
13. Bocca E, Pignataro O, Oldini C, Sambataro G, Cappa C. Extended supraglottic laryngectomy: review of 84 cases. *Ann Otol Rhinol Laryngol.* 1987;96:384–386.
14. Bocca E. Limitations of supraglottic laryngectomy and conservative neck dissection. *Can J Otolaryngol.* 1975;4:403–419.
15. Weinstein GS, Laccourreye O, Brasnu D, Tucker J, Montone K. Reconsidering a paradigm: the spread of supraglottic carcinoma to the glottis. *Laryngoscope,* 1995;105:1129–1133.
16. Herranz-Gonzales J, Gavilan J, Martinez-Vidal J, Gavilan C. Supraglottic laryngectomy: functional and oncologic results. *Ann Otol Rhinol Laryngol.* 1996;105:18–72.
17. Burstein FD, Calcaterra TC. Supraglottic laryngectomy: series report and analysis of results. *Laryngoscope.* 1985;95:833–836.
18. Alonso Regules JE, Blasiak J, de Vilaseca BA. End results of partial horizontal (functional) laryngectomy in Uruguay. *Can J Otolaryngol.* 1975;4:397-339.
19. Spaulding CA, Constable WC, Levine PA, Cantrell RW. Partial laryngectomy and radiotherapy for supraglottic cancer: a conservative approach. *Ann Otol Rhinol Laryngol.* 1988;98:125–129.
20. Brasnu D, Laccourreye H, Dulmet E, Jaubert F. Mobility of the vocal cord and arytenoid in squamous cell carcinoma of the larynx and hypopharynx: an anatomical and clinical comparative study. *Ear Nose Throat J.* 1990;69: 324–330.
21. Laccourreye O, Weinstein GS, Brasnu D, Bassot V, Cauchois R, Jouffre V, Garcia D, Laccourreye H. A clinical trial of continous cisplatin-fluorouracil induction chemotherapy and supracricoid partial laryngectomy for glottic carcinoma classified as T2. *Cancer.* 1994;74:2781-2790.
22. Laccourreye O, Salzer S, Brasnu D, Shen W, Laccourreye H, Weinstein G. Glottic carcinoma with a fixed true vocal cord: Outcomes after neoadjuvant chemotherapy and supracrioid partial laryngectomy with cricohyoidoepiglottopexy. *Otolaryngol Head Neck Surg.* 1996;114:400–446.
23. Piquet JJ, Chevalier D. Subtotal laryngectomy with crico-hyoido-epiglotto-pexy for the treatment of extended glottic carcinomas. *Am J Surg.* 1991;162:357–361.
24. Liu C, Ward PH, Pleet L. Imbrication reconstruction following partial laryngectomy. *Ann Otol Rhino Laryngol.* 1986;95:567–571.
25. Sessions DG. Extended partial laryngectomy. *Ann Otol Rhinol Laryngol.* 1980;89:556–557.
26. Som ML. Cordal cancer with extension to the vocal process. *Laryngoscope.* 1975;85:1298–1307.
27. Biller HF, Ogura JH, Pratt LL. Hemilaryngectomy for T2 glottic cancers. *Arch Otolaryngol.* 1971;93:238-243.

28. Mohr RM, Quenelle J, Shumrick DA. Verticofrontolateral laryngectomy (hemilaryngectomy). Arch Otolaryngol. 1983;109:384–395.
29. Kessler DJ, Trapp TK, Calcaterra TC. The treatment of T3 glottic carcinoma with vertical partial laryngectomy. Arch Otolaryngol Head Neck Surg. 1987;113:1196–1199.
30. Lesinski SG, Bauer, WC, Ogura JH. Hemilaryngectomy for T3 (fixed cord) epidermoid carcioma of larynx. Laryngoscope. 1976: 1563–1571.
31. Biller HF, Lawson W. Partial laryngectomy for vocal cord cancer with marked limitation or fixation of the vocal cord. Laryngoscope. 1986;96:61–64.
32. Kirchner JA, Som ML. Clinical significance of fixed vocal cord. Laryngoscope. 1971;81: 1029–1044.
33. Mendenhall WM, Million RR, Sharkey DE, Cassisi, NJ. Stage T3 squamous cell carcinoma of the glottic larynx treated with surgery and/or radiation therapy. Int J Radiat Oncolol Biol Phys. 1984;10:357–363.
34. Laccourreye H, Laccourreye O, Weinstein G, Menard, M., Brasnu, D. Supracricoid laryngectomy with cricohyoidoepiglottopexy: a partial laryngeal procedure for glottic carcinoma. Ann Otol Rhino Laryngol. 1990;99: 421–426.
35. Burgess LP, Yim DW. Thyroid cartilage flap reconstruction of the larynx following vertical partial laryngectomy: an interim report. Laryngoscope. 1988;98:605–609.
36. Bailey B, Calcaterra TC. Vertical, subtotal laryngectomy and laryngoplasty. Arch Otolaryngol. 1971;93:232–237.
37. Biller HF, Lawson W. Partial laryngectomy for transglottic cancers. Ann Otol Rhinol Laryngol. 1984;93:297–300.
38. Nong HT, Mo W, Huang GW, Chen L. Epiglottic laryngoplasty after extended hemilaryngectomy for glottic cancer. Chin Med J (Engl). 1990;103:925–931.
39. Laccourreye O, Weinstein G, Brasnu D, Troutoux J, Laccourreye H. Vertical partial laryngectomy: a critical analysis of local recurrence. Ann Otol Rhinol Laryngol. 1991; 100:68–71.
40. Guerrier B, Lallemant JG, Balmigere G, Bonnet P, Arnoux B. [Our experience in reconstructive surgery in glottic cancers]. Ann Otolaryngol Chir Cervicofac. 1987;104: 175–179.
41. Vigneau DCH, Passey, JJ, Lacomme, Y. Indications, techniques et resultats carcinologique et fonctionnele. Rev Laryngol. 1988; 109:145–147.
42. Traissac L, Verhulst, J. Indications, techniques et resultats des laryngectomies reconstructives. Rev Laryngol. 1991;112:55–88.
43. Piquet JJ, Desulty A, Decroix G. Crico-hyoido-pexie. Technique operatoire et results fonctionnels. Ann Otolaryngol Chir Cervicofac. 1974;91:681–689.
44. Pech A, Cannoni M, Giovanni A, Thomassin JM, Zanaret M, Goubert JL. La necessaire selection des techniques chirugicales dans le traitment du cancer du larynx. Ann Otolaryngol Chir Cervicofac. 1986;103:565–575.
45. Botazzi D. La laryngectomie subtotale reconstructive selon Labayle: experience clinique sur 21 sujets. Rev Laryngol. 1986;107:207–208.
46. Prades JM, Martin C, Garban T, Perron X, Mayaud R. Les laryngectomies reconstructives: aspects techniques et fontionnels. Ann Otolaryngol Chir Cervicofac. 1987;104:281–287.
47. Marandas P, Luboinski B, Leridant AM, Lambert J, Schwaab G, Richard JM. La chirurgie fontionnelle dans les cancers du vestibule larynge: a propos de 149 cas traites a l'Institut Gustave-Roussy. Ann Otolaryngol Chir Cervicofac. 1987;104:259-265.
48. Junien-Lavillauroy C, Barthez M, Roux O, Geunon P, Tixier C, Morel, D, Ennouri A. La crico-hyoido-pexie: resultats preliminaires et indications therapeutiques (a propos de 41 cas.). JFORL. 1988;37:3–7.
49. Maurice N, Crampette L, Mondain M, Guerrier B. Laryngectomie subtotale reconstructive avec cricohyoidopexie resultats carcinologiques et suites fontionnelles precocoes. Ann Otolaryngol Chir Cervicofac. 1994; 111:435-442.
50. Kronenberger MB, Meyers AD. Dysphagia following head and neck cancer surgery. Dysphagia. 1994;9:236–244.
51. Rouviere H, Tobias MJ, transl. Anatomy of the Human Lymphatic System. Ann Arbor: Edward Brothers Inc; 1938:57.
52. Weinstein GS, Laccourreye O. Supracricoid laryngectomy with cricohyoidoepiglottopexy. Otolaryn Head Neck Surg 1994;111:684–685.
53. Lore JM. An Atlas of Head and Neck Surgery. Philadelphia: WB Saunders Company; 1988: 904.
54. Naudo P, Laccourreye O, Weinstein G, Hans S, Laccourreye H, Brasnu D. Functional outcome and prognosis factors after supracricoid partial laryngectomy with cricohyoidopexy. Ann Otol Rhinol Laryngol. 1997; 106:291–295.

55. Laccourreye O, Weinstein G, Naudo P, Cauchois R, Laccourreye H, Brasnu D. Supracricoid partial laryngectomy after failed laryngeal radiation therapy. *Laryngoscope*. 1996;106:495–498.
56. Crevier-Buchman L, Laccourreye O, Weinstein G, Garcia D, Jouffre V, Brasnu D. Evolution of speech and voice following supracricoid partial laryngectomy. *J Laryngol Otol*. 1995;109:410–413.
57. Piquet JJ, Desaulty A, Decroix G. Crico-hyoido-epiglotto-pexie: technique operatoire et resultats fonctionnels. *Ann Otolaryngol Chir Cervicofac*. 1974;91:681–689.

CHAPTER 9

Advances in Functional Assessment of Patients Treated for Head and Neck Cancer

Gayle Woodson, PhD

Cancer of the head and neck frequently involves functionally important components of the upper aerodigestive tract. As a consequence, tumors in this area commonly present as difficulties in breathing, speaking, or swallowing. Moreover, the treatment of tumors in this area may further compromise function, due to surgical resection of important structures or limitation of function by scarring or radiation changes. Often patients who are successfully cured of head and neck tumors must cope with significant handicaps, such as impaired speech or dependence on a tracheotomy or tube feedings. Because these problems have a significant impact on the quality of life, it is crucial to consider the functions of speech and swallowing along with survival data when assessing the results of different approaches to treating head and neck cancer.

Organ preservation protocols for the treatment of head and neck cancer hold the potential of preserving the anatomy and function of the upper aerodigestive tract. Initial survival data from some studies are encouraging, with cure rates equal to or better than those achieved by major surgical resection, such as laryngectomy, and radiation.[1-3] However, the ultimate value of an organ preservation approach can only be assessed by determining how well the preserved structures function. This requires the use of reproducible and relevant measures of speech and swallowing.

To date, few studies of organ preservation treatment protocols have objectively measured functional results. Despite recent advances in the assessment of speech and swallowing, no standardized criteria have been established for measuring function in patients with head and neck cancer. Recent research has focused on identifying parameters that will be useful in assessing function in these patients. To be clinically useful, tests of function should be relatively easy to perform, reproducible, and relevant to the dysfunction prevalent in the population of interest. The parameters should measure the patient's problems and provide information about the underlying pathophysiology.

Such an approach has been used to measure function in patients treated in the RADPLAT protocol for advanced head and neck cancer.[4] The RADPLAT protocol, described in Chapter 6, involves delivering very high doses of cis-platinum directly into the tumor, via superselective angiography, with simultaneous intravenous administration of a neutralizing agent, sodium thiosulfate. This chemotherapy is combined with conventional radiation therapy. Results to date, in patients with advanced and usually unresectable tumors, indicate a greater than 90% local control rate. Functional studies in these patients have included objective tests of voice and speech, identifying relevant parameters, and analyses of eating status.

VOICE AND SPEECH

A variety of methods for evaluating the voice have been developed and are commercially available for clinical use. However, no standard battery of vocal function tests has been established. This is largely due to the fact that each person has a unique voice and the range of normal human voices is vast. Further, speaking is a voluntary motor task, subject to considerable variability and capable of tremendous enhancement by training. Therefore, it is easy to make a large number of measurements of vocal function, but quite difficult to identify parameters that reflect actual pathology rather than individual differences. This is not unlike selecting the appropriate chemical test to apply to a blood sample. For example, blood glucose is monitored in patients with diabetes, whereas serum creatinine is important in patients with renal impairment.

Many voice assessment techniques are semiquantitative, using interval scales to rate subjective judgments. Other tests are quantitative and objective physical measurements. Functional tests also differ in whether they assess the *sound* of the voice, the physical processes involved in producing that sound, or the effectiveness of communication. Most vocal function tests address the sound of the voice, as this is noninvasive and objective. However, study of only the sound of the voice fails to address important clinical issues.

The chief characteristics of the sound of a voice can be described in terms of pitch, loudness, and vocal quality. Pitch and loudness can be subjectively judged, but these are also direct correlates of physical parameters that can be objectively measured, namely fundamental frequency and sound pressure level, respectively. In contrast, vocal quality has not been directly related to any single specific physical measure. Subjective perceptual analysis is currently the only approach that really addresses how the voice sounds, although research is ongoing to identify the acoustic waveform characteristics that are perceived as differences in voice quality.

Of course, the most important consideration in assessing vocal outcome is patient satisfaction. Patient satisfaction is difficult to quantify, even when a standardized scale or questionnaire is employed, because there is great variability in patients' needs and expectations. Thus, satisfaction cannot realistically be used to compared treatment results among patients. Nonetheless, all other measures of vocal function are useful only to the degree that they reflect the patient's satisfaction with the sound of the voice and how well the voice serves the patient's communication needs. Therefore, objective measures of vocal function should be validated against patients' self-rating of function before they can be adopted for clinical use. This approach has been used to evaluate the relevance of various vocal function parameters in small groups of patients undergoing RADPLAT therapy for head and neck cancer, comparing the correlation of both physical measures and subjective rating scales with patients' perceptions of function.

Perceptual Analysis

In a study of 15 patients treated for head and neck tumors, patients' self-ratings of voice were compared to perceptual ratings generated by a blinded panel of trained listeners.[4]

As controls, the study included five volunteers of comparable smoking and drinking history, but without cancer. Patients and subjects were simply asked to rate speech samples from each patient with respect to five vocal quality parameters, each on a 7-point scale. The overall voice quality rating for each subject was defined as the mean of scores for all parameters.

The results indicated significant concordance between patients' and observers' perceptions. Mean overall voice quality score was 3.4 for "good" voices, 4.3 for "fair" voices, and 5.85 for "bad voices." Mean voice quality score for normal controls was 2.8. Patients treated for laryngeal tumors had a 4.61, within the "fair" range. Patients treated for nonlaryngeal tumors had a mean score or 3.89. Of note, the mean scores included several measurements made within a few months of treatment, when there was still some residual inflammation and edema. Acute measurements were included in the study to ensure that a range of dysfunction was included. Thus, the actual steady-state performance of these patients was better than indicated by these data.

These results underscore the validity of controlled and properly conducted perceptual analysis in assessing the sound of the voice. However, the process is cumbersome and impractical for routine clinical use or application in large studies. Samples must be rated blindly, preferably all during one session, and three or more listeners are needed to establish validity.

Communication Assessment

In the same study, subjects also self-rated overall their communicative ability on a 4-point scale, ranging from class 0 (no oral communication) to class III (normal function).[4] If subjects had some communication dysfunction, but were capable of continuing usual employment and social interactions, the rating was class II. Subjects who had to quit work or could not interact socially because of inability to communicate orally were class I. The results of these self-ratings were compared to the communication score determined by clinicians, using a 9-point communication scale developed for this study., Based on the interview, the clinician rated the subjects' ability to communicate in daily activities. As with perceptual analysis, the communication score demonstrated significant concordance with patient perception.

The clinician's communication rating was 4.3 for class I subjects, 6.07 for class II, and 7.5 for class III. When analyzed for tumor site, the mean communication scores were 6.6 for the patients with laryngeal tumors and 6.7 for those with nonlaryngeal tumors. Thus, although patients with larynx tumors did not *sound* as normal as those treated for nonlaryngeal tumors, communication function was similar in both groups. Both patient groups were significantly different from controls, whose mean score was 9.

Thus, the communication scale appears to be a very valuable clinical measure. It correlates well with patient satisfaction and is much easier to implement than perceptual analysis of vocal function. Hence, it is much more feasible for both routine clinical use and application in large clinical trials.

Acoustic Analysis

Physical measurements and analysis of the sound of the voice are termed acoustic analysis. This assessment approach is extremely objective and reproducible. Measurements of vocal range, the upper and lower limits of pitch and volume, appear to be significant parameters in patients with head and neck cancer. For example, vocal range is severely restricted in patients who use a tracheoesophageal puncture for communication, but much less impaired in patients with larynx tumors treated by RADPLAT.[5]

However, more fine-grained analyses of waveform are of limited use in this patient population. In a study of 15 RADPLAT patients, acoustic measures including shimmer, jitter, harmonic-to-noise ratio, and standard deviation of the fundamental frequency were not significantly correlated with either patient self-ratings or the perceptual ratings by observers.[4] In part, this is because the acoustic determinants of perceived vocal quality have not been identified, and the patients and observers may have attended to other characteristics of the acoustic signal. However, a more significant limitation to the use of acoustic analysis in this population is its decreasing validity as the severity of hoarseness increases. In very noisy voices, analysis software programs become unreliable. In aperiodic voices, no fundamental frequency can be identified, which invalidates other standard measures. In fact, a recent consensus conference concluded that, in very hoarse voices, such as those of head and neck cancer patients, perceptual analysis is the only assessment tool available for the study of voice quality.[6]

Aerodynamic Measures

Aerodynamic measurements quantify air pressure and volume changes over time. Such measures are good indicators of the physical status of the vocal mechanism and the degree of effort involved in voice production. These measures are highly significant, because many head and neck cancer patients are relatively unconcerned by the sound of their voice but are quite disturbed when increased effort is required to produce that sound.

Subglottic pressure during phonation reflects the degree of expiratory effort and the tightness of glottic closure required to produce sound. It should be interpreted in the context of the loudness of the utterance, as greater pressure is normally required to generate louder sounds.

Simultaneous measurement of both phonatory airflow and subglottic pressure permits calculation of *laryngeal resistance*. In a study of 15 RADPLAT patients, laryngeal resistance was the objective measure that correlated best with patient satisfaction. Further, laryngeal resistance was on average twice as high in patients who complained of voice fatigue. However, laryngeal resistance is a calculated ratio and not a direct measure; thus it should be interpreted carefully. For example, a laryngeal abnormality such as scarring may result in increased stiffness, which would increase resistance. But the same abnormality may also impair glottic closure, which would decrease resistance. Further, patients often compensate for scarring by closing the glottis tightly, which would result in increased resistance. Thus, laryngeal resistance is the composite result of many variables and should be interpreted in the context of physical examination of the larynx during phonation, preferably using stroboscopy.

A more promising measure is *phonation threshold pressure* (PTP), the minimum subglottic pressure that can support phonation.[6] It is an excellent indicator of vocal fold stiffness. In studies of RADPLAT patients compared to patients with near-total laryngectomy or tracheo-esophageal puncture speech, PTP was a good indicator of both vocal quality and communication function.

EATING

Patients with head and neck cancer frequently have impairment of eating, either temporarily or permanently. This may involve problems with chewing and/or swallowing. The patient may be unable to ingest the food or may have aspiration into the tracheobronchial tree. Lesser degrees of impairment may result in a restriction of the types of food the patient can eat. With more profound impairment, the patient becomes dependent on tube feedings.

The loss of the ability to eat normally is a devastating handicap. Eating food per se is very pleasurable and dining is a very important social activity. For most patients, being able to eat is more important than being able to speak. Thus, the evaluation of eating function is crucial in assessing the result of treatment of head and neck cancer.

Modified barium swallow is currently accepted as the most comprehensive means of evaluating the swallowing mechanism and detecting aspiration. Nonetheless, this approach is difficult to use in large clinical trials. The examination is time consuming and can involve considerable radiation exposure for the patient. Additionally, extraction of objective data by making temporal and spatial measurements from the recording is tedious. Further, the clinical significance of these parameters remains to be established. It is likely that future research may result in automated or more streamlined methods of analysis and that specific parameters may be identified as being particularly useful. If so, then modified barium swallow would become an even more important means of assessing swallowing function.

Another approach to assessment is to document eating status by tracking weight changes and mode of food intake. In 47 patients treated by RADPLAT for advanced head and neck cancer, weight and eating ability were documented before treatment and at various intervals after treatment. All patients had advanced head and neck cancer. Tumors were unresectable in most patients, and in the others, surgical resection would have severely impacted on voice or swallowing. Weight change after treatment was expressed as a percentage of the pretreatment weight. On the average, weight immediately after treatment was 90% of the pretreatment weight, indicating that subjects tended to lose weight during therapy. This is not surprising, considering the effects of nausea, mucositis, and catabolic stress. Weight loss was not significantly correlated with tumor size, tumor site, nodal status, or the presence or absence of a feeding tube.

Weight stabilized after treatment at 88%, 92%, and 90% at 6, 12, and 18 months, respectively. This indicates that, although patients did not regain to the pretreatment weight level, food intake was sufficient to maintain weight long-term.

The ability to eat was also tracked, determining whether the patient ate a normal diet, mechanically modified diet, or was dependent on tube feedings. Before treatment, the ability to eat was significantly affected by the size of the tumor, but not by the site, as patients with large tumors were more likely to require tube feedings during therapy. At 18 months after treatment, 69% of patients were enjoying a normal diet. Nineteen percent modified their diet, ingesting soft or liquid food; 12% remained dependent on tube feedings. The data indicate that the RADPLAT protocol preserved eating function in a high percentage of patients with advanced tumors.

CONCLUSION

In summary, technological advances have resulted in the availability of a large number of methods for measuring speech and swallowing function. These developments should be of great interest to clinicians caring for patients with head and neck cancer, because tumors in this region can have a profound effect on talking and eating. However, it is essential to identify functional tests that are truly relevant in these patients. The impact on speech is most reliably evaluated by using a standardized scale to assess communication function and by the objective measures of vocal range, laryngeal resistance, and threshold phonation pressure. Useful indices of swallowing function can be obtained by tracking mode of feeding, type of diet, and weight.

REFERENCES

1. Wolf GT, Hong WK, Fisher SG, et al. Induction chemotherapy plus radiation compared with surgery plus radiation in patients with advanced laryngeal cancer: the Department of Veterans Affairs laryngeal study group. *N Engl J Med*. 1991;324:1685–1690.
2. Robbins KT, Vicario D, Segren S, et al. A targeted supradose chemoradiation protocol for advanced head and neck cancer. *Am J Surg* 1994;168:419–422.
3. Robbins, IT, Fontanesi J, Wong FS, et al. A novel organ preservation protocol for advanced carcinoma of the larynx and pharynx. *Arch Otol*. 1996;122:853–857.
4. Woodson GE, Rosen CA, Murry T, et al. Assessing vocal function after chemoradation

for advanced laryngeal carcinoma. *Arch Otol.* 1996;122:858–864.

5. Allegretti J, Woodson GE, Murry T, et al. Vocal function in patients treated for advanced laryngeal cancer. Presented at the Fourth International Conference on Head and Neck Cancer; July 1996; Toronto, Ontario.

6. Tietze I. Workshop of acoustic voice analysis [summary statement]. Iowa City Ia: National Center for Voice and Speech; 1996.

CHAPTER 10

Oral Communication After Laryngectomy

R.E. (Ed) Stone, Jr, PhD

"Then, I came to receive; Now I stay to give."—a patient

If the ensuing discussion were to stay within the "recent advances" confines of the title of this book very few topics would emerge—maybe heat and moisture exchangers, acoustic comparison of alaryngeal voice options and new artificial larynges. Almost every other topic would be reiteration of existing knowledge. But medical personnel usually receive so little training in post-laryngectomy rehabilitation that presentation of new topics would be meaningless without at least an introductory overview of established knowledge about oral communication after laryngectomy. Thus, this chapter reviews, maybe in a new way, older topics as well as presents some of the newer issues. Hopefully, it will benefit both the new as well as more seasoned practitioners.

INTERVENTION BEGINS WITH PRE- AND POSTOPERATIVE CONSULTATION

The necessity of pre- and postoperative consultation for successful laryngectomee rehabilitation is a theme that permeates the world literature.[1-9] In addition to adequate treatment of the disease leading to removal of the larynx, successful rehabilitation is largely influenced by the extent to which the patient and family are informed of the disease, curative treatment, and rehabilitation opportunities. Most otolaryngologists feel that they fully and adequately inform their patients.[10] Yet, Salmon[11] pointed out only about a third of health care consumers (HCCs) feel they are well prepared for laryngectomy. Laryngectomee consultations also do not routinely include the patient's immediate support personnel. Only a fourth of the spouses interviewed by Salmon reported receiving preoperative contact or information and slightly more than 10% reported they felt adequately prepared. Further, she found that only half of the laryngectomees received any information about being a laryngectomee from their physician or surgeon other than education about the surgical procedure. Only one third of the patients she interviewed were taught about the pathologic condition and prognosis for laryngeal cancer.

Salmon found that less than half of the laryngectomized patients in the United States receive preoperative consultation with nurses, an average of 10 contacts amounting to less than 1 hour. Rarely was the patient's spouse involved in these contacts. Less than one third of the laryngectomees reported preoperative contact with speech rehabilitation personnel (speech-language pathologists, esophageal speakers, artificial larynx users, and spouses of other laryngectomees). Spouses of the patients were involved in these contacts less than 10% of the time.

Although some patients are more inquisitive than others, a few may want to attend only to information that might allay their fears. Most patients experience seven fears associated with cancer and laryngectomy:

➤ fear of cancer,
➤ fear of surgery outcome,
➤ fear of the verbal silence,
➤ fear of recurrence,
➤ fear of unemployment,
➤ fear of economic devastation, and
➤ fear of loss of status in the family unit.

Most often news of the need for a laryngectomy is delivered to the patient when the spouse is present. Seldom, however, are the needs of the spouse considered in spite of their fears that their partner:

➤ might not survive the surgery,
➤ might not be cured of the cancer,
➤ might never talk again,
➤ might not psychologically adjust following surgery, and
➤ their fear of inappropriately responding to their laryngectomized partner.

Of those who are given consultation, many possibly do not process the messages and feel inadequately prepared for assuming this new aspect of their lives.

Resolution of the problem of poor preparation may be possible. One solution may lie in cross-training the health care team. Thus, several team members could repeat and reiterate what another member might already have said, but at another time when the patient and his or her family possibly are more receptive. Critical pathways could be developed to incorporate planned repetition of consultations. The team may include not only the physician/surgeon and nursing services but also speech pathology, a laryngectomized visitor and spouse,[12] nutritional services,[13] a social worker, and a vocational counselor for patients of employable age.[14,15] Rather than give pathways here, each team might develop its own time-lines and assignments. At least three questions might guide the development:

➤ Who is to carry the responsibility for initial presentation of given concepts and when?
➤ Which members are to assess patient's understanding? and
➤ What courses of action are to be taken to correct deficits in the consumers understanding.

The speech pathologist's role on the team ideally begins preoperatively and continues most intensely of all the members for several months postoperatively. Thus, a person in this specialty might be the logical person to assume leadership of the team; however, the surgeon generally is the one who takes the lead, at least during the pre- and immediate postoperative period until the patient's discharge from the hospital. Because of their training in anatomy and physiology, early inclusion of speech pathologists may allow for sharing information to supplement that given by the physician and nurses. This consultation, which is supplemental in nature, would include the anatomical alterations and the everyday consequences[16-18] brought by the surgery such as:

➤ personal health adjustments,
➤ effects on olfaction and taste and communication.

Primary or lead responsibilities of the speech pathologist (not referred to here as speech-language pathologist because the laryngectomized patient's language functions are not altered by the surgery and there is no need for language rehabilitation) center around communication. Preoperative visits by the speech pathologist generally serve to:

- establish rapport for postoperative rehabilitation,
- assure the patient that speech pathologists have ways of "making the patient talk,"
- outline, in generalities, various postoperative communication options,
- informally qualify the patient for rehabilitation in terms of:
  - motivation;
  - cognitive abilities;
  - available support personnel;
  - physical abilities such as hearing acuity, vision acuity, reading and writing skills, manual dexterity; and
  - integration into the laryngectomized community.

Consequently, the patient as well as the surgeon benefits from the speech pathologist's involvement. Preoperatively, the surgeon's expectations and decisions for type of surgery to do may be influenced by the outcomes of the speech pathologist's preoperative visit(s). For example, the speech pathologist can give educated guesses about the patient in terms of probable rehabilitation success for speech with and without augmentation via voice prostheses. Speech pathologists, thus, could influence the decision for primary or secondary placement of tracheo-esophageal fistula. Benefit to the patient comes from knowing that someone will continue to care about him or her after he or she is assisted off the surgical table and that learning to speak again will not be done in a rehabilitative vacuum. The spouse who is involved in the speech pathology consultation(s) achieves relief by knowing there is someone other than the surgeon who is approachable for coordinating continuity of surveillance of the need for additional care and who can be called on if questions arise. Further, spousal comfort is derived from knowing that a professional is planning on a long-term commitment (beyond a mere once-per-month follow-up visit) and cares about the patient's and partner's quality of life after surgery.

Postoperative consultation from the speech pathologist involves an active rehabilitative function. It is during this time that various options for postoperative communication can be explored in greater detail.

ORAL COMMUNICATION OPTIONS

The separation of the GI tract from the respiratory tract is mandated by the need to prevent aspiration. Unfortunately, this results in construction of new anatomy to facilitate breathing through an orifice other than the mouth or nostrils. Creation of a permanent tracheostomy is traditional. Accordingly, air that is inhaled and then exhaled through the stoma cannot be used for speech purposes. Alternate processes are needed.

After the first few days of paper and pencil communication, oral forms of communication and additional topics can be implemented in sequential fashion:

- pantomimed speech using oral gestures,
- alaryngeal whisper,
- artificial larynx (AL) use,
- speech with standard esophageal voice (SEV) production,
- speech aided with prostheses,
- assistance from other devices, and
- use of heat and moisture exchangers that may indirectly benefit communication by enhancing the likelihood of social acceptance and effective use of tracheostomal speaking valves.

Pantomimed Speech Using Oral Gestures

Many patients seem to naturally evolve into use of the lips and tongue for communication to supplement or replace immediate postoperative graphic forms of communication. One might call this "mouthed" speech in which no acoustic events are produced (silent whisper).

Alaryngeal Whisper

Having established articulatory function without expiratory effort (silent whisper), voiceless whisper can be encouraged. Accordingly, the patient is instructed to use increased force or contact of the articulators (also without expiratory effort). This is done to elicit intra-oral air pressure that, when the articulators are released, results in the creation of audible sound for plosive consonants. Once [p], [t], and [k] are established, work can begin on developing voiceless affricate and sibilant sounds using compromise of the oral cavity to increase oral pressure that, in turn, results in air flow through narrowed channels with accompanying frication. Speech resembles what laryngeal speakers might do if talking while holding their breath with the glottis closed.

Many clinicians feel such communication is not advisable because it may encourage development of constricted oropharyngeal space and incline the patient to establish voiceless "Donald Duck" speech (pharyngeal speech, sometimes erroneously called buccal speech). Personal experience, however, indicates that patients can be taught through modeling and instruction to avoid this. The advantage of getting the patient "on the air" with oral communication during the immediate postoperative period while still under the services of the speech pathologist prepares the way for quick utilization of the artificial larynx.

Artificial Larynx Use

Approximately 2 to 5 days after surgery patients usually can be introduced to the artificial larynx (AL). These devices provide an audible sound source for the speech tract either by directing sound into the oral cavity through a tube inserted into the mouth (intra-oral type) or through the tissues of the cheeks or the side of the neck (electric neck type). The array of electric and pneumatic types of available instruments has been described by Blom.[19] The International Association of Laryngectomees (International Association of Laryngectomees, c/o Mary Jane Renner, 7440 N. Shadeland Ave., Indianapolis, IN 46250; 317-570-4568), provides literature that includes most of the United States distributors of artificial larynges. Probably the most commonly used AL is the Servox™, distributed by representatives of the Siemens Corporation. Teaching the use of ALs is illustrated through video tape by Salmon,[11] along with presenting a curriculum of instruction. The Siemens Corporation also has recommended guidelines for instruction in the use of the artificial larynxes that were developed by this author and later modified by one of their representatives (C. Thomas Beneventine, 58 Woodstock Dr., Wayne, NJ 07470-3548). These are illustrated in a videotape, "Speech Options after Laryngectomy," available from Siemens Hearing Instruments, Inc. (Siemens Hearing Instruments, Inc., 16 Piper Lane, Prospect Heights, IL 60070). Every laryngectomee at the Vanderbilt Medical Center is provided an artificial larynx that is ordered as part of the person's necessary hospital supplies. Daily instruction and guided practice in its use continues until discharge from the hospital.

Most recently, two new ALs have emerged on the market. One is the Optivox™ which features a set of replaceable outer shells of various colors that easily can be changed to provide color coordination with the user's attire. It is available from Bivona Medical Technologies (5700 West 23rd Ave., Gary, IN 46406). This company also recently introduced for free distribution a kit of supplies to laryngectomees. There, patients will find voice restoration products, attachment aids for tracheostomal valves, and other supplies helpful in maintaining healthy airways.

Another new artificial larynx, TruTone™, has been developed by Griffin Laboratories and is distributed by several companies, the first known to this author being Lauder Enterprises (11115 Whisper Hollow, San

Antonio, TX 78230-3690). Its uniqueness centers around using a single button to activate the device that also varies pitch continuously over an adjustable range of frequencies. This allows the laryngectomee to incorporate prosodic features to a greater extent than is possible with other devices and thus to reduce the monotonic speech characteristics associated with most ALs. Usually patients can learn to use pitch variation in just one to a few sessions when presented with the challenge to do so and instruction. Some clinicians, however, may feel that enhancement of AL use via pitch change is beyond the basics and view this feature as unnecessary and they will resist use of this advanced feature.

Pneumatic ALs funnel the exhaled air from the stoma which vibrates a diaphragm to produce a sound. Sound is directed into the oral cavity through a tube placed in the mouth. This provides an alternative to attempting to transmit sound through tissues of the neck, which may be stiffened as a result of surgery and radiation. Popular pneumatic devices include the Tokyo (Artificial Speech Aid, 3002-8 12th St., Harlan, IA 51537) and the DSP 8 (Memacon, Pres. Kennedylaan 263 P.O. Box 56, Velp 6200, Netherlands). The "Taiwan tube" is another inexpensive pneumatic artificial larynx popular with laryngectomees in Hong Kong.[21] The most standard intra-oral AL is the Cooper-Rand (distributed by Luminaud Co., 8688 Tyler Blvd, Mentor, OH 44060) electric intra-oral device. It is composed of a housing that contains a battery and circuitry that is small enough to be carried in a shirt pocket and has controls to regulate both pitch and loudness levels of the tone. The tone generator with its activation switch is at one end of a wire cord connecting it to the circuitry. Attached to the tone generator is a short tube that is placed in the mouth similarly to that of a pneumatic AL. Regardless of type, all ALs merely provide a sound to the speech mechanism, making what normally would be whispered speech more audible. The patient is responsible for producing various vowels and consonants for intelligible speech by changing mouth, tongue, and lip postures as done preoperatively. Laryngectomees who also have encountered glossectomies may find the use of ALs helpful even though deprived of one of their articulators.

Patient acceptance of ALs appears to be influenced by the models of use that are presented, their motivation for self-improvement, and the degree of positive feedback suggesting effectiveness of communication. The better the models, the greater the acceptance. The greater the degree of patient acceptance of his or her post-op status, the greater the level of acceptance of AL use. Individuals who have high expectations of themselves and high expectations for success in other forms of communication, however, usually are not satisfied with the visual distraction and the robotic sound associated with most ALs. The empirically derived validity of such contentions, however, is yet to be demonstrated except for a few isolated investigations of acceptance.[22] In some series of patients as few as 20% will use an artificial larynx even in cases of esophageal voice treatment failure, when tracheo-esophageal prosthesis is contraindicated, when the esophageal voice has an insufficient volume, or when presented with the need to converse in noisy environments.[22] Our own experiences suggest a high percent of patients will settle for the use of an AL in lieu of attempting other forms of oral communication.

STANDARD ESOPHAGEAL VOICE AS AN OPTION

The gold standard of postlaryngectomy communication against which other forms of communication are often compared has been called "burp speech" or esophageal voice. It possibly is the most biologically natural one and is often used by children to embarrass their parents. This voluntary burping or belching uses the sound created at the junction of the pharynx with the esophagus (P-E segment). This sound is then modified by the resonating cavities of the throat, mouth, and nose and by movement of the articulators (e.g., tongue, teeth, velum, and lips). Although the history of laryngectomy and the development of artificial larynges are well documented,[23] the first patient to use esophageal voice is not documented. Snidecor,[24] however, references an early work of Czermak with the title of "Ueber die Sprache bei luftdchter Verschliessung des Kehlkopfen" (About the Speech at Airtight Closure of the Larynx) written in 1859. Evidence that speech following laryngectomy occupied the attention of rehabilitationists is reflected by the existence of texts dated in the early 1900's.[25-28] Other early references can be traced back to Seeman's work in 1924.[29] Interestingly, emphasis on standard esophageal voice production historically followed artificial larynx usage and tracheoesophageal/pharyngeal fistulization. The first laryngectomy done for treatment of cancer (performed by Billroth in 1873 and reported by Billroth and Gussenbauer in 1874) involved fitting the patient with a pneumatic artificial larynx[23] that introduced sound into the pharynx through a surgically created fistulous tract. Guttman[30] was motivated to advocate tracheoesophageal/pharyngeal puncture (TEP) as a procedure to facilitate speech in the laryngectomized after a patient self-inflicted a TEP with a hot ice-pick.[23] This patient was a butcher with a knowledge of the anatomic relationship between the trachea and esophagus. His intolerance for both the artificial larynx and esophageal voice led him to seek a different manner for introducing air into the esophagus for speech and was presented as a case study at a medical conference in Chicago in 1935. To prevent aspiration, the fistula was plugged with a goose quill when not speaking (Moore, JP, personal communication, 1997).

Esophageal voice production depends first upon putting air into the esophagus (not the stomach), which acts as a reservoir. If air is inadvertently ingested into the stomach the delay in eructation of that air for creation of voice is inappropriately prolonged. Swallowing air, therefore, is not a suitable insufflation technique. Two major methods of acceptable air intake have evolved that reduce the risk of stimulating a swallow reflex.

Pumping Methods of Air Intake

Air pressure developed above the PE segment that exceeds the closing forces of the PE segment and the intraluminal pressure in the esophagus will result in flow of intra-oral air caudally into the esophagus. This increased pressure can be developed by compromising the intra-oral volume through elevating the jaw from a dropped to a closed position (given the lips and velopharyngeal port are closed). This *mouth squeeze* process forms the basis for air charges associated with consonant sounds such as [p] and [b] and possibly [t] and [d]. The first recognized publication highlighting the effectiveness of consonant production to effect air charge of the esophagus is attributed to Moolinaar-Bijl[31] and Helbert Damstè who completed a dissertation on this subject under her mentorship in the 1950s. Yet, Stetson was an advocate of this technique as early as 1937. This process often is referred to in the literature as *consonant injection*.

Air charge in the absence of consonants must be accomplished by other means. One such process is done by reducing the volume between the tongue and palate. This action can be facilitated by envisioning use of the tongue to flatten a balloon held in the mouth with the neck of the balloon pointed posteriorly. As air is squeezed out of the balloon by elevation of the tongue, air is pumped into the oropharynx and down the hypopharynx, through the PE segment and into the esophagus. This has been described as a *tongue lock* method by McClear[32] in the instructional booklet published by the now nonexistent National Hospital for Speech Disorders. Similarly, the tongue may be pulled in a pistonlike action to drive air caudally into the esophagus. This method is referred to as a *glossopharyngeal press*.

In any event, effective air charges are not accomplished by instructing the patient merely to swallow air. Shipp[33] contrasted air charging and vegetative swallowing and pointed out that swallowing is done more slowly and with different muscle activation sequences. Further, swallowing can only be done a limited number of times in rapid succession without producing a spasmlike condition in the throat. There is evidence, however, which suggests that, even with nonswallow air charges, some air does enter the stomach. Snidecor and Isshiki[34] reported one superior speaker could expel a volume of 615 cc of air over a 26-second period. This volume dramatically exceeds the volume of the esophagus. Winans, Reichback, and Waldrop[35] found that better esophageal speakers tended to have greater pressures in the stomach than poorer speakers.

Inhalation Method of Air Charge

In addition to pumping the air down, patients may suck air into the esophagus. Thus, there are both "pumpers" and "suckers." Some patients utilize all forms of air intake. The "suckers" use a quick inhalation maneuver to drop the resting pressure in the thorax and consequently in the esophagus as well as in the trachea. Successful injection of air by this method requires an open PE segment or at least one that has less closing pressures than 14.7 psi. One of the most effective "inhalers" is demonstrated by Lanpher in a videotape she presents with Dugay.[36]

Isshiki[37] reviewed research on the aerodynamics of various air charges indicating mean volumes per air charge range between 7.92–19 cc, mean flow rate of air intake between 68–70 cc/sec, and mean time of injection from 130–250 milliseconds.

The effectiveness of communication that patients achieve depends somewhat on the instruction they receive after the ability to charge air has been accomplished. This instruction generally involves a curriculum that leads the patient into sustaining esophageal voice for progressively longer speech units. Training can begin as soon as the nasogastric feeding tube is removed (sometimes before) prior to the patient's discharge from the hospital. Pressures and tissue strain encountered for speaking should be less than for those involved when swallowing a bolus of food. Thus, the risk of speech inducing an undesired fistulous tract during the healing process is not a factor if instruction is given to avoid unnecessary efforts. Generally, the patient is encouraged to shape eructated sound into one-syllable words with the addition of articulatory gestures of the speech mechanism (hence the benefit of early speech instruction soon after surgery that is encouraged by use of the artificial larynx). After the ability to charge air and make sound consistently has been established, two aspects of nurturing a patient's speech characterize the rehabilitation process. They usually receive attention concurrently. One aspect deals with speech proficiency. Mastering length of response is part of proficiency. It is developed with incorporation of sound generation into longer and longer speech units by encouraging the patient to practice word lists in which the number of syllables is progressively increased and lists of increasingly longer phrases. Other speech proficiencies worthy of attention include developing pitch and loudness variability for prosodic features of speech and encouraging linguistic stress and juncture.[36,38]

The other aspect of speech rehabilitation concerns nurturing speech acceptability. In the pursuit of proficiency, many patients develop unwanted behaviors that must be eliminated in the pursuit of acceptability. These include:

▶ multiple air charge attempts to accumulate a large volume of air (multiple air charges),
▶ facial grimacing (usually associated with the various pumping methods of insufflation),
▶ noises associated with air charging such as lip smacks and clunking noise as air enters the esophagus,

- long latency$_I$ between the desire to charge air and accomplishment of the feat,
- stomal blast derived from air exiting the stoma accompanying eructation of sound from the esophagus, and
- long latency$_{II}$ between accomplishment of air charge and the ensuing sound production.

The degree to which patients experience success in developing esophageal voice by traditional air charge methods of pumping or sucking varies between 5%[39] one month after surgery to at least 70%[40] with increased time postoperatively. A few clinicians have instructional programs in which 80% of patients learn to use effective and efficient esophageal voice production for everyday speaking purposes. Such patients include public school teachers, ministers, and sales personnel. Yet, not everyone is sufficiently motivated,[22] and some patients cannot make sound,[41] or for other reasons[42,43] choose not to use standard esophageal voice production. These individuals led to the development of current trends in prosthetically aided esophageal voice.

TEP AIDED ESOPHAGEAL VOICE AS AN OPTION

Creation of a fistula or tunnel between the trachea and esophagus through the posterior tracheal wall restores communication between the GI tract and respiratory tract. Consequently, if the stoma is occluded, exhaled air flows from the lungs into the esophagus. This air passing upward through the PE segment vibrates the tissues lining the segment for the creation of esophageal voice. Unfortunately, liquids can also find the way from the pharynx into the fistulous tract and into the trachea and lungs. History is long and rich with surgical innovations to develop structures whereby the tract can prevent aspiration of liquids but still allow the patient to admit air into the esophagus for exciting the surgical residuals for sound generation. Maves[18] reported that Conley utilized two procedures in 1959 to effect a lined fistulous tract, one using esophageal mucosa and the second an autogenous vein graft. Problems of leakage and stenosis were the bases of disappointment. Asai, in 1965,[45] Miller,[46] and Montgomery[47] used multistaged procedures to develop two stomas, one for breathing and one for directing air into the hypopharynx. These employed a separate stage to create a communicating dermal tube between the stomas so that pulmonary air could be used for speech. Both Staffieri[48] and Serafini[49] created a phonatory neoglottis using a tracheo-hypopharyngeal shunt by bringing pharyngeal mucosa over the amputated trachea and creating a "button hole" to act as the vibrating source. Staffieri's procedure still enjoys limited acceptance in Europe. Komorn[50] developed a tracheoesophageal shunt using pharyngeal mucosa that carried pulmonary air to the esophagus below the PE segment. Although some of his patients developed excellent esophageal voice others were troubled with the same problems as those of Conley. Amatsu[51] created a side-to-side anastomosis with the trachea and esophagus using a flap of membranous trachea. Unfortunately the results included tracheal stenosis and aspiration.

From the creation of a silastic prosthesis by Blom starting around 1978 and the efficient surgical approach by Singer for establishing communication of the trachea to the esophagus into which the prosthesis is fit, many variations of prostheses have evolved.[52,53] Some are to be changed by the patient when the prosthesis becomes defective. Others (called in-dwelling prostheses) are to be replaced by the speech pathologist or physician. The in-dwelling prostheses have a larger inside diameter than some patient-replaceable devices and generally require lower driving pressures. The two most popular in-dwelling devices in the United States are the Blom/Singer distributed by In-Health and the Provox distributed by Bivona. One of the factors that limits the life span of these devices involves colonization of *Candida albicans*, which interferes with good closure of the one-way valve. Toward a solution of this problem, daily use of an antifungal medication such as Nystatin or Mycelex is recommended.

The major advantages of prosthetically aided speech include earlier establishment of oral communication, longer speech units, greater pitch and intensity variation, and less instructional time. Kischk and Gross[54] found that placement of the TE fistula at the time of laryngectomy, rather than as a later secondary approach, gave better speech results. They discovered that 70% of patients who initially were given prosthetically aided speech later gave up the method after developing standard esophageal voice production, even though prosthetic speech was recognized as having superior characteristics.

ASSISTANCE FROM OTHER DEVICES

Although attempts are being made to render a permanent tracheostoma passé,[55,56] neck-breathing remains the bane of existence for most laryngectomees. Breathing through the stoma deprives the trachea and lungs from the humidification provided by the nose. Subsequently, viscosity of mucus is increased and ciliary action is decreased. The sound associated with attempts to expel the collections of mucus through the stoma (stomal cough) is offensive to the ears of most people. Its uniqueness draws unwanted attention to the laryngectomee. Additionally, cleaning the stomal area of expelled mucus is a nuisance and is repugnant to both the patient and his observers. Further, patients who use prosthetic aided voice by occluding their stoma with a finger or thumb find stoma care is extremely important. Even with the best of care, there are times when stomal occlusion is not desired or possible, for example, when the hands are dirty or are otherwise occupied with objects.

Tracheostoma Valve

To be free of digital occlusion, Blom devised a device known as the tracheostoma valve, which is distributed by In-Health. The valve is held in a housing secured by adhesive to the skin around the stoma. The valve permits ingressive air as well as egressive flow unless the flow rate on exhalation is elevated. High flow rates obstruct the device and divert air through the tracheoesophageal prosthesis. Sensitivity adjustments can be made to the valve so that inadvertent closure is avoided when the patient increases strength of exhalation but does not want to produce voice, as when exercising. Whereas Blom originally designed a "flapper" valve to offset the flow that was made popular through distribution by In-Health, Bivona Medical Technologies distributes a similar mechanism as well as a spring-loaded valve.

In any event, the patient who is able to wear a tracheostoma valve enjoys the benefits of hands-free speech. There are patients, however, whose skin does not tolerate any of the available adhesives inherent in attaching this valve. Other patients present with uneven topography of the anterior neck (surgical crevasses, prominent clavicular heads, and protruding sternocleidomastoid muscles) which obviates adequate adherence of the device.

Various adhesives are available in addition to these supplied in the valve kits provided by distributors. Mastisol (Ferndale Laboratories) comes in ampules that, when broken, delivers adhesive with no mess and seems to have good adherence properties. Skin Bond (Smith-Nephew) is a rubber-based product that some patients find irritates the skin less than other adhesives and can be used for several days without loss of holding power. In addition to trying different glues, clipping the attachment of the sternocleidomastoid muscles at the clavicles sometimes is helpful in producing a flatter surface for attaching the valve. When deep crevices are left as a surgical residual, little can be done to effect adequate seal of the valve housing to the skin. This led clinicians at Mayo Clinic to the development of a different housing called the Barton-Mayo Button[57] distributed by Bivona Medical Technologies. This housing for the tracheostoma valve is part of a short tube inserted through the stoma into the trachea. Use of this device has the added advantages of keeping the stoma of adequate size (that sometimes becomes constricted due to circumferential scar tissue) and the self-retention feature avoids the task of applying adhesives.

Humidifiers

Problems surrounding the increased tenacity of mucus have been shown to be ameliorated by humidification. Laryngectomees who keep their environment at about 40% relative humidity generally cough less often and less vigorously. Yet, most well rehabilitated laryngectomees are not captive to an environment that can be so well controlled. Sales personnel, teachers, housewives, and so on often find themselves in locations that are well below recommended humidities.

The Swedish company, Gibeck (Gibeck, Inc., 10640 E. 59th St., Indianapolis, IN 46236-8334) packages, under the rubric of Stoma-Vent 2 (Lary-care, P.O. Box 160982, Austin, TX 78716), a housing to be worn over the stoma that contains a corrugated paper filter. The filter takes up moisture from exhaled air and yields that moisture back into inhaled air. Blom, in 1990, developed an attachment for his tracheostoma valve that houses a foam sheet specially treated with chlorhexidine and lithium-chloride. The former substance serves to inhibit bacterial growth; the other chemical is used to enhance moisture collection from exhaled air. He also made this available for those laryngectomees who did not wear the hands-free valve. Both are distributed by In-Health (InHealth Technologies, 1110 Mark ave., Carpinteria, CA 93013-2918). Bivona Medical Technologies (57000 W. 23rd Ave., Gary, IN 46406-2617) distributes a similar appliance called a heat and moisture exchanger (HME) called The Provox Stomafilter that was developed and is manufactured by Atos Medical AB in Horby, Sweden. Recent study of the effectiveness in humidification, air flow resistances, and costs associated with the use of these HMEs is presented by Grolman, Blom, Branson, Schouwenourg, and Hamaker.[58] Filter material and size seem to determine the HME's moisture output efficiency and the resistance to flow. The various filters and housings contribute significant differences in the daily costs ranging from around $500 to $1300 per year.

PATIENT SUPPORT: LOST CORD CLUBS

The opening section of this chapter pointed out that laryngectomees, spouses, and families usually desire some affiliation with others who have traveled the rehabilitation road ahead of them. The first organization of laryngectomees helping other laryngectomees developed out of the efforts of Warren Gardner in 1951. By 1953, the International Association of Laryngectomees (IAL) had been formed as an autonomous agency supported by the American Cancer Society (ACS). As summarized in the video presentation *Peer-Support for Laryngectomized Persons*,[12] this organization played a major role in sponsoring annual meetings for laryngectomees and annual voice institutes for training teachers of alaryngeal voice production. The majority of these institutes were directed by Dr. James Shanks, Indiana University School of Medicine. This man, alone, has been responsible for providing group and individual instruction to over 5,000 laryngectomees. As a member of the IAL, he has been a major influence in making the IAL truly international by holding workshops on nearly every continent of the world. Recent years have brought a shift in financial priorities of the ACS away from laryngectomee support. State divisions and local units of the ACS recently have had to assume greater responsibility for providing assistance to laryngectomees. Florida, California, and Texas have developed statewide laryngectomee organizations where county and local groups may network with other groups with similar missions.

The Florida Laryngectomee Association has sponsored annual voice institutes since 1982. Patterned after the models of the early IAL voice institutes, the trainees may be speech-language pathologists seeking continuation of education. Other trainees may be laryngectomized individuals with superior rehabilitation who desire to provide assistance to professional speech pathologists in teaching alaryngeal speech or others who desire to give informed counsel and service to new laryngectomees in hospital and home visitations. Another vital group attending the institutes is composed of laryngectomees who seek to improve their own speaking—sometimes seeking to make their first sounds. Trainees providing therapy to fledgling laryngectomees are supervised during individual therapy sessions twice daily. During therapy, rap sessions are concurrently held for the spouse of any laryngectomized participant in the institute. The curriculum also provides rap sessions led by laryngectomees for their peers. Leadership of the institute is provided by an advisory board made up of members of the state organization and health care providers. Funding is derived from charging the professional attendees a tuition fee and from contributions from the state division of ACS and from individual gifts. The faculty of the institute volunteer their time and services. Personnel involved in the institutes return to their local organizations with renewed commitment and with knowledge and skills to share with other local laryngectomees. Local organizations throughout the country carry a variety of names including *Lost Cord Club of (city), New Voice Club,* or *Anamilo Club* and usually have monthly meetings that are sponsored to some degree by local county units of the ACS, which serve as a point of contact for new laryngectomees and for professionals who want to request a laryngectomized visitor. Not every laryngectomee desires affiliation with other laryngectomees, but most do. A few want to continue their affiliation long after their greatest need of assistance has abated. One such individual demonstrated his accomplished rehabilitation in the comment, "Then I came to receive. Now I stay to give."

REFERENCES

1. Brouwer B, Snow GB, van Dam FS. Experiences of patients who undergo laryngectomy. *Clin Otolaryngol.* 1979;4:108–118.
2. Pruszewicz A, Gasiorek J, Obrebowski A, Czerwinski A. Value of psychological rehabilitation in the process of development of alaryngeal speech after laryngectomee [in Polish]. *Otolaryngologia Polsk.* 1979;33:533–539.
3. Blanchard, SL. Current practices in the counseling of the laryngectomy patient. *J Com Disord.* 1982;15:233–241.
4. deMaddelena H, Pfrang H, Schchohe R, Zenner HP. Speech intelligibility and psychosocial adaptation in various voice rehabilitation methods following laryngectomy [in German]. *Laryngo-rhino-Otologie.* 1991;70:562–567.
5. Mathieson CM, Stam HJ, Scott JP. Psychosocial adjustment after laryngectomy: a review of the literature [Review]. *J Otolaryngol.* 1990;331–336.
6. Lacroix A, Jacquemet S, Assal JP. Patients' experience with their disease: learning from the differences and sharing the common problems. *Patient Educ Counsel.* 1995;26:301–312.
7. Bussi M, Albertini D, Bogetto F, Lombardo P, Maina G, Ravizza L, Cortesina G. Effects of total laryngectomy on the quality of life: a study on certain psychological aspects [in Italian]. *Acta Otorhinolaryngol Ital.* 1994;14:627–632.
8. Sakai T. Psychosomatic analysis of laryngectomized patients. *Nippon Jibiinkoki Gakkai Kaiho (Journal of the Oto-Rhino-Laryngological Society of Japan).* 1994;97:1412–1422.
9. Gonzales Martinez MT, del Canizo Alvarez A. Psychological alterations in patients with cancer of the larynx before and after laryngectomy [in Spanish]. *Acta Otorhinolaryngol Espan.* 1993;44(3):175–178.
10. Johnson JT, Casper J, Lesswing NJ. Toward the total rehabilitation of the alaryngeal patient. *Laryngoscope.* 1979;89:1813–1819.

11. Salmon S. Pre- and postoperative conferences. In: Keith RL, Darley FL, (eds). *Laryngectomee Rehabilitation*, 2nd ed. San Diego, Calif: College-Hill Press; 1986:226–290.
12. Bowman S, Lauder E. Peer support for the laryngectomized. In: Shanks JC, Stone RE Jr, eds. *Help Employ Laryngectomized Persons* [video tape No. VC3810]. Stillwater, Okla: National Clearinghouse of Rehabilitation Disorders, Oklahoma State University; 1983.
13. Logemann J, Rollins SS, Yuska C. Becoming a laryngectomee: multidisciplinary professional support. In: Shanks JC, Stone RE Jr, eds. *Help Employ Laryngectomized Persons* [video tape No. VC4060]. Stillwater, Okla: National Clearinghouse of Rehabilitation Disorders, Oklahoma State University; 1983.
14. Richardson JL, Rainey JL. Employment after laryngectomy. In: Shanks JC, Stone RE Jr, eds. *Help Employ Laryngectomized Persons* [video tape No. VC4022]. Stillwater, Okla: National Clearinghouse of Rehabilitation Disorders, Oklahoma State University; 1983.
15. Holley B. Counseling the head and neck cancer patient: laryngectomy. *Prog Clin Biol Res*. 1983;121:215–225.
16. Pearson BW. From suspicious of laryngeal cancer to laryngectomy. In: Shanks JC, Stone RE Jr, eds. *Help Employ Laryngectomized Persons* [video tape No. VC4079]. Stillwater, Okla: National Clearinghouse of Rehabilitation Disorders, Oklahoma State University; 1983.
17. York, Keith RL. Personal health adjustments following laryngectomy. In: Shanks JC, Stone RE Jr, eds. *Help Employ Laryngectomized Persons* [video tape No. VC3740]. Stillwater, Okla: National Clearinghouse of Rehabilitation Disorders, Oklahoma State University; 1983.
18. Maves MD. Surgical help for alaryngeal voice. In: Shanks JC, Stone RE Jr, eds. *Help Employ Laryngectomized Persons* [video tape No. VC 4079]. Stillwater, Okla: National Clearinghouse of Rehabilitation Disorders, Oklahoma State University; 1983.
19. Blom ED. Helping the laryngectomee through the use of artificial larynges. In: Shanks JC, Stone RE Jr, eds. *Help Employ Laryngectomized Persons* [video tape No. VC 3409]. Stillwater, Okla: National Clearinghouse of Rehabilitation Disorders, Oklahoma State University; 1983.
20. Salmon S. Using the artificial larynx: a presentation on instruction. In: Shanks JC, Stone RE Jr, eds. *Help Employ Laryngectomized Persons* [video tape No. VC 3640]. Stillwater, Okla: National Clearinghouse of Rehabilitation Disorders, Oklahoma State University; 1983
21. Chalstrey SE, Bleach NR, Cheung D, van Hasselt CA. A pneumatic artificial larynx popularized in Hong Kong. *J Laryngol Otol*. 1994;108: 852–854.
22. Motta S. Phonatory rehabilitation via esophageal voice and the laryngophone [in Italian]. *Acta Otorhinolaryngol Ital*. 1992;12:237–243.
23. Keith RL, Shanks JC. Historical highlights: laryngectomee rehabilitation. In: Keith RL, Darley FL, eds. *Laryngectomee Rehabilitation*. San Diego, Calif: College-Hill Press; 1968.
24. Snidecor J. *Speech rehabilitation of the laryngectomized*. Springfield, Ill: CC Thomas, 1969.
25. Schaer A. Cited by: Snidecor, JC. (1969). *Speech Rehabilitation of the Laryngectomized*. Springfield, Ill: CC Thomas; 1969:243.
26. Gutzmann M. Cited by: Snidecor JC. *Speech Rehabilitation of the Laryngectomized*. Springfield, Ill: CC Thomas; 1969:225.
27. Hendrick J. Cited by: Snidecor, JC. *Speech Rehabilitation of the Laryngectomized*. Springfield, Ill: CC Thomas; 1969.
28. Stetson RH. Can all laryngectomized patients be taught esophageal speech? *Trans Am Laryngol Assn*. 1937;59:59–71.
29. Damsté PH. Anatomic and physiological bases of esophageal voice. In: Shanks JC, Stone RE Jr, eds. *Help Employ Laryngectomized Persons* [video tape No. 3532]. Stillwater, Okla: National Clearinghouse of Rehabilitation Disorders, Oklahoma State University; 1983.
30. Guttman MR. Tracheopharyngeal fistulization: a new procedure for speech production in the laryngectomized patient. *Trans Amer Laryng Rhinol Otol Soc*. 1935;41(2):1926. Cited by: Snidecor JC. *Speech Rehabilitation of the Laryngectomized*. Springfield, Ill: CC Thomas; 1969:59.
31. Moolinaar-Bijl AJ. Connection between consonant articulation and the intake of air in oesophageal speech. *Folia Phoniatrica (Basel)*. 1953;5:212–216.
32. McClear JE. *Esophageal Voice Production*. New York: National Hospital for Speech Disorders; 1960.
33. Shipp T. EMG of pharyngoesophageal musculature during alaryngeal voice production. *J Speech Hear Res*. 1970;13:184–192.
34. Snidecor J, Isshiki N. Vocal and air use characteristics of a superior male esophageal speaker. *Folia Phoniatrica*. 1965;17:217–232.

35. Winans CS, Reichback EJ, Waldrop WF. Esophageal determinants of alaryngeal speech. *Arch Otolaryngol.* 1974;99:10–14.
36. Lanpher AG, Dugay MJ. Developing excellence using esophageal voice. In: Shanks JC, Stone RE Jr, eds. *Help Employ Laryngectomized Persons* [video tape No. 3610]. Stillwater, Okla: National Clearinghouse of Rehabilitation Disorders, Oklahoma State University; 1983.
37. Isshiki N. Airflow in esophageal speech. In: Snidecor JC, ed. *Speech Rehabilitation of the Laryngectomized.* Springfield, Ill: Charles C Thomas; 1969:137–150.
38. Weinberg B. Characteristics of esophageal speech. In: Shanks JC, Stone RE Jr, eds. *Help Employ Laryngectomized Persons* [video tape No. VC3635]. Stillwater, Okla: National Clearinghouse of Rehabilitation Disorders, Oklahoma State University; 1983.
39. St. Guily JL, Angelard B, ed-Bez M, Julien N, Debry C, Ficheus P, Gondret R. Postlaryngectomy voice restoration: a prospective study in 83 patients. *Arch Otolaryngol-Head Neck Surg.* 1992;11:252–255.
40. Quer M, Burgues-Vila J, Garcia-Crespillo P. Primary tracheoesophageal puncture vs esophageal speech. *Arch Otolaryngol-Head Surg.* 1992; 118:188–190.
41. Novak A. Objective parameters of the quality of the esophageal voice [in Czech]. *Ceskoslovenska Otolaryngologie.* 1982;31:275–279.
42. Buchanan G. Research opportunities at the Institute of Laryngology and Otology, London. *Can J Otolaryngol.* 1975;4:846–849.
43. Martin D. Barriers to speaking with esophageal voice. In: Shanks JC, Stone RE Jr, eds. *Help Employ Laryngectomized Persons* [video tape No. 3609]. Stillwater, Okla: National Clearinghouse of Rehabilitation Disorders, Oklahoma State University; 1983.
44. Kimura T, Asai R, Hattori H. Voice pattern after Asai's laryngoplasty. *Nippon Jibinkoka Gakkai Kaiho.* 1969;72(2):444–445.
45. Asai R. Laryngoplasty after total laryngectomy. *Arch Otolaryngol.* 1972;95:114–119.
46. Miller A. First experiences with the Asai technique for vocal rehabilitation after total laryngectomy. In: Snidecor JC, ed. *Speech Rehabilitation of the Laryngectomized.* Springfield, Ill: CC Thomas; 1969:50–57.
47. Montgomery WW, Toohill RJ. Voice restoration after laryngectomy. *Arch Otolaryngol.* 1967;88:499–506.
48. Staffieri M. Functional total laryngectomy: surgical technic, indication and results of a personal technic for glottis-plasty with reconstruction of the voice [in German]. *Monatschrift fur Ohrenheilkunde und Laryngo-Rhinologie.* 1973;107:77–89.
49. Serafini I. Total laryngectomy with restoration of normal phonation and breathing: first results (4 cases) [in French]. *Ann Oto-Laryngol Chirurgie Cervico-Faciale.* 1970;87:509–518.
50. Komorn RM. Vocal rehabilitation in the laryngectomized patient with a tracheoesophageal shunt. *Ann Otol Rhinol Laryngol.* 1974;83:445–451.
51. Amatsu M. A new one-stage surgical technique for postlaryngectomy speech. *Arch Otorhinolaryngol.* 1978;220(1–2):149–152.
52. Perry A. Surgical voice restoration procedures. *Sem Speech Lang.* 1986;7:31–42.
53. Heaton JM, Parker J. Indwelling tracheooesophageal voice prostheses post-laryngectomy in Sheffield, UK: a 6-year review. *Acta Oto-Laryngol.* 1994;114:675–678.
54. Kischk BT, Gross M. Comparative evaluation of the voice prosthesis after laryngectomy [in German]. *HNO.* 1995;43:304–310.
55. Hagen R, Schwab B, Marten S. Nasotracheal airway-oropharyngeal alimentary canal: a microvascular technique for reconstruction of the upper airway after total laryngectomy. *Ann Otol Rhino Laryngol.* 1995;104:317–322.
56. Crevier-Buchman L, Laccourreye O, Weinstein G, Garcia D, Jouffre V, Brasnu D. Evolution of speech and voice following supracricoid partial laryngectomy. *J Laryngol Otol.* 1995;109:410–413.
57. Barton D, DeSanto L, Pearson BW, Keith R. An endostomal tracheostomy tube for leakproof retention of the Blom-Singer stomal valve. *Otolaryngol Head Neck Surg.* 1988;99:38–41.
58. Grolman W, Blom ED, Branson RD, Schouwenburg PK, Hamaker RC. (1997, submitted). an efficiency comparison of four heat and moisture exchangers used in the laryngectomized patient.

CHAPTER 11

Rhabdomyosarcoma of the Head and Neck in Children

Alberto S. Pappo, MD, and William M. Crist, MD

Accounting for 5% of all pediatric tumors, rhabdomyosarcoma (RMS) is the most common soft tissue sarcoma in children and adolescents.[1] Prior to introduction of combined modality therapy (including radiotherapy, surgery, and multiagent chemotherapy) fewer than one third of children with RMS survived, compared to about 70% today.[2-5] This cure rate equals or exceeds that for most other common childhood cancers and can be attributed to widespread use of risk-adapted (ie, based on prognostic factors), multimodal therapy, improvements in tumor classification (ie, better systems for histologic classification aided by immunohistochemistry and development of cytogenetic and molecular diagnostic techniques), refinements in staging, and the introduction of improved supportive care.[5,6] Because of the relative rarity of RMS and its heterogeneity, national cooperative group studies have been essential to progress in studies of biology and therapy. By pooling ideas and patients, the Intergroup Rhabdomyosarcoma Study Group (IRSG, established in 1972) was able to design and expeditiously conduct a series of large randomized trials that were designed to answer questions regarding optimum therapy.[7] About three quarters of newly diagnosed children and adolescents with RMS from the United States enter these trials and similar national and international trials are ongoing in Europe. Treatment results of the IRSG trials have been shown to reflect overall results from the United States by comparisons with the data from the Surveillance, Epidemiology, and End Results Section of the National Cancer Institute (SEER), which closely resemble results reported from Europe as well.[1] RMS is clinically and biologically heterogeneous. Tumors of the embryonal histiotype (60% of cases) are associated with a loss of heterozygosity at 11p11.5. Alveolar rhabdomyosarcomas (20%) are characterized by a t(2;13), which fuses the *PAX3* gene to the *FKHR* gene, or (rarely) a t(1;13), which fuses the *PAX7* gene to *FKHR*.[8-12] Within histologic groups, patients with tumors that are more advanced at diagnosis fare less well than do those with localized, completely resected tumors (group I) or those with microscopic residual tumor only (group II) (Table 11–1).[5,7,13] Also, patients within the same clinical group may fare very differently depend-

Table 11-1. IRS clinical grouping for rhabdomyosarcoma

Group I: *Localized disease, completely resected*
(Regional nodes not involved—lymph node biopsy or dissection is required except for the head and neck lesions)
- (a) Confined to muscle or organ of origin
- (b) Contiguous involvement—infiltration outside the muscle or organ of origin, as through fascial planes. *Notation:* This includes both gross inspection and *microscopic confirmation of complete resection.* Any nodes that may be inadvertently taken with the specimen must be negative. If the latter should be involved microscopically, then the patient is placed in Group IIb or IIc (see below).

Group II: *Total gross resection with evidence of regional spread*
- (a) Grossly resected tumor with microscopic residual disease.
(Surgeon believes that he has removed all of the tumor, but the pathologist finds tumor at the margin of resection *and* additional resection to achieve clean margin is not feasible.) *No evidence of regional node involvement.* Once radiotherapy and/or chemotherapy have been started, re-exploration and removal of the area of microscopic residual does not change the patient's group.
- (b) Regional disease with involved nodes, completely resected with no microscopic residual.
Notation: Complete resection with microscopic confirmation of no residual disease makes this different from Groups IIa and IIc. Additionally, in contrast to Group IIa, regional nodes (which are completely resected, however) are involved, but the most distal node is histologically negative.
- (c) Regional disease with involved nodes, grossly resected, but with evidence of microscopic residual and/or histologic involvement of the most distal regional node (from the primary site) in the dissection.
Notation: The presence of microscopic residual disease makes this group different from Group IIb, and nodal involvement makes this group different from Group IIa.

Group III: *Incomplete resection with gross residual disease*
- (a) After biopsy only
- (b) After gross or major resection of the primary (>50%)

Group IV: *Distant metastatic disease present at onset*
(Lung, liver, bones, bone marrow, brain, and distant muscle and nodes)
Notation: The above excludes *regional* nodes and adjacent organ infiltration which places the patient in a more favorable grouping (as noted above under Group II).

ing on site or origin of the tumor. For example, virtually all patients with group III (macroscopic residual tumor) tumors arising in the orbit are cured with irradiation and relatively nonintense multiagent chemotherapy. In contrast, patients with group III tumors arising in the retroperitoneum have a much less favorable outcome.[14] Therefore, extent of disease, tumor histology, and site of tumor origin are especially important factors for consideration in determination of choice for therapy and for predicting prognosis.[14]

Accounting for 35% of all cases, the head and neck region is the most common primary anatomic location for pediatric RMS.[5,7,13] (Fig 11-1). The diagnosis and treatment of tumors within this anatomic region require individual discussion because the biology of rhabdomyosarcoma in this site differs from that of other anatomic regions; therefore, issues important for treatment design are especially relevant to this tumor site. For example, patients with relatively advanced tumors of the orbit (group III) are highly curable without extremely intensive chemotherapy, yet issues regarding local therapy and its effects on cosmesis and organ function (eg, vision and hearing) are of special importance for children with tumors arising in this site.[5] It is of interest that RMS arising in the head or neck generally have embryonal histology, contrasting sharply with those arising in the extremities (usually alveolar).[15] Also, metastatic disease is exceedingly rare at

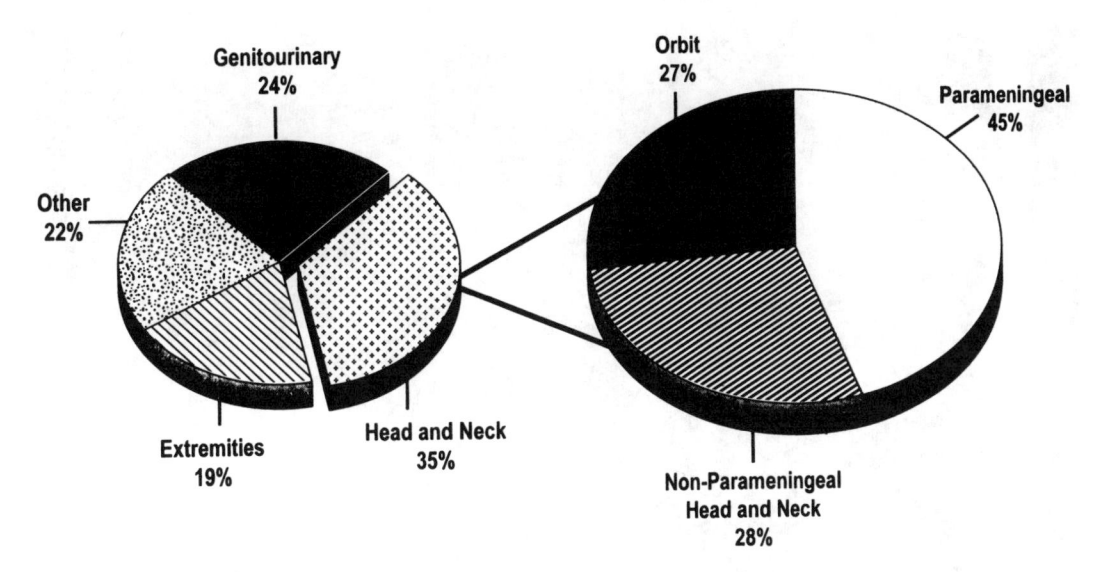

FIG 11-1. Distribution of patients according to primary site in the first, second, and third IRS trials.[5,7,13]

diagnosis in patients with orbital and nonparameningeal head and neck tumors, whereas tumors arising from an extremity or from the trunk are much more frequently metastatic at the time of diagnosis.[5]

Within the head and neck, three distinct regions require separate discussion due to the unique clinical features, widely different prognostic implications, and differences in necessary therapy of the tumors in these regions. We discuss separately the clinical features and therapy of tumors arising in the orbit, parameningeal region (nasopharynx, nasal cavity, paranasal sinus, middle ear, mastoid, pterygoid fossae, and orbit with intracranial tumor or bone destruction), and other nonparameningeal head-neck sites, comparing and contrasting these groups as appropriate.

ORBITAL RHABDOMYOSARCOMA

Clinical Features

Orbital RMS accounts for one fourth of RMS arising in the head and neck and for approximately 9% of all cases of pediatric RMS (Fig 11–1). In a review of 132 patients with localized orbital and eyelid tumors, the median age at diagnosis was 6 years and 84% of these children had embryonal tumors.[16] Because tumors in this site generally cannot be resected without unacceptable cosmetic results, most patients (70%) with orbital RMS present with unresectable disease (clinical group III). Yet, despite the relatively advanced stage at presentation, prognosis for these patients is excellent (~90% of patients with localized disease are cured).[16] Metastatic disease is an uncommon feature at presentation; lymphatic spread at diagnosis is also rare. Patients with orbital tumors are usually diagnosed early in the course of their disease; they commonly present with proptosis or (rarely) with ophthalmoplegia (Fig 11–2). Initial diagnostic investigations should include computed tomography (CT) or magnetic resonance imaging (MRI) of the primary site and cranial contents. The search for distant metastases should include bone marrow examination, CT of the chest, and bone scan. Orbital tumors associated with intracranial extension or bone destruction are considered to be parameningeal in origin. Therefore, cerebrospinal fluid examination should be performed in these children because they are at high risk of intracranial extension, which requires more intensive treatment.

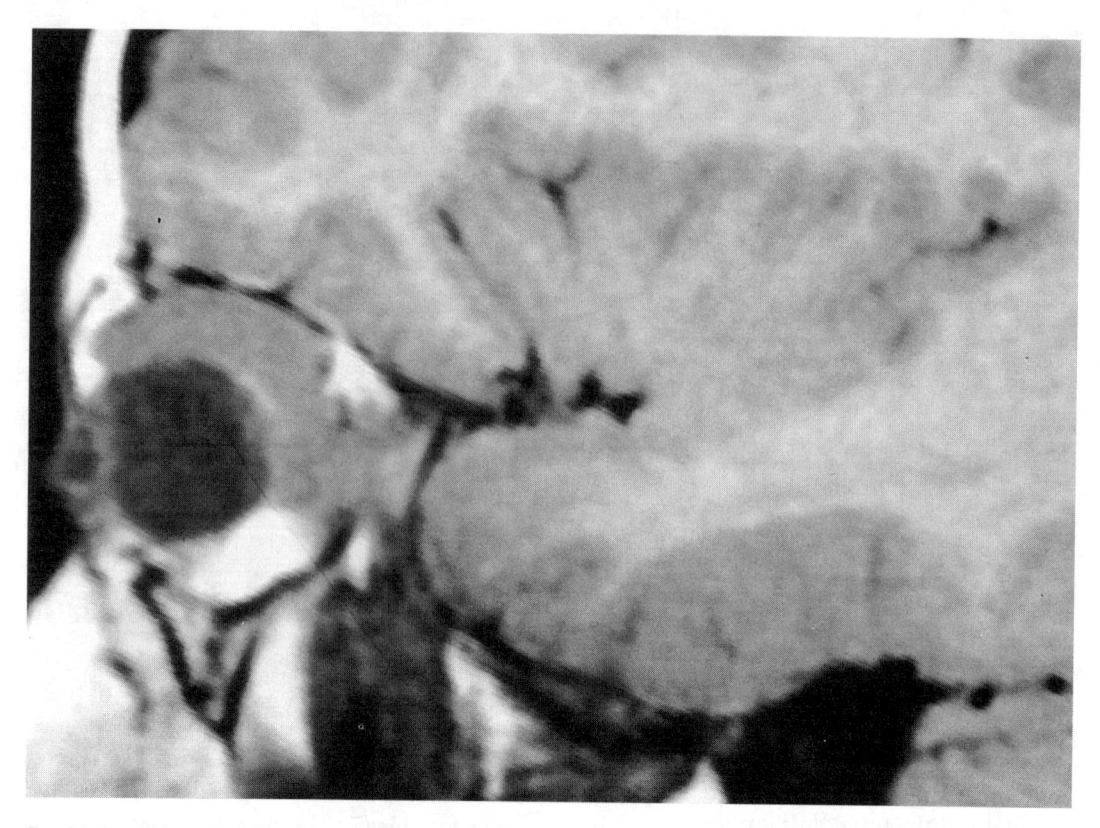

FIG 11–2. This sagittal T$_1$-weighted MR image through the orbit of a 5-year-old girl shows a soft tissue mass (embryonal RMS) arising from the right lacrimal gland that extends pre- and postseptally. The bony orbit and adjacent intracranial structures are intact.

Therapeutic Considerations

The treatment of orbital RMS has changed significantly over the past 30 years. In the 1950s, prognosis for children with this tumor was poor, and orbital exenteration was the only potentially curative procedure employed.[17] In the 1960s, Sagerman and Cassaday documented that radiotherapy could potentially control and cure this tumor without the need for exenteration in a significant number of patients.[18,19] In Sagerman's report, 68% of 31 children survived 2 years after diagnosis and the local tumor control rate was 90%.[18] Demonstration in the 1960s of single-agent chemotherapy (eg, vincristine, dactinomycin, and cyclophosphamide [VAC]) activity against rhabdomyosarcoma led to their combined use in both the adjuvant and neoadjuvant settings.[2,20] During this period, reports by Abramson, Heyn, and Donaldson documented the value of using multiagent chemotherapy with radiotherapy to avoid extensive surgery and to prolong disease-free survival in patients with orbital RMS.[21-23]

Results of the first and second Intergroup Rhabdomyosarcoma Studies showed that patients with orbital RMS could be cured without the need for exenteration and that prognosis was excellent after moderately intensive therapy consisting of VAC ± doxorubicin (ADR) and radiotherapy (Table 11–2).[7,13] The 5-year survival rates for patients in IRS-I and IRS-II were 89% and 93%, respectively.[7,13] The successor study (IRS-III) identified patients with orbital non-alveolar group II or II tumors as a favorable prognostic subgroup; therefore, these patients were spared randomization to the

Table 11-2. Summary of patient groups, therapy, and outcome for children with head and neck rhabdomyosarcoma enrolled in Intergroup Rhabdomyosarcoma Study Group trials[5,14]

	IRS-I (1972–1978)*		IRS-II (1978–1984)†		IRS-III (1984–1991)‡	
	Treatment	5-yr Survival (%)	Treatment	5-yr Survival (%)	Treatment	5-yr Survival (%)
Clinical Group I						
Parameningeal	VAC±RT × 2 yr	100	VA±C × 1–2 yr	—	VA × 1 yr	93§
Orbit	VAC±RT × 2 yr	100	VA±C × 1–2 yr	100		
Other head and neck	VAC±RT × 2 yr	100	VA±C × 1–2 yr	86		
Clinical Group II						
Parameningeal	VA±C+RT × 1–2 yr	70	VA±C+RT × 1 yr	92	VA±ADR+RT × 1 yr	81"
Orbit	VA±C+RT × 1–2 yr	95	VA±C+RT × 1 yr	91	VA+RT × 1 yr	
Other head and neck	VA±C+RT × 1–2 yr	73	VA±C+RT × 1 yr	84	VA+RT × 1 yr	91**
Clinical Group III						
Parameningeal	VAC±ADR+RT × 2 yr	45	VAC±ADR+RT × 2 yr	66	VAC±ADR±VP16/CDDP	74#
Orbit	VAC±ADR+RT × 2 yr	88	VAC±ADR+RT × 2 yr	90	VA+RT × 1 yr	
Other head and neck	VAC±ADR+RT × 2 yr	64	VAC±ADR+RT × 2 yr	76	VA+RT × 1 yr	91**
Clinical Group IV						
Parameningeal	VAC±ADR+RT × 2 yr	11	VAC±ADR+RT × 2 yr	29	VAC±ADR/CDDP±VP16	30&
Orbit	VAC±ADR+RT × 2 yr	50	VAC±ADR+RT × 2 yr	0		
Other head and neck	VAC±ADR+RT × 2 yr	25	VAC±ADR+RT × 2 yr	40		
Overall Results						
Parameningeal		47		69		74
Orbit		89		92		95
Other head and neck		55		81		78

V vincristine; A, dactinomycin; C, cyclophosphamide; ADR, doxorubicin; CDDP, cisplatin; VP16, etoposide; RT, radiotherapy.
* All patients were randomized by Clinical Group only; prognostically important subgroups were not recognized until IRS-II and IRS-III.
§ Overall results for all patients with Clinical Group I favorable histology enrolled in IRS-III.
** Overall results for all patients with Clinical Groups II and III head and orbital sites enrolled in IRS-III. Patients with neck primaries were treated more intensively with VAC±ADR/CDDP±VP16.
# Overall results for all patients with parameningeal tumors enrolled in IRS-III (80% of patients had Clinical Group III disease).
& Overall results for all patients with parameningeal tumors enrolled in IRS-III.
" Overall results for all Clinical Group II patients enrolled in IRS-III.
† Radiotherapy for patients with parameningeal tumors at increased risk for meningeal relapse included the whole brain and spinal axis in combination with triple intrathecal chemotherapy.
‡ Whole brain radiotherapy was avoided in patients with limited intracranial extension (base of skull erosion, cranial nerve palsy) in IRS-III but triple intrathecal therapy was routinely give to these patients.

intensive and more toxic therapy that was used for patients with other group III tumors.[5] Patients with orbital nonalveolar tumors received less intensive therapy consisting of vincristine and dactinomycin for 1 year and local radiotherapy (45 Gy). Results from this trial showed that omission of cyclophosphamide did not appear to compromise treatment outcome (5-year survival, 91%).

However, a report from the IRS-IV suggests that failure-free survival is significantly lower with less intense therapy compared to more intensive approaches (ie, three-drug combinations and higher doses of radiation). The failure-free survival at 3 years in this preliminary report from IRS-IV was 100% for such patients compared to 83% in IRS-III ($p = 0.0096$).[24] Survival is not worse at the present time because some patients who fail therapy are rescued with retrieval regimens. Until further data are collected and longer follow-up is available, we recommend that children with localized unresectable nonalveolar orbital rhabdomyosarcoma be treated with at least two drugs (vincristine and dactinomycin) for 1 one year in combination with local radiotherapy.

Treatment approaches for orbital RMS have varied in other multi-institutional studies. For example, French investigators use a primary chemotherapy approach for these patients, reserving radiotherapy and surgery for patients who fail to achieve a complete response to chemotherapy. In a report from the Malignant Mesenchymal Study 84, 31 patients with nonmetastatic mesenchymal tumors of the orbit and eyelid were treated with an ifosfamide-based regimen.[25] Twenty-two patients were initially treated with chemotherapy alone, and 9 received combination therapy with chemotherapy and radiation. The local control rate for the entire cohort was 62% ± 9%. Eleven local recurrences were observed; 10 of these were among children who were treated without local irradiation. However, 9 of 11 patients achieved a second remission following additional therapy including irradiation or surgery; 2 of these 9 children failed locally a second time. Survival after primary chemotherapy, however, does not seem to be compromised because 4-year actuarial survival is 86% ± 7%, a result similar to that reported from the IRS trials. Nevertheless, despite the fact that nearly 40% of the children in this study were spared local therapy with radiation or surgery, longer follow-up is needed prior to recommending this approach outside a study setting.

PARAMENINGEAL RHABDOMYOSARCOMA

Clinical Features

Parameningeal RMS accounts for 16% of all cases of RMS and is the most common anatomic location of disease in the head and neck region (Fig 11–1). Within the parameningeal region, the most common primary sites include the nasopharynx, the middle ear-mastoid area, and the paranasal sinuses. In a review of 230 patients with parameningeal RMS who were treated in four major cooperative studies over a 10-year period, the median age at diagnosis was 6 years, with a male predominance.[26] Nearly 70% of these tumors are of embryonal histology and 69% of the patients have high-risk features (ie, clinical or radiologic evidence of intracranial extension, cranial nerve palsy, or base of skull erosion).[26] In this review, the tumor extended beyond the tissue of origin in more than 90% of cases and 40% of patients had tumors larger than 5 cm. Lymphatic involvement was reported in 17%.

Tumors in the parameningeal region commonly produce nasal or sinus obstruction with discharge, which may be sanguinous or mucopurulent. Cranial nerve palsy, which usually involves the sixth, seventh, or eighth nerve, may be present at diagnosis. Headaches, vomiting, and/or hypertension may result from intracranial extension.[27] Extension of tumor into the maxillary sinuses can cause swelling of the cheek and loss of sensation in the lips due to invasion of the trigeminal nerve. Tumor extension into the orbit can cause exophthalmos and strabismus, whereas inferior extension of the tumor can lead to submucous swelling in the palate and gingival spaces.[27] Tumors in the pterygomaxillary space can remain asymptomatic for long periods of time and may manifest as trismus or pain and altered sensation in the region served by the trigeminal nerve.[27] Initial workup for patients with nonorbital parameningeal RMS should include cranial CT and/or MRI of the face and brain (Fig 11–3) to evaluate location and extent of the primary tumor and to determine if there is intracranial extension and/or base of the skull erosion. Cytology of the cerebrospinal fluid is recommended for patients at high risk for intracranial extension. The workup for metastases should include imaging of lungs and bones as well as bone marrow aspirate and biopsy.

Therapeutic Considerations

Because the majority of patients with parameningeal tumors have unresectable disease at time of presentation, the role of surgery in this neoplasm is usually limited to obtaining adequate tissue for histologic analysis. Local control measures include administration of radiotherapy with adequate meningeal and tumor margins. Multiagent chemotherapy is routinely used to eradicate micrometastases. The treatment of parameningeal RMS has changed significantly over the past quarter century. Children with parameningeal tumors in the first IRS study were treated with chemotherapy consisting of VAC or VADRC; they also received local radiotherapy, which included the primary tumor volume and a 2-cm tumor margin beginning at week 6 of therapy.[7] Preliminary analysis from this study revealed that 20 of 57 patients (35%) with parameningeal tumors developed evidence of direct meningeal extension either at diagnosis or within the first 12 months of initiating therapy.[28] Ninety percent of these patients died as a consequence of this complication.

Patient characteristics associated with a high risk of direct meningeal involvement included erosion of the base of the skull, cranial nerve palsy, and intracranial extension in contiguity with the primary tumor (Fig 11–3). Detailed analysis of these patients revealed that 42% of them received lower doses of radiotherapy than prescribed by protocol. In

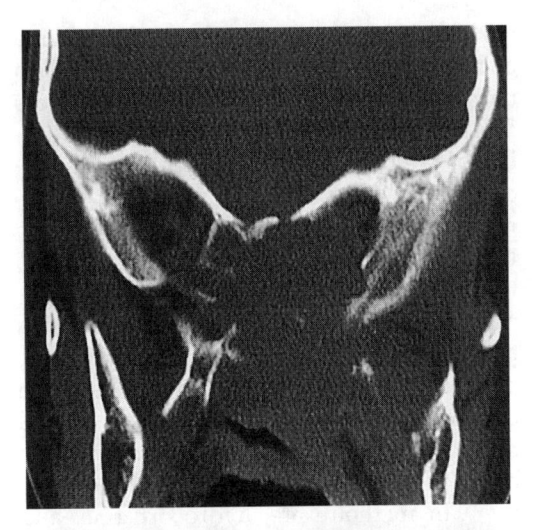

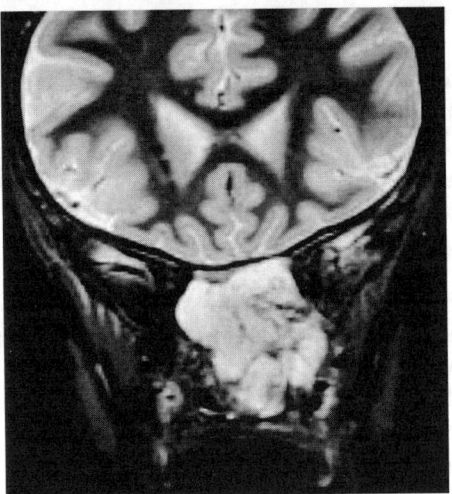

FIG 11–3. *Top*: This coronal CT (filmed with bone windows) through the midface of a 6-year-old girl with nasopharyngeal RMS demonstrates extensive bony erosion by the large, predominantly left-sided mass arising from the posterior nasopharynx. There is invasion of the left maxillary sinus, the left orbit, cribriform plate of the ethmoid sinus, and the body of the sphenoid bone. *Bottom*: However, coronal T_2-weighted MR image through the same level shows the dura to be intact and the adjacent frontal lobes to be uninvolved.

addition, in 58% of the patients, the volume of tumor that was irradiated was too small to encompass all sites of primary disease. These findings suggest that dose, volume, and timing of radiotherapy can adversely influence clinical outcome in these patients. For this reason, the protocol was modified in 1977 to include radiation therapy starting at day 0 to the entire cranial neuraxis as well as the primary tumor for patients who presented with these high-risk features.[29] In addition, patients at extraordinary risk (ie, those with bony erosion at the base of the skull, cranial nerve palsies, or direct extention into the brain) also received intrathecal chemotherapy with methotrexate, hydrocortisone, and cytarabine for 18 to 24 months. The prescribed meningeal dose was 30 Gy for children at least 5 years of age (24 Gy for those younger than 5 years), with a boost of 20–25 Gy to the primary tumor. Analysis of 68 patients treated in this manner revealed significant improvements in 3-year disease-free survival and survival compared to children treated before 1977 (57% vs 33% and 68% vs 41%, respectively).[29] In addition, the incidence of meningeal relapse decreased significantly from 28% to 6%.

In an attempt to limit the amount of radiotherapy, patients with base of skull erosion and cranial nerve palsy but without evidence of intracranial extension were spared the use of whole brain radiotherapy in the IRS-III trial. Radiotherapy for these patients also began at day 0 and doses ranged from 40–55 Gy, depending on the age of the patient. The irradiated volume consisted of the primary tumor with a 5-cm margin, including a 2-cm margin of adjacent meninges. The 5-year progression-free survival in IRS-III was 69% compared to 61% in IRS-II, suggesting that this treatment modification did not compromise outcome.[30] A similar conclusion was reached by Italian investigators who treated patients with parameningeal RMS who had high-risk features with systemic chemotherapy, intrathecal chemotherapy, and limited volume radiation.[31] This approach was successful in preventing meningeal extension of tumor. In IRS-IV, the use of intrathecal therapy has been reserved for patients who have positive cerebrospinal fluid cytology, whereas whole brain radiotherapy is limited to patients who have multiple sites of parenchymal brain disease.

Chemotherapy for parameningeal RMS is intended to decrease the incidence of distant metastatic disease and, perhaps, improve local control. In the third IRS trial, addition of agents such as doxorubicin, cisplatin, and etoposide to standard VAC chemotherapy failed to improve progression-free survival or survival for patients with unresected tumors.[5] However, overall survival at 5 years was 74%.[26] The 5-year survival rate was significantly better for patients who presented with low- vs high-risk features (97% ± 3% vs 61% ± 7%).[26] The most frequent type of relapse was local failure (65%); in eight patients, the tumor recurred in-field, and 3 cases were considered to be marginal failures.

Results from the third IRS study are superior to those reported by other large cooperative trials. Reasons for these improved results may include relatively fewer patients with large tumors (51%) and a lower percentage of patients with lymphatic involvement.[26] However, it is likely that differences in treatment philosophies may have influenced clinical outcome. For example, investigators from the International Society of Pediatric Oncology (SIOP) used a primary chemotherapeutic approach with an ifosfamide-based regimen followed by second line chemotherapy with doxorubicin and cisplatin. Radiotherapy comprised a relatively small volume (1-cm margin), and doses ranged from 45–46 Gy.[26] In addition, radiotherapy was routinely administered only to patients older than 5 years who had high-risk features. These differences in treatment philosophy are important because 95% of relapses in this study were local. Further, one third of patients did not receive initial radiotherapy and one third of local relapses in irradiated patients were considered to be marginal failures, suggesting that the irradiated volume was too small.[26] Despite the high incidence of local recurrence in this study, the 5-year survival rate was similar for irradiated and unirradiated patients. German investigators used a VAC-VADRC regimen with routine administration of radiotherapy to all patients. However, radiotherapy was delayed until day 42 or day 90 in high-risk or low-risk patients, respectively.[26] Delaying radiotherapy might permit tumors to become therapy-resistant, and quality control (ie, central review) for radiotherapy was applied only in the IRS trials.

In summary, it is recommended that all children with parameningeal tumors receive local radiotherapy and systemic chemotherapy. In low-risk patients, radiotherapy can be safely delayed until week 6 or 9 of therapy. The radiation volume should encompass the primary tumor with a 2-cm margin, and the minimal tumor dose should be 50 Gy. For high-risk patients, wider tumor margins and early initiation of radiotherapy should be strongly considered. To further improve outcome for patients with parameningeal tumors, hyperfractionation of radiotherapy and optimization of chemotherapy should be explored.

NONPARAMENINGEAL HEAD AND NECK RHABDOMYOSARCOMA

Clinical Features

This anatomic designation comprises tumors that arise in the oral cavity, larynx, parotid gland, cheek, scalp, and soft tissues of the neck.[32] Approximately 10% of all RMS arise in this anatomic region and approximately 28% of head and neck RMS are located in the nonorbital nonparameningeal head and neck area (see Fig 11–1). In a review of 74 patients with head and neck[32] RMS who were treated on the first IRS trial, the median age at diagnosis was 7.5 years and no sex predominance was noted. Two thirds of the patients had tumors with embryonal histology, and 18% had pathologically proven loco-regional nodal involvement. The most common anatomic locations within the nonparameningeal region included the soft tissues of the neck followed by the parotid and cheek area and the oral cavity (Fig 11–4). Nearly half of all patients present with grossly or completely resected disease, while 45% have unresectable disease at diagnosis. Tumors confined to superficial sites such as the scalp and cheek are more often completely resected, whereas tumors in the oral cavity, parotid gland, and oropharynx more often present with unresectable disease. There is a higher incidence of alveolar histology in tumors of the scalp and cheek (46%) when compared to tumors arising in the oropharynx and parotid (6%). Tumors in this anatomic location usually present as a painless enlarging mass that tends to remain localized; metastatic disease at diagnosis is seen in fewer than 10% of patients with nonparameningeal tumors.

Assessment of extent of disease at diagnosis should include CT or MRI of the primary tumor and chest and a search for metastatic disease in bone and bone marrow as well. Particular attention should be paid to the regional lymph nodes to ascertain whether the tumor is metastatic or is arising primary in the head or neck. In addition, extension of tumor into the parameningeal area should alert the physician to treat patients with therapy designed for patients with parameningeal primary tumors.

Therapeutic Considerations

Therapy for nonparameningeal head tumors is similar to that for patients with orbital tumors. In the first two IRS trials, patients with orofacial and laryngopharyngeal RMS had a 3-year survival rate of 83%. Therapy for these patients was assigned according to Clinical Group and consisted of chemotherapy with vincristine and dactinomycin ± cyclophosphamide ± doxorubicin. Local radiotherapy was added for patients with groups II and III disease (Table 11–2). In the IRS-III study, patients with Groups II or III nonparameningeal orbital and head tumors were treated with vincristine and dactinomycin for 1 year and local radiotherapy. At 5

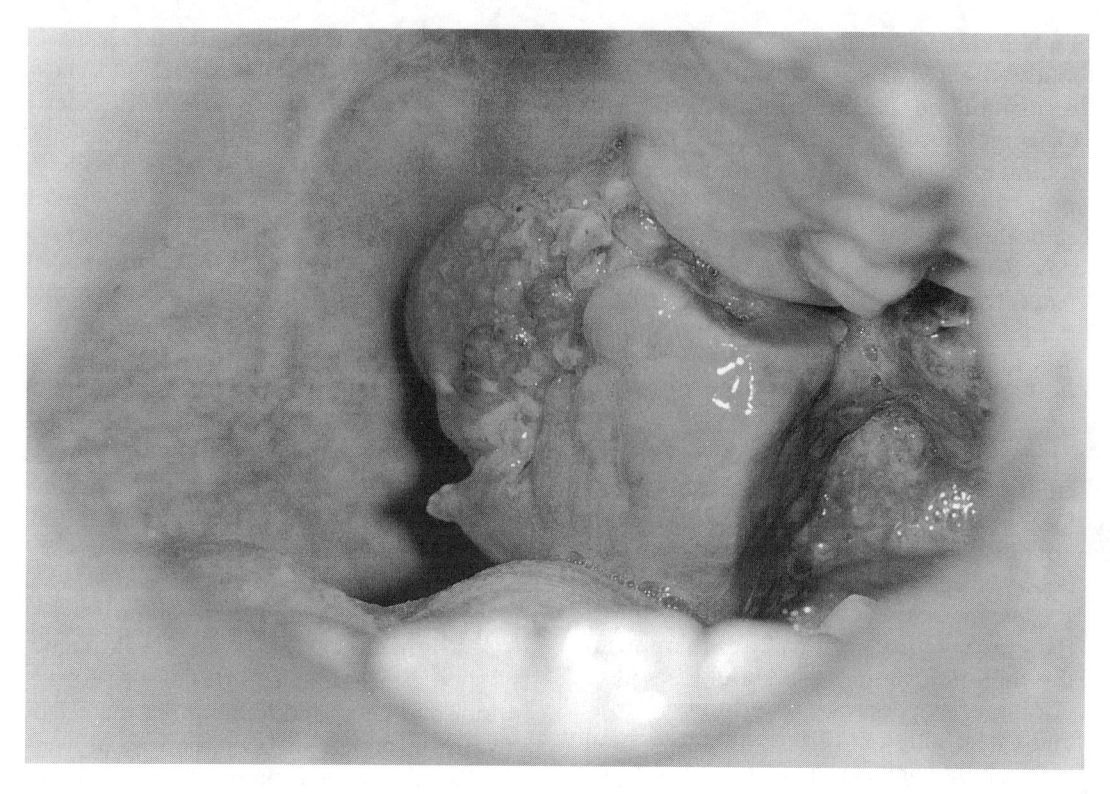

FIG 11–4. Anterosuperior view with opened mouth of an 11-year-old boy with an alveolar RMS of the left alveolar ridge.

years, progression-free survival and survival for these patients was 78% ± 4% and 91% ± 3%, respectively, compared to 85% ± 4% and 91 ± 3% in IRS-II, which used a more intensive treatment regimen. Therefore, limiting therapy to two drugs without compromising survival is feasible in patients with nonparameningeal head tumors.

Compared to patients with head tumors, patients whose primary disease arises in the neck have a worse prognosis (54% relapse-free at 3 years in the first IRS trial). Therefore, these patients have been treated more intensively in subsequent IRS trials (see Table 11–2). In the third Intergroup Trial, patients with unresected (group III) neck primaries were randomized to the same intensive treatment as other patients with group III tumors (ie, VAC ± doxorubicin, cisplatin, and etoposide, and local radiotherapy). The two more intensive regimens did not improve outcome for children in this category with group III disease (overall 5-year progression-free survival and survival rates, 65% ± 3% and 65% ± 3%, respectively).

ACUTE AND DELAYED EFFECTS OF THERAPY

Because multimodal therapy has clearly improved survival for patients with head and neck RMS, late complications related to therapy have become apparent. In addition, acute side effects have become more marked as more intensive therapy has been used to boost cure rates for patients with advanced disease (ie, group III, unfavorable site and group IV). Acute and late effects of therapy are reviewed below according to tumor site within the head and neck.

Acute Complications

The toxic death rate in patients treated in IRS studies have been as high as 12% for certain regimens.[5] The causes of death have included sepsis during episodes of myelosuppression, cardiac complications, metabolic derangements, and hemorrhage secondary to thrombocytopenia. The incorporation of ifosfamide-based regimens into the frontline treatment of RMS has been associated with a 14% incidence of renal toxicity including overt Fanconi's syndrome.[33] Factors that contribute to the development of this complication include hydronephrosis, age younger than 3 years, and doses of ifosfamide >72 g/m^2.[33]

Severe mucositis has been a common complication in patients with parameningeal RMS. It is especially severe after concomitant radiation and chemotherapy. Many of these patients require placement of gastrostomy tubes while receiving therapy in order to ensure appropriate caloric intake.[34]

Delayed Effects

Among 162 patients with head and neck RMS who were treated on the IRS-II and IRS-III trials and survived more than 5 years after diagnosis, 20% were receiving growth hormone therapy. Cataracts were documented in 16 patients, and hearing impairment was found in 50% of those who were tested. Asymmetry or hypoplasia of the irradiated body part, sometimes requiring reconstructive surgery, was seen in 30% of children and 40% had dental malformations.[35]

Second malignant neoplasms are uncommon events following successful therapy of RMS, but they have been documented in 22 of 1770 patients enrolled in IRS-trials.[36] Bone sarcomas followed by acute nonlymphoblastic leukemia were the most common malignancies. Treatment-related secondary myeloid leukemia has been reported in patients who received epipodophyllotoxin and/or alkylating agent-containing regimens.

For patients with orbit RMS, a review from the first IRS study revealed that decreased or absent vision was documented in 89% of survivors. Keratoconjunctivitis, photophobia, and conjunctivitis were evident in about one third of patients. Cataract formation was seen in 90%, bony hypoplasia in 60%, and decrease in statural growth in 61% of patients.[37]

Patients with parameningeal primaries have a high prevalence of hypothalamic-pituitary dysfunction. It is characterized by decreased statural growth, thyroid dysfunction, and elevated basal FSH and LH levels. Ascending transverse myelitis was observed in 3% of patients over a 10-year period. It was characterized by flaccid quadriparesis at a high cervical or thoracic level. This complication is no longer observed because the number of intrathecal injections has been decreased to four in more recent IRS trials.[34]

Nonorbital head and neck rhabdomyosarcomas are associated with a high incidence of dental malformations, caries formation, and endocrine sequelae.[34]

FUTURE DIRECTIONS

Improvements in risk-based, multimodal therapy have substantially increased cure rates for patients with head and neck RMS over the past 25 years (Fig 11–5). Acute and late effects of therapy remain a serious concern for many patients and 20% to 30% of patients continue to die from recurrent tumor. Therefore, more effective and safer therapy is needed for many patients. The use of hyperfractionated irradiation and conformal radiotherapy is being explored in an attempt to improve local control while reducing the morbidity of therapy.[5,38] Reductions in the dose of radiation are also being considered for patients with tumors in selected favorable primary sites such as the orbit. Avoidance of external beam radiotherapy by combining surgery and brachytherapy has been recently explored in a limited number of patients.[39] Advances and refinements in microsurgical techniques and craniofacial sur-

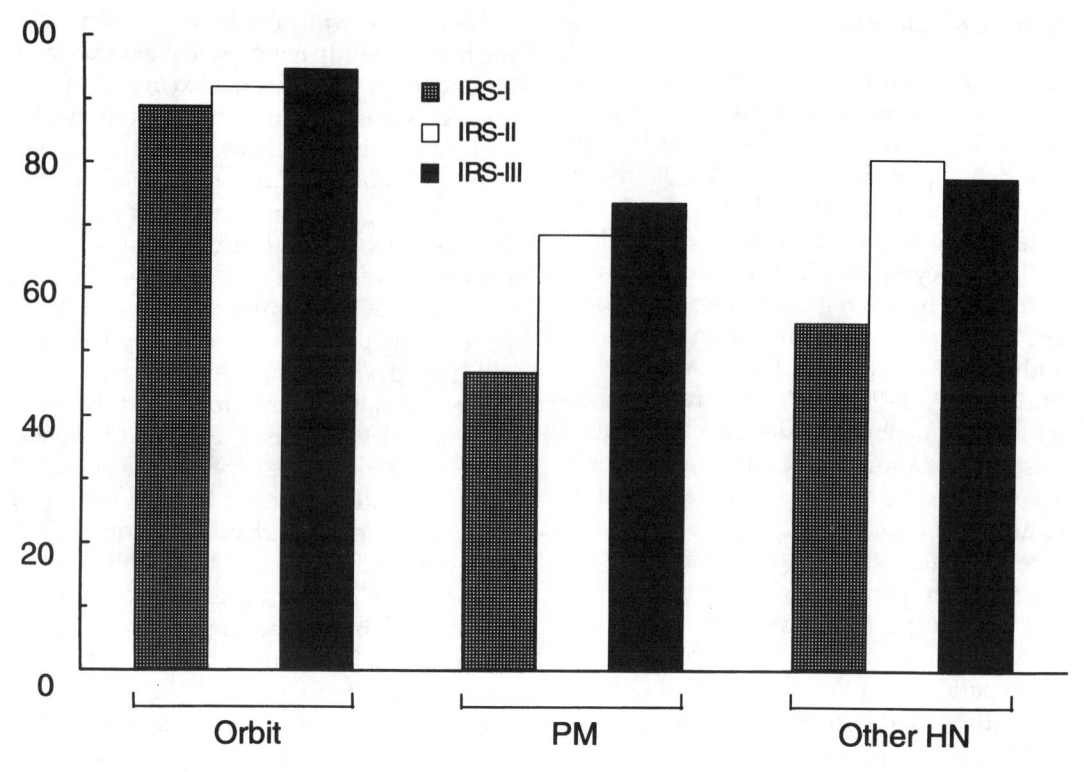

FIG 11–5. Comparison of 5-year survival estimates for patients with orbital, parameningeal (PM), and nonorbital nonparameningeal head and neck tumors (other HN) who were enrolled in three consecutive IRS studies (IRS-I–IRS-III).[5,7,13]

gery may allow increased use of second-look surgeries in selected patients who achieve a very good response to initial chemotherapy.[40] New agents are being evaluated in an effort to develop more effective and less toxic combination chemotherapy.[41,42] Hemopoietic growth factors are being used to diminish myelosuppresison and serious infections and to permit use of increased dose intensity.[43] Finally, the recent identification of some of the genes that are involved in tumorigenesis holds promise for development of new relatively tumor-specific therapies (eg, ribozymes and antisense oligonucleotides to tumor RNA).

ACKNOWLEDGMENTS

We wish to thank Amy Frazier for editorial assistance.

Supported in part by grants CA-23099 and CA-21765 from the National Cancer Institute, Bethesda, Maryland, and by the American Lebanese Syrian Associated Charities (ALSAC), Memphis, Tennessee.

REFERENCES

1. Pappo AS, Shapiro DN, Crist WM, Maurer HM. Biology and therapy of pediatric rhabdomyosarcoma. *J Clin Oncol.* 1995;13: 2123–2139.
2. Pratt CB, Hustu HO, Fleming ID, Pinkel D. Coordinated treatment of childhood rhabdomyosarcoma with surgery, radiotherapy, and combination chemotherapy. *Cancer Res.* 1972;32:606–610.
3. Lawrence W, Jegge G, Foote F. Embryonal rhabdomyosarcoma. *Cancer.* 1964;17:361–376.
4. Pinkel D, Pickren J. Rhabdomyosarcoma in children. *JAMA.* 1961;175:293–298.

5. Crist W, Gehan EA, Ragab AH, et al. The Third Intergroup Rhabdomyosarcoma Study. *J Clin Oncol.* 1995;13:610–630.
6. Crist WM, Kun LE. Common solid tumors of childhood. *N Engl J Med.* 1991;324:461–471.
7. Maurer HM, Beltangady M, Gehan EA, et al. The Intergroup Rhabdomyosarcoma Study—I. *Cancer.* 1988;61:209–220.
8. Shapiro DN, Sublett JE, Li B, et al. Fusion of PAX3 to a member of the forkhead family of transcription factors in human alveolar rhabdomyosarcoma. *Cancer Res.* 1993;53:5108–5012.
9. Davis RJ, D'Cruz CM, Lovell MA, et al. Fusion of PAX7 to FKHR by the variant t(1;13) (p36;q14) translocation in alveolar rhabdomyosarcoma. *Cancer Res.* 1994:54:2869–2872.
10. Scrable H, Witte D, Shimada H, et al. Molecular differential pathology of rhabdomyosarcoma. *Genes Chromosom Cancer.* 1989;1:23–25.
11. Horn RC, Enterline HT. Rhabdomyosarcoma: a clinicopathological study and classification of 39 cases. *Cancer.* 1958;11:181–191.
12. Newton WA, Jr, Soule EH, Hamoudi AB, et al. Histopathology of childhood sarcomas, Intergroup Rhabdomyosarcoma Studies I and II: clinicopathologic correlation. *J Clin Oncol.* 199;6:67–75.
13. Maurer HM, Gehan EA, Beltangady M, et al. The Intergroup Rhabdomyosarcoma Study—II. *Cancer.* 1993;71:1904–1922.
14. Crist WM, Garnsey L, Beltangady MS, et al. Prognosis in children with rhabdomyosarcoma: a report of the Intergroup Rhabdomyosarcoma Studies I and II. *J Clin Oncol.* 1990;8:443–452.
15. Andrassy RJ, Corpron CA, Hays D, et al. Extremity sarcomas: an analysis of prognostic factors from the Intergroup Rhabdomyosarcoma Study III. *J Pediatr Surg.* 1996;31:191–196.
16. Wharam M, Beltangady M, Hays D, et al. Localized orbital rhabdomyosarcoma. *Ophthalmology.* 1987;94:251–254.
17. Porterfield J, Zimmerman L. Rhabdomyosarcoma of the orbit: a clinicopathologic study of 55 cases. *Virchow's Arch.* 1962;335:329–344.
18. Sagerman RH, Tetter P, Ellsworth RM. Orbital rhabdomyosarcoma in children. *Trans Am Acad Ophthalmol Otolaryngol.* 1974; 78: 602–605.
19. Cassady Jr, Sagerman R, Tretter P, Ellsworth R. Radiation therapy for rhabdomyosarcoma. *Radiology.* 1968;90:116–120.
20. Wilbur J. Combination chemotherapy for embryonal rhabdomyosarcoma. *Cancer Chemother Rep.* 1974;58:281–284.
21. Donaldson SS, Castro JR, Wilbur JR, Jesse RH Jr. Rhabdomyosarcoma of head and neck in children. Combination treatment by surgery, irradiation, and chemotherapy. *Cancer.* 1973; 31:26–35.
22. Heyn R, Holland R, Newton WJ, Tefft M, Breslow M, Hartmann J. The role of combined modality therapy in the treatment of rhabdomyosarcoma in children. *Cancer.* 1974;34: 2128–2142.
23. Abramson DH, Ellsworth RM, Tretter P, et al. The treatment of orbital rhabdomyosarcoma with irradiation and chemotherapy. *Ophthalmology.* 1979;86:1330–1335.
24. Wharam MD, Anderson JR, Laurie F, Glicksman AS, Maurer HM. Failure-free survival for orbit rhabdomyosarcoma patients on Intergroup Rhabdomyosarcoma Study IV (IRS-IV) is improved compared to IRS-III. *Proc Am Soc Clin Oncol.* 1997;16:518a. Abstract 1864.
25. Rousseau P, Flamant F, Quintana E, Voute PA, Gentet JC. Primary chemotherapy in rhabdomyosarcomas and other malignant mesenchymal tumors of the orbit: results of the International Society of Pediatric Oncology MMT 84 study. *J Clin Oncol.* 1994;12:516–521.
26. Benk V, Rodary C, Donaldson SS, et al. Parameningeal rhabdomyosarcoma: results of an international workshop. *Int J Radiat Oncol Biol Phys.* 1996;36:533–540.
27. Flamant F, Luboinski B, Couanet D, McDowell H. Rhabdomyosarcoma in children: clinical symptoms, diagnosis, and staging. In: Maurer HM, Ruymann FB, Pochedly C, eds. *Rhabdomyosarcoma and Related Tumors in Children and Adolescents.* Boca Raton, Fla: CRC Publications; 1991:91–124.
28. Tefft M, Fernandez C, Donaldson M, Newton W, Moon T. Incidence of meningeal involvement by rhabdomyosarcoma of the head and neck in children: a report of the Intergroup Rhabdomyosarcoma study (IRS). *Cancer.* 1978;42:253–258.
29. Raney RB Jr, Tefft M, Newton WA, et al. Improved prognosis with intensive treatment of children with cranial soft tissue sarcomas arising in nonorbital parameningeal sites. A report from the Intergroup Rhabdomyosarcoma Study. *Cancer.* 1987;59: 147–55.
30. Ortega J, Fryer C, Gehan E, et al. Efficacy of reducing tissue volume irradiation in children with cranial (CR) parameningeal (PM) rhabdomyosarcoma (RMS). A report for the Intergroup Rhabdomyosarcoma Study (IRS)

III. *Proc Am Soc Clin Oncol.* 1990;9:296. Abstract 114.
31. Gasparini M, Lombardi F, Gianni M, Massimino M, Gandola L, Fossati-Bellani F. Questionable role of CNS radioprophylaxis in the therapeutic management of childhood rhabdomyosarcoma with meningeal extension. *J Clin Oncol.* 1990;8:1854–1857.
32. Wharam MD Jr, Foulkes MA, Lawrence W Jr, et al. Soft tissue sarcoma of the head and neck in childhood: nonorbital and nonparameningeal sites. *Cancer.* 1984;53:1016–1019.
33. Raney B, Ensign L, Foreman J, et al. Renal toxicity of ifosfamide in pilot regimens of the Intergroup Rhabdomyosarcoma Study for patients with gross residual tumor. *Am J Pediatr Hematol Oncol.* 1994;16:286–295.
34. Raney RB Jr. Rhabdomyosarcoma and related tumors of the head and neck in childhood. In: Maurer HM, Ruymann FB, Pochedly C, ed. *Rhabdomyosarcoma and Related tumors in Children and Adolescents.* Boca Raton Fla: CRC Publications; 1991:319–332.
35. Raney R, Asmar L, Vassilopoulou-Sellin R, et al. Late sequelae in 162 patients with non-orbital soft-tissue sarcoma of the head and neck: report from Intergroup rhabdomyosarcoma studies (IRS) II and III. *Proc Am Soc Clin Oncol.* 1995;14:454. Abstract 1459.
36. Wharam MD, Beltangady MS, Heyn RM, et al. Pediatric orofacial and laryngopharyngeal rhabdomyosarcoma. *Arch Otolaryngol Head Neck Surg.* 1987;113:1225–1227.
37. Heyn R, Ragab A, Raney RB Jr, et al. Late effects of therapy in orbital rhabdomyosarcoma in children. A report from the Intergroup Rhabdomyosarcoma Study. *Cancer.* 1986;57: 1738–1743.
38. Donaldson SS, Asmar L, Breneman J, et al. Hyperfractionated radiation in children with rhabdomyosarcoma results of an Intergroup Rhabdomyosarcoma Pilot Study. *Int J Radiation Oncol Biol Phys.* 1995;32:903–911.
39. Schouwenburg P, Voute P, Blank L, Kupperman D, BeBoer J. Local treatment with ablative surgery, moulage and reconstructive surgery, "the amore protocol." *Med Pediatr Oncol.* 1994;23:188. Abstract 0–76.
40. Posnick J, Polley J, Zuker R, Chan H. Chemotherapy and surgical resection combined with immediate reconstruction in a 1-year old child with rhabdomyosarcoma of the maxilla. *Plast Reconstr Surg.* 1992;89:320–325.
41. Houghton P, Shapiro D, Houghton J. Rhabdomyosarcoma: from the laboratory to the clinic. *Pediatr Clin North Am.* 1991;38:349–364.
42. Houghton P, Chesire P, Myers L, Stewart C, Synold T, Houghton J. Evaluation of 9-dimethyaminomethyl-10-hydroxycamptothecin against xenografts derived from adult and childhood solid tumors. *Cancer Chemother Pharmacol.* 1992;31:229–239.
43. Ruymann FB, Vietti T, Gehan E, et al. Cyclophosphamide dose escalation in combination with vincristine and actinomycin-D (VAC) in gross residual sarcoma. A pilot study without hematopoietic growth factor support evaluating toxicity and response. *J Pediatr Hematol Oncol.* 1995;17:331–337.

CHAPTER 12

State of the Art Techniques for Mandibular Reconstruction

Wayne B. Colin, DMD, MD, and Bruce H. Haughey, MB, ChB, FRACS, FACS

The continuity defect of the mandible has long been a challenge to the reconstructive surgeon. The etiology of the defect may be a planned part of a resection for a neoplasm, infection, or osteonecrosis or present as a congenital defect or gunshot wound. No matter what the cause, the goals and principles of reconstruction are similar for each mandibular defect, in an attempt to return a patient to his or her premorbid state of oromandibular function. Although the currently preferred technique for repairing the discontinuous jaw defect is the osseous microvascular free tissue transfer, other options can be considered in a stepwise approach to mandibular reconstruction. The mandible contributes to multiple functions of the upper aerodigestive tract including respiration, swallowing, speech, mastication, oral sphincter competence, and cosmesis. It also supports the muscles of the oral cavity, pharynx, and neck so that acute loss of the upper airway may result from certain mandible fractures. Chronic compromise of the upper airway may be precipitated by mandibular osteotomy[1] or segmental resection without reconstruction[2] resulting in sleep apnea.

MANDIBULAR ANATOMY

Several unique anatomical features of the mandible must be considered in the reconstruction of the continuity defect: the temporo-mandibular joint (TMJ), teeth, occlusion, and inferior alveolar nerve (IAN). The jaw articulates with the skull base on paired condyles attached in tandem by the mandibular arch, all of which support dental occlusion. The loss of a condyle or an entire joint will result in both a cosmetic and functional deformity. The jaw and chin will deviate to the affected side, and an open bite or crossbite malocclusion may be seen on the contralateral side with anticipated poor mastication. Subsequent scarring in the wound bed may cause trismus. As a result of the deviation and decreased range of motion, arthralgia of the contralateral joint may occur.

Teeth expose the supporting bone to the constant threat of oral bacterial invasion by breaching the oral mucous membrane. Periodontal and apical dental infections are in direct contact with the mandibular alveolar bone and may predispose patients to more generalized gnathic infections. The eradication of infected dental tissues prior to or concurrent with a segmental mandibular reconstruction is important to prevent contamination of a bone graft and supporting hardware.

The mandible contains the IAN which provides sensation to the lower lip and chin. Loss of sensation may produce inadvertent lip biting, drooling, scalding of tissues on hot food, and real or perceived deficits of speech. The total intraosseous course of the IAN is 8 cm with a proximal entrance at the mandibular foramen and a distal exit at the mental foramen.[3] Planning of a mandibular osteotomy site for tumor access, proximal or distal to the nerve foramina, will spare sensation to the lip and chin, by not traversing the nerve trunk.[4]

CONTINUITY DEFECTS OF THE MANDIBLE

Characteristic patterns of anatomical and functional deformity are associated with unrepaired or poorly reconstructed mandibulectomy defects. For the purposes of discussion, mandibulectomy defects can be summarized into essentially three types: anterior-symphyseal, lateral-body, and ramus/condyle.[5] Combined, subtotal, and rarely total mandibulectomy defects are seen, usually from resections with intrinsic bone malignancy (eg, osteosarcoma). The functional deficits have a clear association with the extent of the soft tissue resection, especially the tongue, although the location and extent of the bony defect will certainly contribute to the problem.[6]

The symphyseal resection produces the so-called "Andy Gump" deformity, named after the comic strip character with no chin. The unrepaired resection shows a patient with an unsupported and anesthetic lip and chin, severe retrogenia, incompetent lips, and malocclusion. Functional problems may include drooling, speech deficits, impaired deglutition, and possible respiratory compromise due to loss of the genial tubercle, which provides anchorage for the origin of the tongue and floor of mouth musculature.

The lateral defect of the body of the jaw is less problematic than the anterior defect. Despite sparing the symphysis, cosmesis of the chin is still affected by drift of the mandible and dentition to the resected side. A hollowed appearance is seen over the mandibulectomy site as the neck and buccal tissues collapse and scar onto the deep tissues. Unless a coronoidectomy is performed, the proximal bone segment bearing the condyle will rotate superiorly and medially by the unopposed tension of the temporalis muscle. Unrecognized, this might cause a functionally disturbing protrusion in the retromolar and tonsillar area. The remaining jaw deviates to the affected side with wide opening of the mouth. This occurs because of separation of the ipsilateral condyle from the remainder of the jaw with loss of force from the lateral pterygoid muscle. Unless repaired, the resected IAN produces anesthesia in the mental and incisive nerve dermatomes. When the IAN is transected or resected with immediate or subsequent reconstruction by primary anastomosis or with an interpositional nerve graft, functional sensation is predictably anticipated.[7]

Defects of the posterior mandible cause loss of height and support around the TMJ. Resection of the posterior ramus, condyle, and meniscus will impart common cosmetic and functional problems. A resection including the condyle (disarticulation) will cause loss of vertical dimension of the posterior mandible resulting in open bite occlusion contralateral to that joint and gradual shift of the jaw to the affected side. Depending on the extent of soft tissue removed from the pterygomandibular region, the inferior alveolar, mylohyoid, and lingual nerves are also at risk in such resections. Loss of the meniscus, along with the condyle, would not change the postablative findings, but would require an awareness for reconstructive treatment planning. Resection of the condyle, meniscus, and glenoid fossa might reveal all of the findings mentioned, with possible exposure of the middle cranial fossa dura.

PRINCIPLES AND TECHNICAL GOALS OF MANDIBULAR RECONSTRUCTION

Mandibular reconstructive surgery endeavors to restore the pretreatment level of function to the patient by recreating the bone structures removed by the ablation. The specific strategies of planning mandibular reconstruction are to:

1. Optimize the patient's medical condition prior to the procedure.
2. Plan and execute an oncologically sound resection with preservation of the TMJ relationships and cranial nerve branches, if appropriate.
3. Close soft tissue deficits of the oral mucous membrane prior to the bony reconstruction.
4. Rebuild the osseous defect with bone stock imported on a vascular pedicle.
5. Secure the reconstruction with excellent fixation, sufficient to overcome loading forces across the osteotomies.
6. Reconstruct the teeth with a bone-supported dental prosthesis.

The specific technical tactics for continuity defects of the jaw are to:

1. Restore mandibular continuity.
2. Restore alveolar bone height.
3. Restore osseous bulk.
4. Reconstruct the lower facial contours.
5. Maintain these characteristics over time.[8]

PREOPERATIVE EVALUATION AND MANAGEMENT

Patients who require a segmental mandibulectomy often have one or more major systemic illnesses. Tobacco and ethanol abuse, the usual etiologic factors for head and neck cancer, are commonly coupled with malnutrition and may contribute to derangements of the pulmonary, cardiac, vascular, hepatic, renal, or hematopoietic systems. General medical clearance is mandatory prior to surgery both for risk assessment and intervention and anesthesia treatment planning. A percutaneous endoscopic gastrostomy (PEG) tube may be placed several weeks ahead of the anticipated procedure. This is especially helpful for patients who require pharyngectomy/glossectomy with the mandibulectomy. Dental evaluation is also necessary to remove any infectious sources, plan for dental rehabilitation, and prepare for radiation. Social service input is helpful for subsequent home care.

Site-specific problems of the neck are usually related to prior surgery and/or radiation. Fifteen percent of treated head and neck oncology patients have occult hypothyroidism, which if untreated could precipitate a perioperative cardiopulmonary event or result in delayed or failed wound healing.[9] Radiation-induced atherosclerosis may cause subtotal occlusion of the carotid vasculature with possible cerebral ischemia after manipulation of the head and neck.[10] If a microvascular anastomosis is planned in a neck that has been previously dissected, careful clinical evaluation of the neck for potential venous connections is essential. If both sides of the neck have been entered, the patient should be considered for a carotid and/or aortic angiogram to aid in the search for appropriate recipient arteries. Anticipated pre-existing soft tissue deficits of the cervical skin and oral and oropharyngeal mucous membrane also need to be quantified and included in the treatment planning.

A variety of donor sites, which offer differing degrees of bone and soft tissue quantity and quality, is available for free tissue. Because there are wide variations from patient to patient at the same donor site, careful review of the individual and all his or her potential sites is warranted prior to formulating a final operative plan. Although the fibula osseocutaneous free flap is currently the favored donor site, significant arterial or venous peripheral vascular disease or deformity due to prior fracture would mitigate against its use. A lower extremity angiogram or magnetic resonance angiogram elucidates the possibility of a dominant peroneal artery, aids in documenting the extent of atherosclerosis, and helps select the leg with the longest pedicle.[11] The iliac crest donor site might be ruled in or out according to soft tissue bulk or whether prior groin surgery has traversed the deep circumflex iliac vessels. Simultaneous harvest and resection also favors the fibula and iliac donor sites, but not the scapular donor site. If the minimization of blood loss is an important issue, the iliac crest donor site must be avoided due to its sanguinous harvest. Early ambulation can be expected after dissection of the scapula bone flap, but less so with the fibula or iliac crest harvests.

One of the goals of a reconstruction is to replicate the native facial symmetry and projection. We recommend a lateral cephalogram and axial CT scan as a template to help with contouring the donor bone to the recipient defect.[12]

THE RESECTION

The optimal mandibular reconstruction begins with a well planned and executed resection. This requires that the resecting surgeon, who may not be the reconstructive surgeon, know the operative plan and make technical adjustments especially in anticipation of a free tissue transfer. In this way inadvertent injury to potential recipient neck vessels can be avoided. However, the retention of neck vessels at the expense of negative resection margins is strongly condemned, as is any oncological compromise. Ideally, two arteries are available to choose from the external carotid system and both the external jugular veins and the internal jugular vein tributaries are usable. Our favored recipient vessels with the fibula free flap are the branches of the linguo-facial trunk, the external carotid artery trunk, and, for veins, the external jugular vein or a tributary into the internal jugular vein or both. The transverse cervical vessels are also spared in the event that the other vessels are not usable.

We find that the most optimal cosmesis comes from a curved transverse incision, allowing a visor flap of cervical skin and chin to be elevated off the mandible. Thus the split lower lip and chin is avoided. In the retraction of the visor flap, care should be exercised with the mental nerve so as not to cause an inadvertent avulsion injury. Alternately, an IAN lateralization, as is performed for dental implant insertion in the atrophic jaw, will allow greater soft tissue retraction, ultimately sparing sensation in the mental dermatome.[13]

Prior to performing the mandibulectomy, we stabilize the mandibular remnants to assure TMJ alignment, function, occlusion, and to maintain the true size of the bony defect.[14] There are many methods by which this can be accomplished. In our hands, the favored approach is the use of a reconstruction plate that is contoured to the lateral surface of the jaw. The resection is performed, the flap brought into the field, the precontoured plate is secured by the predrilled, pretapped screw holes. This realigns the condyles and dentition and holds the osseous reconstruction in rigid fixation. One caution with this method is to remove the mental protuberance before applying the plate so as to avoid prognathism, especially if implants are being inserted.

Tumor-free tissue margins should be confirmed prior to beginning the reconstruction. In a recent study using clinical judgment and radiographs, only a 2% rate (4/182) of positive mandibular margins was encountered despite the fact that 45% (82/182) of the resected mandibles were pathologically positive.[15] This means that some of the bony resection margins were unnecessarily large, but readily compensated for with the microvascular reconstruction. Adequacy of the mandibular resection margins can be performed by frozen section study of the periosteum, the IAN, and cytology of the cancellous bone. Another report compared frozen section to permanent section evaluation of the marrow space and showed that frozen section evaluation was able to correctly determine the adequacy of the bone margins in 97% (32/33).[16] This is reassuring because this intraoperative assay could help prevent leaving a positive marrow margin and might avoid the major disadvantage of having to remove a new mandible reconstruction contaminated with tumor.

ORAL SOFT TISSUE RECONSTRUCTION

Adequate oral soft tissue closure is essential for a successful reconstruction. Inadequate soft tissue surface area will produce a wound closed under tension resulting in dehiscence, a contaminated reconstruction, and fistula formation. Native tissue quality may be poor because of infection, radiation, or cicatrix, further reinforcing the need for soft tissue reconstruction.

Deficiencies of oral soft tissue quantity or quality are overcome at the same time as the reconstruction by the use of a vascularized free tissue transfer. A common donor vascular pedicle will provide both viable bone, varying degrees of soft tissue, and soft tissue mobility around this pedicle. The exact choice depends on the location of the deficit, the extent of the hard and soft tissue to be replaced, the mobility requirements of the soft tissue component, and the availability of recipient vessels in the neck. Alternatively, a regional myocutaneous or osseomyocutaneous flap, such as the trapezius/spine of scapula flap, might be considered.[17] Finally, local flaps such as tongue, buccal, or palate flaps may be available,[18] but these, with the exception of the buccal flaps, have a minor role in the current armamentarium of reconstruction because they use specialized tissues at the expense of oral and oropharyngeal function.[19]

THE RECONSTRUCTION: TIMING AND THERAPEUTIC OPTIONS

The timing of the mandibular reconstruction, the type of repair, and the appropriate donor site are issues that must be addressed before embarking on a course of therapy. Strong indications for an immediate bony reconstruction are an anterior arch defect or a concurrent large soft tissue defect. Indications for a secondary reconstruction are a patient with multiple comorbidities rendering a high risk of complications.

Once it is determined that the patient will benefit from the immediate reconstruction, choices remain between a vascularized or nonvascularized bone graft or an alloplast (see Fig 12–1, Options for Mandibular Reconstruction). Local wound conditions are pivotal in this decision making because a mandibulectomy bed compromised by salivary contamination, prior radiation, significant soft tissue deficits, or large mandibulectomy defects, especially the symphysis, will respond predictably and well to the vascularized bone and soft tissue reconstruction. Our current practice is to perform an immediate reconstruction of the mandibular and soft tissue defect with a microvascular osseocutaneous free tissue transfer because this approach is highly successful in experienced hands (96% success rate in 322 cases of oromandibular reconstruction),[20] large resections can be performed with predictably tumor-free margins,[15] and there is a lower cost with fewer complications associated with a single procedure compared to a staged one.[21,22] Immediate reconstruction in the radiated patient is highly predictable, with healing of the osteosynthesis sites and infrequent loss of the soft tissue component.[23]

An alternative to the osseocutaneous free tissue transfer is the pedicled osseomyocutaneous regional flap. Examples of this are the sternocleidomastoid muscle borne clavicular graft, temporalis calvarial graft, pectoralis major rib graft, latissimus rib graft, serratus rib graft, or trapezius scapular spine graft. Unfortunately, the pedicled bone grafts have a less predictable ability to survive or form a solid osteosynthesis.[24] This may be due to several factors: the bone becomes separated from the vascular field of the primary soft tissue flap, tension or compression on the vascular leash, and harvest of bone too distant from the appropriate angiosome.

A nonvascularized free cortico-cancellous bone graft is another method for mandibu-

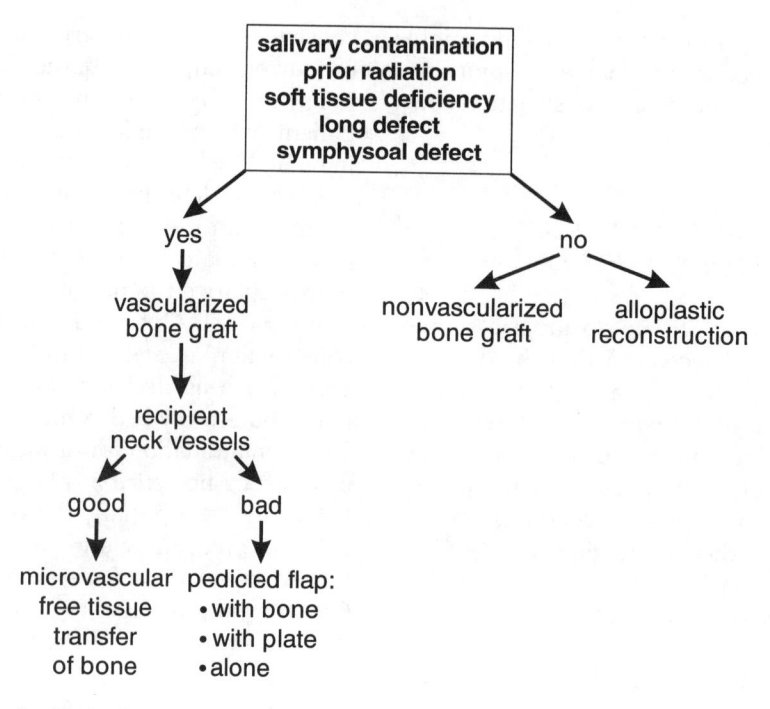

```
                 salivary contamination
                 prior radiation
                 soft tissue deficiency
                 long defect
                 symphysoal defect
                  /            \
                yes             no
                 |             / \
          vascularized   nonvascularized  alloplastic
          bone graft      bone graft     reconstruction
                 |
            recipient
          neck vessels
            /      \
          good     bad
            |       |
     microvascular  pedicled flap:
     free tissue    • with bone
     transfer       • with plate
     of bone        • alone
```

FIG 12–1. Options for mandibular reconstruction.

lar reconstruction. This technique is unfavorable for primary reconstruction because at least 50% will fail due to contamination by saliva.[25] However, when used as a secondary reconstruction technique, the successes approach 100%.[26] This requires the strict avoidance of entry into the mouth and adequate fixation of the graft. Possible soft tissue rehabilitation with a myocutaneous flap or hyperbaric oxygen therapy might be indicated if the recipient site was previously radiated. An appropriate course of hyperbaric oxygen therapy (100% oxygen at 2.4 atmospheres for 90 minutes per session with 20 preoperative and 10 postoperative treatments) will raise the PO_2 of radiated tissue to within 80% of nonradiated tissue allowing for improved hard and soft tissue wound healing.[8]

The alloplastic fixation appliances should be viewed as temporary space holders. They are useful for maintenance of the occlusion and preventing the cosmetic deformity of midline deviation. However, many of these appliances will eventually fail by way of loosening, infection, extrusion, or fracture, especially in a dentate individual capable of high chewing forces. Early postoperative failures of implanted stainless steel appliances tend to be the result of flap dehiscence with plate exposure either intraorally or externally. Late complications are usually due to hardware failure.[27]

In response to some of these failures, and due to the attenuation of therapeutic radiation by stainless steel,[28] a more refined bone reconstruction plating technique has been developed. The THORP plating system[29] (Synthes, Paoli, Pennsylvania) and the next generation Leibinger Titanium Locking Screw Mandibular Reconstruction Plating System (Howmedica Leibinger, Inc, Dallas, Texas) differ from conventional reconstruction plates by the mechanism that secures the plate to the bone. Conventional plating attempts stability by pressure between the plate and the lateral surface of the jaw due to compression from the screw head. The THORP and Leibinger systems rely on rigid fixation between the head of the screw and the plate, which obviates the need for intimate contact between the plate and the bone. It also avoids pressure resorption of bone under the plate with subsequent screw loosening. A stainless steel or THORP plate covered by a soft tissue flap will fail 20% of the time, but the bulk of the failures will be seen with anterior reconstructions.[30] The other drawback to plate reconstruction is that it will not support dental implants.

PREFERRED DONOR SITES FOR VASCULARIZED OSSEOUS MANDIBULAR RECONSTRUCTION

Fibula

The fibula is currently a favored donor site for composite bone and skin mandibular reconstruction. Originally described in 1975 by Taylor,[31] the bone stock is long (commonly 25 cm), straight, strong, and expendable and easily accessed. The blood supply is from the peroneal artery via multiple segmental periosteal vessels and an endosteal nutrient vessel. The former permits multiple wedge ostectomies, cut in a subperiosteal plane, without injury to the blood supply. The vascular pedicle is from 6–10 cm in length with vessels that are at least 2 mm in diameter. The vascular anatomy is fairly constant, but a preoperative vessel study is still recommended. This is done both to avoid a dominant peroneal artery[11] and to prevent a technically difficult anastomosis of a peroneal vessel riddled with atherosclotic plaques. Angiography is also helpful in choosing the leg with the longest peroneal pedicle.

Oral and cutaneous soft tissue defects, or both, may be replaced by a skin paddle, which is fed by septocutaneous or musculocutaneous perforating vessels from the peroneal pedicle. Early in the experience with this flap the cutaneous component was felt to be unreliable.[32] However, careful Doppler identification of the septocutaneous perforating vessels or modification of the dissection to include a cuff of soleus and flexor hallucis longus muscle will reliably supply the skin paddle.[33] The skin paddle donor site usually needs to be closed with a skin graft.

Advantages to this donor site include a bloodless harvest because of application of a tourniquet and a harvest concurrent with the tumor extirpation. Donor site morbidity is minimal provided that 8 cm of distal fibula are preserved for stability of the ankle. Measured mild deficits of strength at the ankle and mild decreased range of motion for ankle flexion and extension have been recorded subsequent to fibula harvest.[34] The prevalence of ipsilateral ankle pain also increased with time from 1.6% to 11.5 % over 5 years from 247 fibulectomy sites.[35]

Iliac Crest

The iliac crest free flap is another common donor site for reconstruction of composite oromandibular defects. Several different vascular pedicles originate in the groin, but the consistent supply of the deep circumflex iliac artery (DCIA) to the iliac crest was described in 1979.[36] Multiple transmuscular perforating vessels from the DCIA supply the overlying groin skin in an array separate from the superficial circumflex iliac pedicle. The ascending branch of the DCIA supplies the internal oblique muscle which when harvested with the bone flap offers a muscle component for mucosal replacement and bone coverage.[37] The bone stock, which may be up to 14 cm in length, is naturally well contoured for reconstruction of the ipsilateral hemimandibular defect.[38] Similar to the fibula flap, the iliac free flap maintains a segmental blood supply from the DCIA that allows for multiple contouring osteotomies. The vascular pedicle is 6 cm in length and the artery from 1–3 mm in diameter.

Advantages of this osseocutaneous donor site are the volume of bone and soft tissue that can be reliably revascularized, although in certain patients this bulk is a detriment. A composite flap for replacement of cheek/neck skin, mandible, and oral lining can be harvested simultaneously with the oromandibular ablation. The potential disadvantages of this donor site include a sanguinous harvest, incisional hernia, abdominal wall weakness, hip pain, limping, and pain along the lateral thigh due to injury of the lateral femoral cutaneous nerve. The technique can cause injury to the femoral nerve, peritoneal contents, or hip joint.

Scapula

The scapula free flap remains useful for mandibular reconstruction, especially when confronted with a moderate length bone defect and a large or multidimensional soft tissue defect. First reported clinically in 1982,[39] the scapular flap takes its origin from the circumflex scapular pedicle. The subscapular pedicle branches from the axillary vessels and gives rise to both the thorcodorsal trunk to the serratus anterior and latissimus dorsi muscles and the circumflex scapular system.[40-43] The latter is parent to three branches of surgical interest: a deep branch to the periosteum along the lateral border of the scapula, a horizontal fasciocutaneous branch to the scapular paddle, and a vertical fasciocutaneous branch to the parascapular paddle. A separate angular branch supplies the tip of the scapula as a takeoff of the thorcodorsal vessels. When harvested at the origin of the subscapular pedicle, the vascular leash is at least 6 cm in length with a large (3–4 mm) diameter vessel. The lateral border of the scapula can be up to 3 cm in thickness with 10 to 12 cm of length, which may be extended by including the tip of the scapula with the angular vessel. The segmental blood supply to the periosteum allows for osteotomies enabling the construction of a curved neomandible.[44] For massive composite defects, the "mega" flap, consisting of tissues of both the circumflex scapular and thorcodorsal branches, can be obtained on one vascular pedicle.

The merits of this flap are its versatility: simultaneous harvest of multiple skin, muscle, and bone components based on a single pedicle; a good color match for head and neck recipient sites; and the ability to harvest large areas of skin. There is usually little donor site morbidity as long as the patient is prescribed physical therapy. The major disadvantage is that the flap harvest requires positioning the patient on at least a 45° angle, with the scapula up, which makes a two-team approach more awkward.

FIXATION OF THE RECONSTRUCTION

Our favored approach is the use of the Leibinger mandibular reconstruction plate, similar in concept to the THORP system.[29] This is contoured to the lateral bony cortex prior to the resection and employs screws with the potential for osseointegration and expanding screw heads. Rigid fixation occurs at the plate and screw interface rather than relying on compression of the plate against the bone (Fig 12–2). If the tumor has significantly deformed the lateral aspect of the jaw, a superolateral and inferior border miniplate technique is employed using monocortical screws (Fig 12–3).[45] This technique requires more judgment with the inset of the reconstruction, particularly regarding symmetry, projection, and alignment of the alveolar ridges. If a reconstruction plate cannot be fitted prior to mandibulectomy, a transverse jointed plate and bar system is also available for fixation of the native mandible components.

TMJ RECONSTRUCTION

The goals of TMJ reconstruction are to restore the vertical height of the posterior ramus, support the dental occlusion, and maintain adequate movement of the joint. Reconstructive options are the same as those already discussed: vascularized bone, nonvascualrized bone, or alloplasts. State of the art reconstruction places the disarticulated condyle back into the joint space, secured to the end of the fibular graft.[12] If the condyle must be discarded, the fibula is placed into the joint space with the periosteal soft tissues covering the end of the bone. If not already performed as a part of the resection, an ipsilat-

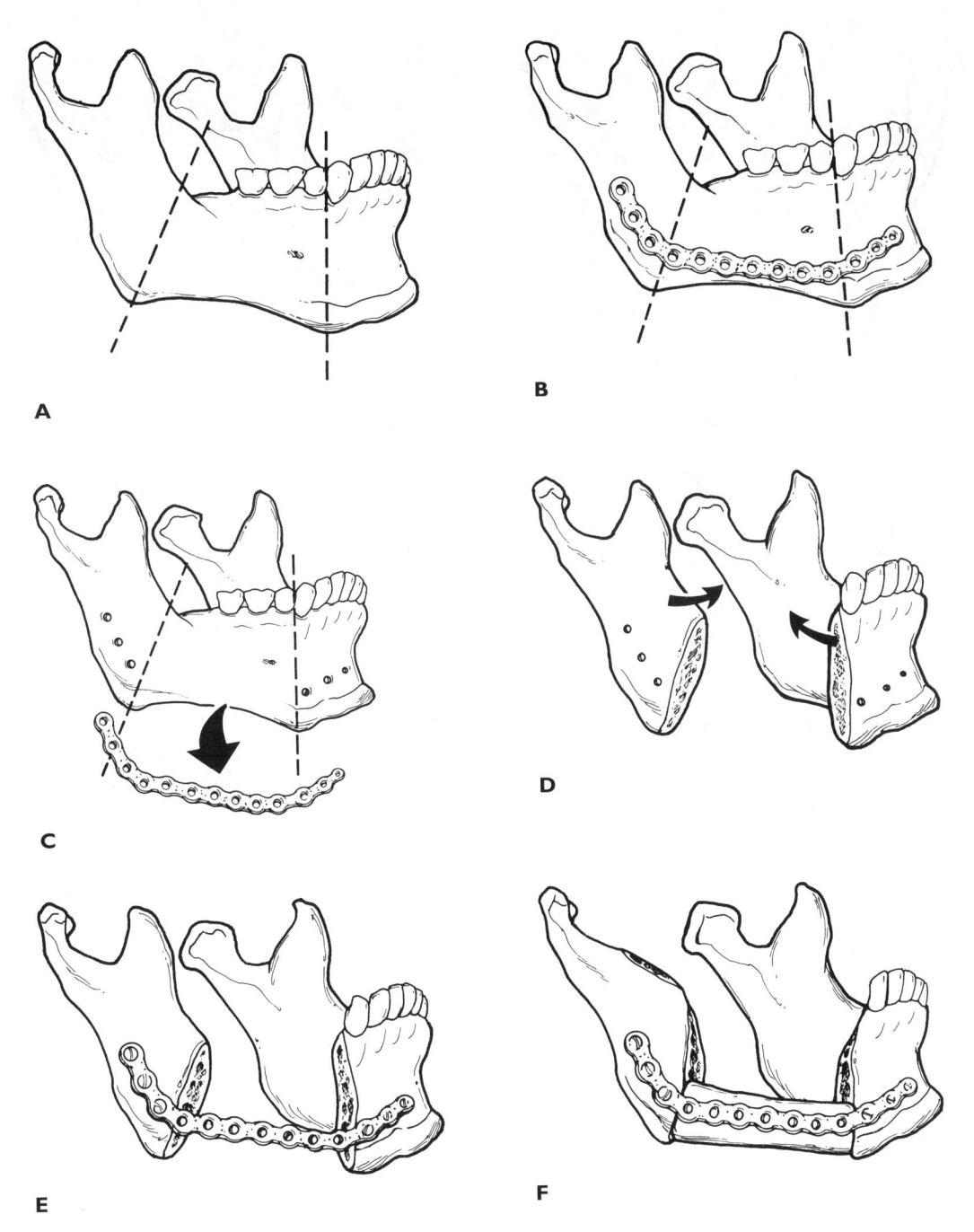

FIG 12–2. The sequence of operative steps for fixation of a segmental mandibulectomy defect with a vascularized bone graft reconstruction using a mandibular reconstruction plate is outlined. A. The margins of the mandibulectomy defect are marked. B. The reconstruction plate is precontoured to match the contour of the native mandible. Drill holes are made in the proximal and distal bone stumps, measured for depth, and screw threads are tapped. C. The contoured plate is removed. D. The resection is performed. The unsupported bone stumps collapse due to the unopposed forces imposed by the soft tissues. E. The dimensions of the native bone defect are recrested, and the occlusion is restored after application of the precontoured plate by way of the previously prepared screw holes. F. The vascularized bone graft is sized to the defect and then secured to the plate by using lag screws. A coronoidectomy is performed to prevent rotational forces at the jaw-graft interface.

FIG 12–2. The sequence of operative steps for fixation of a segmental mandibulectomy defect and vascularized bone graft reconstruction using miniplates, when the buccal surface of bone has been distorted by tumor, is outlined. A. Tumor of the symphysis is depicted which has perforated through the buccal cortical plate of bone. B. The marquis of the mandibulectomy are marked. The stabilizing jig is affixed to the rami of the mandible. C. The resection is performed. The jaw segments remain stabilized relative to each other and, to the occlusion, held by the temporary appliance. D. The vascularized bone graft is osteotomized as necessary to fit with the bone defect and held in fixation using miniplates applied on the buccal and inferior control surfaces of the jaw and reconstruction. E. The stabilizing jig is removed, and bilateral coronoidectomies are performed to prevent undue tension at the jaw-graft interface.

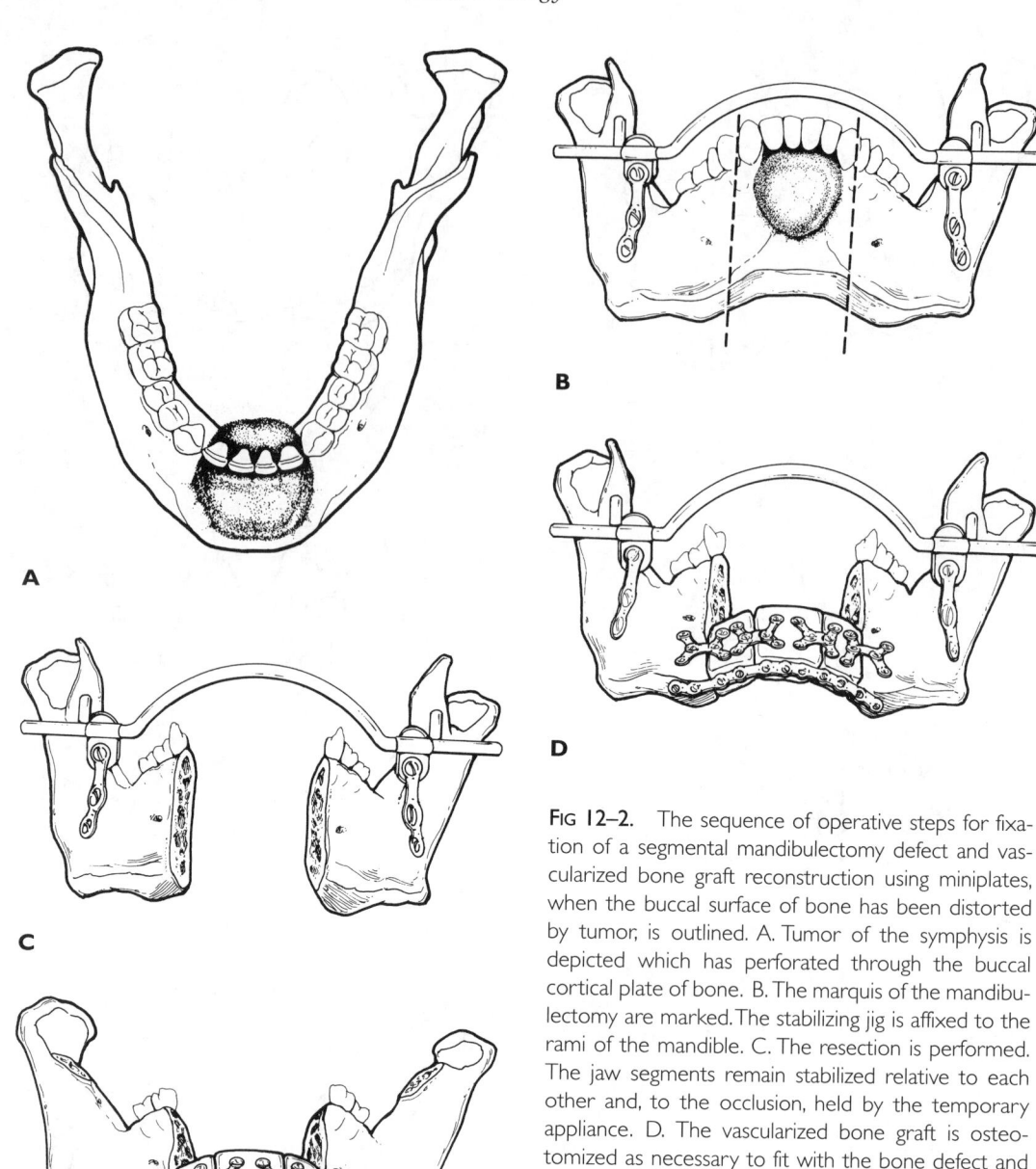

eral coronoidectomy is advocated to avoid the strain of the temporalis muscle against the reconstruction and to minimize postoperative trismus. If the meniscus has been resected along with the condyle, a soft tissue flap, usually temporalis muscle and fiscia, should be interposed between the condylar reconstruction and the skull base to avoid development of a bony ankylosis.[46]

A free costochondral graft is a good reconstructive option for repair of end-stage osteoarthritis, bony ankylosis, or congenital mandible deformity where salivary contamination will not occur.[47] Likewise, corticocancellous bone packed into a cadaveric bone tray may be used for secondary reconstruction of the disarticulation defect with a good result.[8]

A variety of temporomandibular joint alloplastic implants are available. The THORP and Leibinger lock screw systems both have a condylar apparatus. Of greatest infamy is the Proplast-Teflon TMJ implant, which resulted in granulomatous erosion of the skull base, frequent infection, requisite removal of many implants, and withdrawal from the market.[48] We recommend against the use of a condylar or total joint alloplast.

DENTAL RECONSTRUCTION

Complete reconstruction of a mandibulectomy defect includes dental reconstruction. A removable soft tissue borne dental prosthesis is commonly unstable in the mouth due to the abnormal anatomy and radiation induced xerostomia. These problems can be overcome with metallic bone implants. Implants and soft tissues overlying the alveolar ridge can share in stabilizing a removable denture or the implants can completely support the fixed denture. There are two types of dental implants: osseointegrating and transmandibular. Osseointegrating implants effectively "fuse" with the bone due to the material employed, the method of insertion and delayed loading of the implants. Histological evidence of osseointegration is that of bone matrix and osteocytes adjacent to a microscopic layer of titanium oxide without an intervening soft tissue layer.[49] Dental implantation must be considered in the treatment planning of mandible reconstruction if the dental rehabilitation is to be successful. The fibula and iliac crest free tissue transfers are now well documented to accept osseintegrated implants[50] either at the time of the mandibular reconstruction[51] or secondarily.[52] The fibula may be better suited for the edentulous condition; whereas, the iliac free flap is more appropriate for the dentulous state because of the height of each graft relative to the alveolar ridge.[53] The key principles to successful implant placement are:

1. Atraumatic placement by use of low speed irrigating burrs to avoid denaturation of the bone.
2. Delayed loading of the implant for several months.
3. Coordinated treatment planning with the restoring prosthodontist.[54]

Like native teeth, implant-borne prosthetic teeth can be lost due to infection. Less than scrupulous oral hygiene risks infection of the peri-implant gingiva and bone, an infection analogous to periodontitis. Unrecognized or poorly managed, the implant might be lost and the patient exposed to possible osteomyelitis or pathological fracture of the mandibular reconstruction.

An alternative to the osseointegrated implant is the fixed mandibular implant (FMI). This fixture is placed through the inferior border of the native jaw or neomandible and retained due to several screws and multiple parallel transosseus pins. A 20-year experience with this prosthesis showed greater than a 90% long-term success rate. The implant can support a bone-borne fixed prosthesis or stabilize a removable denture. The FMI has now been used to retain dental prostheses after microvascular mandibular reconstruction with equal success in eight reported cases at a mean follow-up of 14 months.[55] The disadvantage to this implant is its lack of versatility or adaptability to novel anatomy, which is better suited to conventional implants.

COMPLICATIONS

The timing of osseocutaneous free tissue transfer complications can be divided into those that occur in the operative/perioperative period (early) or later. Early complications include vascular pedicle occlusion. The etiology is often a technical one related to the anastomosis, geometry of the pedicle, or extrinsic compression, which, if unrecognized, will result in vascular thrombosis and irreversible flap ischemia.[56] Salivary, gastric, or tracheal contamination and purulence also predispose to anastomotic thrombosis.[57] This is rare in experienced hands and may be salvageable by prompt re-exploration.

Subsequent complications may be divided into soft tissue and hard tissue problems. Partial loss of a free flap soft tissue paddle is frequently handled by local wound care. A near total or total loss, especially with concern for contamination of the great vessels or vascular pedicle to a bone flap, necessitates a second flap for coverage. Wound infections are treated in customary fashion by antibiotics and drainage, as appropriate, and fistulae must be carefully diverted away from microvascular pedicles while healing.

Problems with the osseous reconstruction relate to the bone itself or the supporting hardware. A malpositioned reconstruction should be circumvented by appropriate planning, but secondary repositioning of the bone flap has been reported.[14] A nonunion or fibrous union might be managed by observation, antibiotics, application of further hardware, or revision grafting. One always needs to be mindful of recurrent or persistent malignancy in this situation. Osteoradionecrosis of a graft and/or native mandible is treated according to the standard protocols. Loose or exposed bone plate or screws generally will need removal as mobile hardware tends to become infected. The etiology of the hardware failure should be ascertained so as not to overlook the possibility of locally persistent tumor.

COSTS

The reconstruction of the composite oromandibular defect is costly. Recent data[58] (from University of California, Los Angeles) show that the hospital fees, excluding surgeons' fees, for primary free tissue transfer averaged $85,000 using the fibula, scapula, or radial forearm donor sites. When stratified according to donor site the scapula proved to be the most expensive at just over $100,000 due to the duration of the procedure and the length of stay in the ICU. The pectoralis flap and osteocutaneous radial forearm flaps were similar in cost at $60,000; the fibula reconstructions were intermediate at $80,000.

This cost differential between treatment groups is supported by another older report.[21] The authors proposed to control these costs by appropriate selection of the donor site to allow simultaneous graft harvest and tumor ablation, creation of an intermediate care ICU specific for flap monitoring, wound care, and airway observation, encouraging early transfer out of the ICU and discharge of patients with tracheotomy and enteral feeding tubes. Using that approach, in their study, the cost of the last 10 fibula reconstructions was reduced to $65,000 per procedure. Unfortunately for patients, the choice of a "less expensive" procedure may have significant hidden "costs." Although the PMF group was initially less expensive, there were significantly more readmissions for wound-related complications and revisions as compared with the primary free tissue transfer group. Thus, the monetary savings were diminished and quality of life was compromised. Monetary expenditure is just one of many factors in outcome evaluation of head neck cancer patients.

CONCLUSIONS

Immediate reconstruction of the segmental mandibulectomy defect by free tissue transfer is successful, predictable, and beneficial to patients. Other techniques are available if microvascular methods are not an option. The amount of animate and sensate native soft tissue that remains in and around the oral cavity after the resection is also a major factor dictating the functional outcome of the hard tissue reconstruction. Rehabilitation is optimized when dental implants are incorporated into the reconstruction.

REFERENCES

1. Riley RW, Powell NB, Guilleminault C, Ware W. Obstructive sleep apnea syndrome following surgery for mandibular prognathism. *J Oral Maxillofac Surg*. 1987;45:450–452.
2. Panje WR, Holmes DK. Mandibulectomy without reconstruction can cause sleep apnea. *Laryngoscope*. 1984;94:1591–1594.

3. Matsuda Y. Effect of nerve injuries on action potential of inferior alveolar nerve: clinical study. *Shikwa Gakuo.* 1980;80:1591–1611.
4. Attia EL, Bentley KC, Head T, Mulder D. A new external approach to the pterygomaxillary fossa and parapharyngeal space. *Head Neck Surg.* 1984;6(4):884–891.
5. Boyd JB, Gullane PJ, Rotstein LE, et al. Classification of mandibular defects. *Plas Reconstr Surg.* 1993;92:1266–1275.
6. Komisar A. The functional result of mandibular reconstruction. *Laryngoscope.* 1990;100: 364–374.
7. LaBanc JP, Gregg JM. Trigeminal nerve injuries: basic problems, historical perspectives, early successes, and remaining challenges. *Oral Maxillofac Surg Clinics NA.* 1992;4:277–283.
8. Marx RE. The science and art of reconstructing the jaws and temporomandibular joints. In: Bell WH, ed. *Modern Practice in Orthognathic and Reconstructive Surgery.* Philadelphia, Penna: WB Saunders; 1992:1449–1531.
9. Cannon CR. Hypothyroidism in head and neck cancer patients: experimental and clinical observations. *Laryngoscope.* 1994;104(suppl 66): 1–21.
10. Feehs RS, McGuirt WF, Bond MG, et al. Irradiation: a significant risk factor for carotid atherosclerosis. *Arch Otolaryngol Head Neck Surg.* 1991;117:1135–1137.
11. Carroll WR, Esclamado R. Preoperative vascular imaging for the fibular osteocutaneous flap. *Arch Otolaryngol Head Neck Surg.* 1996;122: 708–712.
12. Hidalgo DA. Asthetic improvements in freeflap mandible reconstruction. *Plast Reconstr Surg.* 199;58:574–585.
13. Jensen J, Reiche-Fischel O, Sindet-Pedersen S. Nerve transposition and implant placement in the atrophic posterior mandibular alveolar ridge. *J Oral Maxillofac Surg.* 1994;52:662–668.
14. Li KK, Cheney ML, Teknos TN. The importance of mandibular position in microvascular mandibular reconstruction. *Laryngoscope.* 1996; 106:903–907.
15. Schusterman MA, Harris SW, Raymond AK, Goepfert H. Immediate free flap mandibular reconstruction: significance of adequate surgical margins. *Head & Neck Surg.* 1993;15: 204–207.
16. Forrest LA, Schuller DE, Lucas JG, Sullivan MJ. Rapid analysis of mandibular margins. *Laryngoscope.* 1995;105:475–477.
17. Urken ML. The trapezius system. In: Urken ML, Cheney ML, Sullivan MJ, Biller HF, eds. *Atlas of Regional and Free Flaps for Head and Neck Reconstruction.* New York: Raven Press, 1995:39.
18. Komisar A, Lawson W. A compendium of intraoral flaps. *Head & Neck Surg.* 1985;8:91–99.
19. McConnel FMS, Teichgraeber JF, Adler RK. A comparison of three methods of oral reconstruction. *Arch Otolaryngol Head Neck Surg.* 1987;113: 496–500.
20. Urken ML, Buchbinder D, Weinberg H, et al. Functional evaluation following microvascular oromandibular reconstruction of the oral cancer patient: a comparative study of reconstructed and nonreconstructed patients. *Laryngoscope.* 1991;101:935–950.
21. Kroll SS, Schusterman MA, Reece GP. Costs and complications in mandibular reconstruction. *Ann Plast Surg.* 1992;29:341–347.
22. Kroll SS, Evans GRD, Goldberg D, et al. A comparison of resource costs for head and neck reconstruction with free and pectoralis major flaps. *Plast Reconstr Surg.* 1997;99: 1282–1286.
23. Duncan MJ, Manktelow RT, Zuker RM, Rosen IB. Mandibular reconstruction in the radiated patient: the role of osteocutaneous free tissue transfers. *Plast Reconstr Surg.* 1985; 76:829–840.
24. Conley J. Use of composite flaps containing bone for major repairs in the head and neck. *Plast Reconstr Surg.* 1972;49:522–526.
25. Lawson W, Baek S, Loscalzo LJ, Biller HF, Krespi YP. Experience with immediate and delayed mandibular reconstruction. *Laryngoscope.* 1982;92:5–10.
26. Tidstrom KD, Keller EE. Reconstruction of mandibular discontinuity with autogenous iliac bone graft: report of 34 consecutive patients. *J Oral Maxillofac Surg.* 1990;48: 336–346.
27. Davidson MJ, Gullane PJ. Prosthetic plate mandibular reconstruction. *Otolaryngol Clin NA.* 1991;24:1419–1431.
28. Gullane PJ. Primary mandibular reconstruction: analysis of 64 cases and evaluation of interface radiation dosimetry on bridging plates. *Laryngoscope.* 1991;101(6, Pt 2, Suppl 54).
29. Vuillemin T, Raveh J, Sutter F. Mandibular reconstruction with the titanium hollow screw reconstruction plate (THORP) system: evaluation of 62 cases. *Plast Reconstr Surg.* 1988;82:804–814.
30. Boyd JB, Mulholland RS, Davidson J, et al. The free flap and plate in oromandibular reconstruction: long-term review and indications. *Plast Reconstr Surg.* 1995;122:708–712.
31. Taylor GI, Miller G, Ham F. Free vascularized bone graft: a clinical extension of microvas-

cular techniques. *Plast Reconstr Surg.* 1975; 55:533–539.
32. Hidalgo DA. Fibula free flap: a new method of mandible reconstruction. *Plast Reconstr Surg.* 1989;84:71–79.
33. Schusterman MA, Reece GP, Miller MJ, Harris S. The osteocutaneous free fibula flap: is the skin paddle reliable? *Plast Reconstr Surg.* 1992;90:787–795.
34. Anthony JP, Rawnsley JD, Benhaim P, et al. Donor leg morbidity and function after fibula free flap mandible reconstruction. *Plast Reconstr Surg.* 1995;96:146–152.
35. Vail TP, Urbaniak JR. Donor-site morbidity with use of vascularized autogenous fibular grafts. *J Bone Joint Surg.* 1996;78A:204–211.
36. Taylor GI, Townsend P, Corlett R. Superiority of the deep circumflex iliac vessels as the supply for free groin flaps. *Plast Reconstr Surg.* 1979; 64:595–604.
37. Urken ML, Vickery C, Weinberg H, et al. The internal oblique-iliac crest osseomyocutaneous free flap in oromandibular reconstruction. *Arch Otolaryngol Head Neck Surg.* 1989;115:339–349.
38. Manchester W. Immediate reconstruction of the mandible and temporomandibular joint. *Brit J Plast Surg.* 1965;18:291–303.
39. Gilbert A, Teot L. The free scapular flap. *Plast Reconstr Surg.* 1982;69:601.
40. Nassif TM, Vidal L, Bovet JL, et al. The parascapular flap: a new cutaneous microsurgical free flap. *Plast Reconstr Surg.* 1982;69:591–600.
41. Rowsell AR, Davis DM, Eisenberg N, et al. The anatomy of the subscapular-thorcodorsal arterial system: a study of 100 cadaver dissections. *Brit J Plas Surg.* 1984;37:574–576.
42. Barwick WJ, Goodkind DJ, Serafin D. The free scapular flap. *Plast Reconstr Surg.* 1982;69: 779–785.
43. Urbaniak JR, Koman LA, Goldner RD, et al. The vascularized cutaneous scapular flap. *Plast Reconstr Surg.* 1982;69:772–778.
44. Swartz WF, Banis JC, Newton ED, et al. The osteocutaneous scapular flap for mandibular and maxillary reconstruction. *Plast Reconstr Surg.* 1986;77:530–545.
45. Hidalgo DA. Fibula free flap mandibular reconstruction. *Clin Plast Surg.* 1994;21:25–35.
46. Pogrel MA, Kaban LB. The role of a temporalis fascia and muscle flap in temporomandibular joint surgery. *J Oral Maxillofac Surg.* 1990; 48:14–19.
47. Kaban LB, Perrot DH, Fisher K. A protocol for management of temporomandibular joint ankylosis. *J Oral Maxillofac Surg.* 1990;48: 1145–1151.
48. Kearns GJ, Perrott DH, Kaban LB. A protocol for the management of failed alloplastic temporomandibular joint disc implants. *J Oral Maxillofac Surg.* 1995;53:1240–1247.
49. Branemark R, Skalak R, Branemark PI. Osteointegration and rigid fixation. In: Yaremchuk MJ, Gruss JS, Manson PN, eds. *Rigid Fixation of the Craniomaxillofacial Skeleton.* Boston. Butterworth-Heinemann; 1992:163–175.
50. Moscoso JF, Keller J, Genden E, Weinberg H, Biller HF, Buchbinder D, Urken ML. Vascularized bone flaps in oromandibular reconstruction: a comparative anatomic study of bone stock from various donor sites to assess suitability for enosseous dental implants. *Arch Otolaryngol Head Neck Surg.* 1994;120:36–43.
51. Urken ML, Buchbinder D, Weinberg H, Vickery, Sheiner A, Biller, HF. Primary placement of osseointegrated implants in microvascular mandibular reconstruction. *Otolaryngol Head Neck Surg.* 1989;101:56–73.
52. Listrom RD, Symington JM. Osseointegrated dental implants in conjunction with bone grafts. *Int J Oral Maxillofac Surg.* 1988;17: 116–118.
53. Haughey BH, Fredrickson JM, Lerrick AJ, Sclaroff A, Gay WD. Fibular and iliac crest osteomuscular free flap reconstruction of the oral cavity. *Laryngoscope.* 1994;104:1305–1313.
54. Lukash FN, Sachs SA. Functional mandibular reconstruction: prevention of the oral invalid. *Plast Reconstr Surg.* 1989;84:227–233.
55. Li KK, Cheney ML, Gliklich RE, et al. Fixed mandibular implant after microvascular mandibular reconstruction. *Arch Otolaryngol Head Neck Surg.* 1996;122:1308–1312.
56. Hidalgo DA, Jones CS. The role of emergent exploration in free-tissue transfers: a review of 150 consecutive cases. *Plast Reconstr Surg.* 1990; 86:492–498.
57. Urken ML, Weinberg H, Buchbinder D, et al. Microvascular free flaps in head and neck reconstruction: report of 200 cases and review of complications. *Arch Otolaryngol Head Neck Surg.* 1994;120:633–640.
58. Talesnick A, Markowitz B, Calcaterrra T, Ahn C, Shaw W. Cost and outcome of osteocutaneous free tissue transfer versus pedicled soft-tissue reconstruction for composite mandibular defects. *Plast Reconstr Surg.* 1997: 1167–1178.

CHAPTER 13

Quality of Life, Comorbidity, and Cost-Effectiveness in Head and Neck Cancer Treatment

Ernest A. Weymuller, Jr, MD, Frederic W.-B. Deleyiannis, MD, MPhil, MPH,
Jay F. Piccirillo, MD, FACS, and Bevan Yueh, MD

Although the topics reviewed in this chapter have always been relevant they have been approached with increasing sophistication and emphasis in the last 5–10 years. Perhaps the dominant impetus for this attention is the disquieting truth that in many instances we cannot confidently identify a significant difference between the treatment options available in a given situation. Using the therapeutic endpoints of survival and local regional control, it is true that no multi-institutional study that has included surgery as a form of treatment has demonstrated a significant separation between the control and treatment arms.[1] In such a setting other variables can assume greater significance. Quality of life, comorbidity, and cost-effectiveness have great relevance when considering therapeutic options in the absence of a clear, survival-based mandate. It is thus important to understand the conceptual foundations related to these assessment methods so they may be properly applied in both selecting treatment for a given patient and the development of future studies of head and neck cancer treatment.

The ensuing discussion will be subdivided to highlight each area, a division that is to some degree artificial because final treatment decisions require integration of all the relevant factors. This chapter focuses on the most important advances in the last decade which largely relate to refinement and definition of the parameters used to study these issues.

QUALITY OF LIFE

F.W.-B. Deleyiannis, MD, MPhil, MPH

Whether treatment is palliative or curative, the disabilities associated with treatment for advanced cancer often seem worse to the patient than the untreated cancer, and the traditional outcome measures of treatment efficacy, such as tumor recurrence and survival time, are often meaningless to the patient. What matters is the ability to return to pre-illness function and psychosocial well-being.

Defining the Concept and the Content of Quality of Life

QOL is a multidimensional construct without a universally accepted definition. Ferrans and Powers define QOL as a "person's sense of well-being that stems from satisfaction or dissatisfaction with the areas of his life that are important to him."[2] According to Cella, QOL is a "patient's appraisal of and satisfaction with their current level of functioning as compared to what they perceive to be possible or ideal."[3,4] Crucial to any definition is the recognition that different people have different values which cause aspects of their lives to have different impacts on their QOL.[5]

A range of components have been proposed to define the content of QOL. Aaronson stated that there are minimally four core dimensions of QOL: (1) Functional status (i.e., activity level, vocational activity), (2) physical complaints (eg, somatic sensations, disease symptoms, side effects), (3) psychological distress (eg, anxiety, depression), and (4) social interactions (quality and quantity of relationships with significant others).[6,7] Schipper and Levitt presented a similar classification.[8] Additional factors that have been proposed for inclusion in QOL assessment include financial/economic status, satisfaction with medical treatment, sexuality, spirituality, body image, sleep, and the ability to pursue personal leisure activities (Table 13–1).

Health-related QOL should be conceptually differentiated from health status and overall QOL.[9] Health status refers to the functional, physical, and emotional effects of disease, whereas health-related QOL is a measure of how patients perceive and react to their health status. Overall QOL includes health-related QOL and non-health-related factors, such as family, friends, employment, and other life circumstances.

General Versus Disease-Specific QOL Measures

The increasing use of QOL assessment in clinical research has renewed the discussion concerning the relative advantages of general and disease-specific QOL measures.[10] General measures, such as the Sickness Impact Profile (SIP), the Quality of Well-Being Scale, and Medical Outcomes Study 36-item short-form health survey (SF-36), summarize the general health status of an individual by asking detailed and numerous questions from a spectrum of the components of QOL (Table 13–2).[11-13] They are used for QOL assessment in a broad range of patients, particularly in those patients with chronic disease. The principal advantage of general QOL measures is that they allow a comparison of results across different diseases.

Disease-specific measures are designed to assess specific diagnostic groups or patient populations and include questions about clinical change. Disease-specific measures thus are often more responsive to fluctuations in patient status over time than general measures, but they are less generalizable to other QOL studies. The Karnofsky Performance Status Scale for cancer and the New York Heart Association Functional Classification are examples of disease-specific measures that have been used for decades.[14,15]

To gain the advantages of both types of measures, investigators have recently synthesized both approaches into one measurement strategy, called a "modular approach to QOL assessment."[16] In this approach a set of core disease-specific questions is supplemented by a set of site- or treatment-specific questions. The Functional Assessment of Cancer Therapy (FACT) and European Organization for Research and Treatment of Cancer (EORTC) scales are examples of the modular approach.[16,18]

Methodology

QOL research originates from a long history of theoretical and methodologic research in the social sciences, particularly in the assess-

Table 13-1. Questions asked in the Functional Living Index—Cancer

1. Most people experience some feelings of depression at times. Rate how often you feel these feelings.
2. How well are you coping with your everyday stress?
3. How much time do you spend thinking about your illness?
4. Rate your ability to maintain your usual recreation or leisure activities.
5. Has nausea affected your daily functioning?
6. How well do you feel today?
7. Do you feel well enough to make a meal or do minor household repairs today?
8. Rate the degree to which the cancer has imposed a hardship on those closest to you in the past two weeks.
9. Rate, how often you feel discouraged about your life.
10. Rate your satisfaction with your work and your jobs around the house in the past month.
11. How uncomfortable do you feel today?
12. Rate in your opinion, how disruptive your cancer has been to those closest to you in the past two weeks.
13. How much is the pain or discomfort interfering with your daily activities?
14. Rate the degree to which your cancer has imposed a hardship on you (personally) in the past two weeks.
15. How much of your usual household tasks are you able to complete?
16. Rate how willing you were to see and spend time with those closest to you in the past two weeks.
17. How much nausea have you had in the last two weeks?
18. Rate the degree to which you are frightened of the future.
19. Rate how willing you were to see and spend time with friends in the past two weeks.
20. How much of your pain or discomfort over the past two weeks was related to caner?
21. Rate your confidence in your prescribed course of treatment.
22. How well do you appear today?

Source: Schipper H, Clinch J, McMurray A, Levitt M. Measuring the quality of life of cancer patients: the Functional Living Index—Cancer: development and validation. *J Clin Oncol.* 1984;2(5):472-483. Reprinted with permission of WB Saunders, Philadelphia, Penna.

ment and quantification of subjective experience. The hesitancy to incorporate QOL outcome measures into clinical oncology trials originates partially from a lack of familiarity with this methodology. Several of the more salient methodological issues involved in the designing or selecting of QOL outcome measures address the following questions:

What Should be Measured?

The scope of QOL inquiry is particularly important. Measurement of functional status or physical complaints alone may fail to assess the impact of disease or treatment on patients' entire life whereas global measurements may fail to assess noteworthy functional deficits or complaints. The researcher must strike some balance between the breadth of the domains of QOL and the depth of coverage within domains.

Which type of instrument to use (general versus disease-specific) for a particular study becomes clarified once the researcher has decided the spectrum and depth of QOL domains. Pilot studies will aid in determining the appropriate instrument. Instead of creating an instrument *de novo*, Cella recom-

Table 13–2. Sickness Impact Profile categories and selected items

Behavior Category	Selected Items *
1. Sleep and rest	I sit during much of the day. I sleep or nap during the day.
2. Eating	I am eating no food at all; nutrition is taken through tubes or intravenous fluids. I am eating special or different food.
3. Work	I am not working at all. I often act irritably toward my work associates.
4. Home management	I am not doing any of the maintenance or repair work around the house that I usually do. I am not doing heavy work around the house.
5. Recreation and pastimes	I am going out for entertainment less. I am not doing any of my usual physical recreation or activities.
6. Ambulation	I walk shorter distances or stop to rest often. I do not walk at all.
7. Mobility	I stay within one room. I stay away from home only for brief periods of time.
8. Body care and movement	I do not bathe myself at all, but am bathed by someone else. I am very clumsy in body movements
9. Social interactions	I am doing fewer social activities with groups of people. I isolate myself as much as I can from the rest of the family.
10. Alertness behavior	I have difficulty reasoning and solving problems: for example, making plans, making decisions, learning new things. I sometimes behave as if I were confused or disoriented in place or time: for example, where I am, who is around, directions, what day it is.
11. Emotional behaviors	I laugh or cry suddenly. I act irritably and impatiently with myself: for example, talk badly about myself, swear at myself, blame myself for things that happen.
12. Communication	I am having trouble typing or writing. I do not speak clearly when I am under stress.

* Note: The complete questionnaire includes 136 items.

Source: Bergner M, Bobbitt RA, Carter WB, Gilson BS. The Sickness Impact Profile: development and final revision of a health status measure. *Medical Care.* 1981;19(8):787–805. Reprinted with the permission of Lippincott-Raven Publishers, Philadelphia, Penna.

mends supplementing an existing instrument with relevant and specific items that are not included in the existing instrument.[4]

Who Should Assess QOL?

Data concerning patients' QOL can be obtained from patient self-report or from others such as health care providers or persons close to the patient such as friends or family members. In oncology trials it has historically been the physician who has routinely graded the performance status of the patient. However, several studies document the poor interphysician reliability of performance scores obtained from physician-based observations and, perhaps more importantly, the low level of agreement between scores from patients' self-ratings and ratings determined by physicians.[19,20] Consequently, current opinion endorses patient self-report, either from an interview or questionnaire completed by the patient, as the more reliable and valid source of QOL information.

Self-administered questionnaires should be designed so that questions can be answered by individuals with varying educational backgrounds. Their use excludes patients who cannot read or write for either educational or health reasons. The principal advantage of interviewer-administered questionnaires is the decreased restriction on who and what can be asked. Anderson and colleagues also report that interviewer-administered questionnaires are less likely to under report dysfunction than self-administered questionnaires.[21] The main disadvantage of interviewer-administered questionnaires is that the quality of the data is highly interviewer dependent.

When Should QOL Be Measured?

Specific assessment times are determined primarily by the natural history of the disease, the characteristics of treatment, and the purpose for QOL assessment in a particular study. Cella suggests QOL measurement at four points during the course of treatment and follow-up: (1) Immediately pretreatment, (2) during the middle of treatment, (3) at the end of successful treatment or at the point when the patient is considered as nonresponsive to treatment, and (4) at 6 month follow-up after time point 3.[4]

What Are Some of the Considerations for Response Scales and for the Computation of an Overall QOL Score?

The two principal response scales are Likert-type scales and visual analog scales. Likert scales utilize categorical data and present patients with a set of ordinal items from which they choose the one that best describes their experience. Visual analog scales typically are 10 cm lines with descriptive anchors at the end. Visual analog and hybrid scales theoretically offer patients an increased number of responses. However, many investigators favor Likert scales because the level of abstraction required by Likert scales is less (Table 13–3).

Overall QOL scores are computed in two principal ways: individual items are summed or individual items are summed after being adjusted by a relative weight. Item response scores are typically adjusted by an importance scale. The importance score is then used to calculate a unique patient-specific score for each item.

The Statistical Criteria for Judging QOL Questionnaires

Once a questionnaire has been designed and accepted by patients, the questionnaire must satisfy the statistical criteria of validity, reliability, and responsiveness in order to be accepted for general use.

Validity

Validity refers to the ability to assess what the questionnaire was designed to measure. There are three main types of validity: construct, content, and criterion validity.[22] "Construct validity" refers to how a particular instrument relates to prior expectations or theory. "Content validity" indicates the internal validity of the items of the questionnaire and their role in the overall goal of the questionnaire. The "criterion validity" is a comparison between the results obtained with the new QOL questionnaire against an accepted "gold standard." In QOL research there is not a consensus that a single QOL measure is the "gold standard." Generally, QOL questionnaires that are lengthier and cover more aspects of QOL are considered more valid. There is no accepted rule for the degree of correlation that is required for a test to be considered valid, but a coefficient of correlation (ie, Pearson product-moment correlation coefficient) greater than 0.7 is regarded as very adequate.[23]

Table 13–3. Questionnaire response and importance scales

a.	Circle one number:				
	Not at all	A little bit	Somewhat	Quite a bit	Very much
	0	1	2	3	4
b.	Mark the appropriate position on the line:				
	No pain _____ Extreme pain				
	(10 cm)				
c.	Mark the appropriate position on the line:				
	No pain _____ Extreme pain				
	0 1 2 3 4				
d.	Circle one number:				
	How important is your physical well-being to your QOL?				
	Not at all 0 1 4 3 4 5 Very much				

a. Likert-type scale
b. Visual analogue scale
c. Hybrid scale
d. Importance scale

Reliability

Reliability indicates whether a measuring instrument would repeatedly produce the same results when applied to the same person under the same circumstances. It indicates the reproducibility of data and is established by test-retest results. In clinical trials, QOL measures must have a high degree of reliability to ensure that any observed change is due to the treatment and not to variation in the responses given to QOL questions. A variety of statistical test values, such as correlation coefficients, Kappa values, and standard deviations of repeated measurements, can be used to indicate reliability.[24,25] Similar to validity, a QOL measure with a coefficient of correlation greater than 0.7 is considered to be highly reliable.

Responsiveness

Responsiveness measures the ability of a questionnaire to detect clinical change over time and after clinical intervention. Therefore, responsiveness is proportional to the change in scores determined from a particular questionnaire during and after treatment. A highly responsive QOL instrument can detect small changes in QOL. An overall QOL score should have logical relation to specific oncologic stage. For example, a patient with a stage I cancer ought to have a significantly higher disease-specific QOL score than a patient with a stage IV cancer.

Cancer-Specific QOL Questionnaires

Numerous valid and reliable QOL measures have been developed in oncology. The Karnofsky, Eastern Cooperative Oncology Group (ECOG), and American Joint Committee (AJC) on Cancer Performance Scales are the three most widely used measures (Table 13–4).[14,26,27]

In 1949 the Karnofsky Performance Rating scale was developed to assess the physical well-being of cancer patients receiving chemotherapeutic agents. The scale is physician-administered and is thus based on the physician's subjective determination of the adjustment of the patient to the disease and its treatment effects. It offers little as to the patient's own perception of his

Table 13–4. The Eastern Cooperative Oncology Group (ECOG), Karnofsky and the American Joint Committee on Cancer (AJC) Performance Status Scales of Host (H)

Performance	ECOG Scale	Karnofsky Scale (%)	AJCC
Normal activity	0	90–100	H0
Symptomatic but ambulatory; cares for self	1	70–80	H1
Ambulatory more than 50% of time; occasionally needs assistance	2	50–60	H2
Ambulatory 50% or less of time; nursing care needed	3	30–40	H3
Bedridden; may need hospitalization	4	10–20	H4

Source: Used with permission of the American Joint Committee on Cancer (AJCC), Chicago, Illinois. The original source for this material is the AJCC *Manual for Staging of Cancer*, 4th ed. Philadelphia, Penna: Lippincott-Raven Publishers; 1992.

quality of life. The scale consists of 10 different levels, which describe the functional status of the patient. The large steps between levels and the crudeness of the scale have made it unresponsive to subtle differences in the psychosocial and functional status of patients. Several studies have found its reliability to be as high as 0.89 with good validity, whereas other studies have questioned these conclusions. The ECOG scale, like the Karnofsky Performance Scale, measures only a single item, functional status. The Karnofsky scale and ECOG have been used primarily to determine patient eligibility for enrollment in a particular study and to predict prognosis. Other recently validated cancer QOL measures include the Quality of Life Index (QL-Index), the Functional Living Index—Cancer (FLIC), the FACT scale, and EORTC Questionnaire.[9,17,28,29]

Previous Studies of QOL in Head and Neck Cancer Patients

There have been two types of QOL studies in head and neck cancer: those which report assessment strategies and QOL instruments and those which document QOL in specific patient populations. The purpose for QOL research in head and neck cancer has been threefold: (1) To use QOL as an outcome measure of treatment, (2) to assess the rehabilitation needs of patients, and (3) to determine patients' pre-treatment QOL in order to use QOL as a predictor of prognosis (Table 13–5).

Head and Neck Specific Questionnaires

Five head and neck QOL questionnaires have been developed for use across the broad spectrum of head and neck cancers: List's Performance Status Scale for Head and Neck Cancer Patients, the EORTC Core QLQ-30 Questionnaire with a Head and Neck Module, the University of Washington (UW) QOL Questionnaire, and the FACT Scale with a Head and Neck Module.[18,30-32] Browman et al recently developed and validated The Head and Neck Radiotherapy Questionnaire (HNRQ).[33] One additional QOL questionnaire, Piccirillo's Head and Neck Tumor Outcome Measure, is presently being validated.

List's Performance Status Scale is a *clinician-rated tool* for measuring the unique disabilities of head and neck cancer in the areas of eating and speaking (Table 13–6). Patients receive a functional rating score in three subscales: eating in public, understandability of speech, and normalcy of diet. In each subscale a list of items is arranged in a hierarchy

Table 13–5. Studies of quality of life in head and neck cancer

Study*	Sample Size	Tumor Site**	Treatment	Purpose of Study
Harwood (1983)[38]	129	Larynx	Radiation (113 pts.) Surgery (16 pts.)	Assessment of QOL: radiation versus surgery
Teichgraeber (1985)[44]	51	Oral cavity	Radiation (20 pts.) Surgery (21 pts.) Rad. + Surg. (10 pts.)	Development of a QOL test series for oral cancer patients
McConnel (1987)[45]	15	Tongue/FOM	Surgery (skin graft, tongue flap, or distal flap)	Comparison of oral function by type surgical reconstruction
Komisar (1990)[47]	16	Oral cavity/Oropharynx	Surgery	Assessment of functional results of mandibular reconstruction with a free bone graft or metal plate
Urken (1991)[48]	20	Oral cavity/Oropharynx	Surgery	Assessment of functional results of mandibular reconstruction with free transfer tissue
List (1990)[30]	181	Multiple	Surgery, radiation, and/or chemotherapy	Validation of a new performance scale
Harrison (1992)[34]	30	BOT	Radiation	Assessment of performance status following radiation
Harrison (1993)[35]	40	BOT	Radiation (30 pts.) Surgery (10 pts.)	Assessment of performance status: radiation versus surgery
Bjordal Questionnaire (1992)[31]	126	Multiple	Radiation	Validation of a new QOL
Hassan (1993)[32]	75	Multiple	Surgery and/or Radiation	Validation of a new QOL Questionnaire
Browman (1993)[33]	175	Multiple	Radiation and/or fluorouracil	Validation of a QOL instrument for trials of radiation therapy
DeSanto et al (1995)[50]	172	Larynx	Surgery	Comparison of QOL according to type of laryngectomy: Total vs near-total vs partial
Deleyiannis et al (1996)[36]	13	Orophaynx	Radiation/Surgery and radiation	Assessment of QOL for patients treated for stage III or IV cancer
D'Antonia et al (1996)[51]	50	Multiple	Surgery	Comparison of QOL questionnaires (FACT-H&N, PSS-HN, UWQOL)†
List et al (1996)[52]	151	Multiple	Surgery/Radiation/Chemotherapy	Comparison of QOL questionnaires (FACT-H&N and PSS-HN)
McConnel (1996)[49]	284	Oral Cavity/Oropharynx	Surgery	Assessment of speech and swallowing according to type of reconstruction: primary closure, distal flap, or free flap.

* Listed by principal author and year of publication.
** "Multiple" refers to oral cavity, pharynx, larynx, and other/unknown sites.
"BOT" = Base of tongue. "FOM" = Floor of Mouth.
† FACT-H&N = Functional Assessment of Cancer Therapy–Head and Neck Module; PSS-HN = Performance Status Scale for Head and Neck Cancer; UW-QOL = University of Washington QOL Questionnaire.

Table 13-6. List's performance status scale for head and neck cancer patients

Eating in public
- 100   No restriction of place, food, or companion (eats out at any opportunity)
- 75   No restriction of place, but restricts diet when in public (eats anywhere, but may limit intake to less "messy" foods, eg, liquids)
- 50   Eats only in presence of selected persons in selected places
- 25   Eats only at home in presence of selected persons
- 0   Always eats alone

Understandability of speech
- 100   Always understandable
- 75   Understandable most of the time; occasional repetition necessary
- 50   Usually understandable; face-to-face contact necessary
- 25   Difficult to understand
- 0   Never understandable; may use written communication

Normalcy of diet
- 100   Full diet (no restriction)
- 90   Peanuts
- 80   All meat
- 70   Carrots, celery
- 60   Dry bread and crackers
- 50   Soft, chewable foods (eg, macaroni, canned/soft fruits, cooked vegetables, fish, hamburger, small pieces of meat)
- 40   Soft foods requiring no chewing (eg, mashed potatoes, apple sauce, pudding)
- 30   Pureed foods (in blender)
- 20   Warm liquids
- 10   Cold liquids
- 0   Nonoral feeding (tube fed)

Source: List MA, Ritter-Sterr C, Lansky SB. A performance status scale for head and neck cancer patients. *Cancer.* 1990;66:564–569. Copyright © (1990) American Cancer Society. Reprinted by permission of Wiley-Liss, Inc., a subsidiary of John Wiley & Sons, Inc.

with normal function and total incapacitation receiving scores of 100 and 0, respectively. Reliability and validity were demonstrated in 181 head and neck cancer patients representing a range of diagnoses including cancer of the oral cavity, pharynx, larynx, and other head and neck sites. Harrison et al used List's Performance Status Scale to assess the functional outcome of patients with base of tongue cancer who had been treated with radiotherapy and/or surgery. In his series of 30 patients with squamous cancer of the base of the tongue, patients treated with external beam irradiation plus brachytherapy maintained an excellent quality of life.[34] The mean scores were 83% for eating in public (indicating virtually no restrictions of where to eat), 93% for understandability of speech (virtual normal speech), and 75% for normalcy of diet (some restrictions on types of foods). Functional outcome did not deteriorate with advancing stage, but the relatively small number of patients prevented statistical confirmation of an association between performance status and T stage. In a related study in which 30 patients with squamous cell cancer of the base of tongue treated with primary radiation were compared with 10 patients treated with primary surgery, patients treated with radiation therapy had consistently better performance scores.[35] Because primary radiation therapy and surgery have similar local control and survival rates, the authors stated that these results suggest that radiation therapy should be the preferred treatment for

T1–T3 lesions and that surgery may not be needed for all T4 lesions.

The EORTC QLQ-30 with a head and neck module is a patient self-administered questionnaire. It was found to discriminate between groups of patients before, during, and after treatment with radiation and between acute, subacute, and late disease and treatment-related symptoms and toxicity. For example, problems with soreness in the mouth, swallowing, and salivation/mucus production were worst halfway through the radiation course, whereas change of taste was greatest immediately after completed treatment.[31] The questionnaire's high acceptance and compliance rate among patients adds to its utility as practical QOL instrument.

The UW-QOL questionnaire (Table 13–7) was designed to be specific for head and neck patients.[32] It is patient self-administered and generally can be completed in less than 5 minutes. The questionnaire was administered to 75 head and neck cancer patients on three separate occasions: (1) several days preoperatively, (2) immediately postoperatively, and (3) 3 months postoperatively. Patients were grouped according to their clinical stage (T1,2,3,4). The questionnaire was found to be sufficiently sensitive to detect not only the expected large differences in QOL for T3 and T4 stage cancer after treatment, but also the more subtle changes that may occur in T1 and T2 stage patients. Deleyiannis and coinvestigators administered the UW-QOL questionnaire to a group of 13 patients undergoing combined surgery and postoperative radiation therapy (RT) versus primary RT for advanced curable oropharyngeal cancer. Treatment (whether primary RT [$n = 7$] or combined surgery and postoperative RT [$n = 6$]) was significantly associated with a worsening of QOL. This was particularly true in the QOL domains of chewing and swallowing. Patients who received surgery appeared more likely to suffer from disfigurement and from a worsening of speech but also to have greater pain relief compared to patients who received primary RT.[36]

The HNRQ is interviewer-administered and consists of 22 questions that deal with radiation symptoms related to six domains: oral cavity, throat, skin, digestive function, energy level, and psychosocial status. Each question has seven possible response options listed according to the degree of impairment with a Likert scale. In a prospective, randomized double blind study of concurrent 5FU and radiotherapy in the treatment of advanced head and neck cancer, the HNRQ was able to measure acute morbidity due to radiation therapy and to discriminate between patients receiving 5FU and placebo.[33]

Studies of Head and Neck Cancer QOL

Site-specific and treatment-specific QOL questions comprise the majority of QOL research in head and neck cancer. Particularly in cases where different treatments have nearly equivalent cure rates but different functional problems, questions of QOL have been raised to guide the selection of treatment.

Before any modality, either surgical or radiotherapeutic, becomes the accepted primary treatment of a particular type of head and neck cancer, the long-term effects of that modality on QOL should be known. The results of Larson's retrospective study of 148 patients with cancer of the oral cavity or oropharynx treated only with radiotherapy and free of disease for at least 5 years (median of 119 months) support this particular need.[37] The study reported a 56.3% overall incidence of soft tissue ulceration, osteonecrosis, or spontaneous fracture. Osteonecrosis had occurred within 2 years of radiotherapy in 42% of the patients with radiation-induced osteonecrosis (44 patients), within 3 years in 56%, and within 5 years in 82%. Eighteen of the 44 patients with osteonecrosis required subsequent partial or hemimandibulectomy.

The survival of patients with advanced glottic cancer treated with primary surgery is often reported as being the same for patients treated with primary radical radiotherapy. The perception of a better posttreat-

Table 13–7. The University of Washington (UW) QOL Questionnaire

Name: _____ Pt ID: _____ Date _____

This questionnaire asks about your views about your health and quality of life **during the past seven days**. Please answer the following questions and statements as indicated. If you have any questions, please call Linda Peyton at 206-548-4437.

1. In general, would you say your health is: **(circle one number)**

1	2	3	4	5
Poor	Fair	Good	Very good	Excellent

2. <u>Compared to **one year prior** to the diagnosis of your illness</u>, how would you rate your health in general <u>now</u>? **(circle one number)**

   1   Much worse now than one year prior to diagnosis
   2   Somewhat worse now than one year prior to diagnosis
   3   About the same as one year prior to diagnosis
   4   Somewhat better now than one year prior to diagnosis
   5   Much better now than one year prior to diagnosis

3. **Pain**   check one box ❑

   ❑   I have no pain.
   ❑   There is mild pain not needing medication.
   ❑   I have moderate pain—requires regular medication (codeine or non-narcotic).
   ❑   I have severe pain controlled only by narcotics.
   ❑   I have severe pain not controlled by medication.

   How important is your **pain** to your overall quality of life? **(circle one number)**
   (not important)   1   2   3   4   5   (extremely important)

4. **Appearance**   check one box ❑

   ❑   There is no change in my appearance.
   ❑   The change in my appearance is minor.
   ❑   My appearance bothers me but I remain active.
   ❑   I feel significantly disfigured and limit my activities due to my appearance.
   ❑   I cannot be with people due to my appearance.

   How important is your **appearance** to your overall quality of life?
   (circle one number)
   (not important)   1   2   3   4   5   (extremely important)

(continued)

Table 13–7. *continued*

5. **Activity   check one box** ❑

   ❑ I am as active as I have ever been.
   ❑ There are times when I can't keep up my old pace, but not often.
   ❑ I am often tired and have slowed down my activities although I still get out.
   ❑ I don't go out because I don't have the strength.
   ❑ I am usually in bed or chair and don't leave home.

   How important is your **activity** to your overall quality of life? **(circle one number)**
   (not important)   1   2   3   4   5   (extremely important)

6. **Recreation/entertainment   check one box** ❑

   ❑ There are no limitations to recreation at home or away from home.
   ❑ There are a few things I can't do but I still get out and enjoy life.
   ❑ There are many times when I wish I could get out more but I'm not up to it.
   ❑ There are severe limitations to what I can do, mostly I stay at home and watch TV.
   ❑ I can't do anything enjoyable.

   How important is your **recreation/entertainment** to your overall quality of life? **(circle one number)**
   (not important)   1   2   3   4   5   (extremely important)

7. **Employment   check one box** ❑

   ❑ I work full time.
   ❑ I have a part-time but permanent job.
   ❑ I only have occasional employment.
   ❑ I am retired, not related to cancer treatment.
   ❑ I am retired, due to cancer treatment.
   ❑ I am unemployed.

   How important is your **employment** to your overall quality of life? **(circle one number)**
   (not important)   1   2   3   4   5   (extremely important)

8. **Chewing   check one box** ❑

   ❑ I can chew as well as ever.
   ❑ I can eat soft solids but cannot chew some foods.
   ❑ I cannot even chew soft solids.

   How important is your **chewing** to your overall quality of life? **(circle one number)**
   (not important)   1   2   3   4   5   (extremely important)

9. Swallowing   check one box ❑

   ❑   I can swallow as well as ever.
   ❑   I cannot swallow certain solid foods.
   ❑   I can only swallow liquid food.
   ❑   I cannot swallow because it "goes down the wrong way" and chokes me.

   How important is your **swallowing** to your overall quality of life?
   (circle one number)
   (not important)   1   2   3   4   5   (extremely important)

10. Speech   check one box ❑

    ❑   My speech is the same as always.
    ❑   I have difficulty saying some words but I can be understood over the phone.
    ❑   Only my family and friends can understand me.
    ❑   I cannot be understood.

    How important is your **speech** to your overall quality of life? **(circle one number)**
    (not important)   1   2   3   4   5   (extremely important)

11. Shoulder   check one box ❑

    ❑   I have no problem with my shoulder.
    ❑   My shoulder is stiff but it has not affected my activity or strength.
    ❑   Pain or weakness in my shoulder has caused me to change my work.
    ❑   I cannot work due to problems with my shoulder.

    How important is your **shoulder mobility** to your overall quality of life?
    (circle one number)
    (not important)   1   2   3   4   5   (extremely important)

12. Taste   check one box ❑

    ❑   I can taste food normally.
    ❑   I can taste most foods normally.
    ❑   I can taste some foods.
    ❑   I cannot taste any foods.

    How important is your **taste** to your overall quality of life? **(circle one number)**
    (not important)   1   2   3   4   5   (extremely important)

13. Saliva   check one box ❑

    ❑   My saliva is of normal consistency.
    ❑   I have too little saliva.
    ❑   I have too much saliva.
    ❑   I have no saliva.

    How important is your **saliva** to your overall quality of life? **(circle one number)**
    (not important)   1   2   3   4   5   (extremely important)

(continued)

Table 13–7. *continued*

14. **Dryness of your mouth   check one box** ❑

    ❑   I have no abnormal dryness of mouth.
    ❑   My mouth is a little more dry.
    ❑   My mouth is somewhat more dry.
    ❑   My mouth is much more dry.
    ❑   My mouth is completely dry.

    How important is the **dryness of your mouth** to your overall quality of life? **(circle one number)**

    (not important)   1   2   3   4   5   (extremely important)

15. *Overall quality of life includes not only physical and mental health but also many other factors, such as family, friends, spirituality, or personal leisure activities that are important to your enjoyment of life. Considering everything in your life that contributes to your personal well-being, please rate your overall quality of life by circling the number between 1 and 6 that best applies to you.*

    How would you rate your overall quality of life **during the past 7 days**?

1	2	3	4	5	6
Very poor	Poor	Fair	Good	Very good	Excellent

    Please indicate on the following lines any items (medical or nonmedical) that are important to your quality of life and have not been adequately addressed in the above questions and statements.

    _____
    _____
    _____
    _____

Comment: *The UW QOL questionnaire was designed to be specific for head and neck patients. It is patient self-administered and generally can be completed in less than 5 minutes. The scale consists of nine categories, each describing important daily living dysfunction or limitations patients complain of as part of head and neck cancer or its treatment effects. Each of the nine categories has several options which allow patients to describe their current functional status. The highest level or "normal" function is assigned 100 points, whereas the lowest level or greatest dysfunction is scored 0 points. Each category contributes equally in the final score of the questionnaire of 900 points. We have recently added a set of questions to assess the importance of each domain and to provide a global rating of overall QOL.*

ment QOL, even in situations where radiation therapy has a less likely chance of cure, may lead patients to choose radiotherapy instead of surgery. Harwood's comparison of posttreatment QOL between radiotherapy and surgery illustrates the importance of using a QOL measurement for treatment selection for laryngeal cancer patients.[38] In his series of 129 patients (113 patients treated with radiotherapy and 16 treated with surgery) in every parameter of rating of voice (volume, pitch, ability to communicate, rate of speech), with the exception of dryness of throat, successfully irradiated patients had better ratings than the surgical patients. Moreover, less than half of the laryngectomy patients were working following treatment, whereas more than 80% of the irradiated patients were working.

Numerous investigators have recently conducted trials using induction chemotherapy plus radiotherapy in patients with locally advanced head and neck cancer.[39-42] Induction chemotherapy has not been shown to improve survival rates, but it may play an important role in preserving laryngeal function. Consequently, investigators are interested in identifying the chemotherapy regimens that have the most complete response rate, highest rate of organ preservation, longest survival, and lowest toxicity. The effects of chemotherapy on QOL can be assessed in a number of QOL domains. A standard QOL questionnaire (such as Browman's HNRQ) for chemotherapy trials in head and neck cancer would aid comparisons of toxicity across different studies and drug regimens.

A common purpose of QOL measurement is to assess the rehabilitation needs and the rehabilitative outcome of reconstructive surgery. Perhaps the most extensive use of functional parameters in rehabilitative analysis has been for patients with oral cancer.[43-45] Teichgraeber et al. in 1985 compared three groups of patients with oral cancer who had received radiation alone (20 patients), surgery alone (21), or combined therapy (10). Radiotherapy patients had the best speech and swallowing function; patients treated with combined therapy had the worst function. In comparing oral reconstruction techniques, patients with intraoral skin grafts had the best speech results. Patients with tongue flap reconstruction had better speech results than patients treated with primary closure, but the patients with primary closure had the best deglutition scores. The uneven distribution of the oral lesions by site and the limited number of patients necessitate that the results of this study be confirmed in a larger prospective study. In 1987 McConnel, Teichgraeber, and Adler used a similar protocol to compare three types of oral cavity reconstruction: skin grafts, hemitongue, and myocutaneous flaps.[45] Speech and swallowing were studied in 15 surgical patients with T2 or T3 tongue and/or floor of mouth lesions. The study demonstrated that tongue mobility was the most significant variable in determining postoperative speech results and that patients with split-thickness skin grafts had the best speech and swallowing.

Komisar published the first studies of the functional result of mandibular reconstruction for patients who underwent composite resection of oral pharyngeal cancer.[46,47] The functions of deglutition, mastication, and cosmesis were compared between the reconstructed and nonreconstructed patients. There was no significant difference in deglutition. Mastication was poorer and cosmesis was improved in the reconstructed patients. Reconstructed patients also had a greater number of hospitalizations secondary to complications from the reconstructive procedure. Kosimar concluded that aggressive surgical reconstruction of the mandible does little to improve the QOL of patients with oral pharyngeal cancer.

In 1991 Urken et al demonstrated the functional advantages of free tissue transfer in oromandibular reconstruction.[48] Urken compared 10 patients who underwent one-stage oromanbibular reconstruction using the iliac crest-internal oblique free flap and dental rehabilitation with enosseous implants to 10 patients with similar soft tissue and bone defects who received no bony reconstruction of the mandible. In almost all functional and psychosocial categories reconstructed patients had higher scores. The average length of hospitalization of reconstructed patients was not significantly longer than nonreconstructed patients. Also reconstructed patients achieved a functional level nearer to their predisease state and were able to resume employment and social activities more frequently than nonreconstructed patients. Urken's study represents the type of critical analysis of posttreatment function that is necessary for the evaluation of surgical therapies. However, this study did not address pretreatment status and should be repeated in a prospective fashion.

In 1996 McConnel and coworkers reported the results of their multi-institutional, 10-year prospective study that compared the speech and swallowing outcomes of 284 patients who were surgically treated for oral and oropharyngeal cancer and reconstructed with primary closure, distal flaps, or free flaps.[49] Patients were matched on both the site of resection and the extent of resection, and multivariate analysis was used to control for differences in preoperative function. Primary defect closure resulted in better oropharyngeal swallowing efficiency, speech intelligibility, and speech articulation than either distal or free flap reconstruction. These results challenge the current theories in oral and oropharyngeal reconstruction which advocate the replacement of resected soft tissue with skin or muscle flaps to preserve swallowing and speech function.

The Future

The present and future challenge of head and neck cancer research is to routinely incorporate QOL outcome measures in clinical trials and to use QOL as a guide to treatment selection. To improve QOL assessment in future studies, the authors reiterate three recommendations proposed by Gill and Feinstein.[9] First, ask patients to give two global ratings, one for overall QOL and the other for health-related QOL. Second, for each QOL domain being measured ask the patient to rate the importance as well as the severity of the problems in that domain. Third, allow the patient to add supplemental items.

Prospective randomized clinical trials are regarded as the optimal means to evaluate the efficacy of proposed treatment. The Radiation Therapy Oncology Group (RTOG) has recently incorporated the UW QOL Questionnaire and Cella's FACT scale with a head and neck module into ongoing clinical trials. Each questionnaire is being separately monitored for responsiveness. Hopefully, a compact scale fusing these two instruments will evolve.

THE IMPORTANCE OF COMORBIDITY IN STAGING UPPER AERODIGESTIVE TRACT CANCER

Jay F. Piccirillo, MD, FACS*

Because a patient's general health status is an important determinant of treatment and prognosis, any interpretation of outcome should also include an analysis of comorbidity.[53,54] The participants at a recent (September 1996) National Cancer Institute Strategic Staging Symposium concluded that future multi-institutional studies in head and neck cancer should include specific measures of comorbidity as stratification variables. Measures that were determined to be "readily available and easy to obtain" included medical comorbidity (options the Kaplan-Feinstein Index or the Charlson Comorbidity Index); performance status (Karnofsky Performance Status); and a measure of alcohol and tobacco use.[55]

Comorbidity is defined as the presence of non-neoplastic disease in patients with cancer. The American Joint Committee on Cancer and the International Union Against Cancer state the following objectives for a cancer staging system: (1) aiding in treatment planning, (2) providing estimates of

---

*This section is abstracted with permission of Rapid Science Publishers and the authors: Publiano FA, Piccirillo JF. The importance of comorbidity in staging upper aerodigestive tract cancer. Current Opinion in Otolaryngol Head Neck Surg. 1996;4:88–93.

prognosis, (3) assisting in treatment evaluation, (4) improving communication between treatment centers, and (5) facilitating continued cancer research.[27] The presence of comorbidity directly influences treatment planning and estimates of prognosis. Severe comorbidity can have a prognostic impact by decreasing survival and altering therapy. A patient who is "too sick" to tolerate preferred treatment may be given a less aggressive or even palliative treatment. Therefore, the importance of comorbidity in cancer of the upper aerodigestive tract is its potential impact on both outcome and treatment selection.

The impact of comorbidity is most clearly evident in cancers that are not rapidly fatal. For example, if the overall 5-year survival in a hypothetical cancer patient is 70%, then the likelihood that the patient will die of comorbid conditions is greater than in patients with more malignant tumors. Thus, when including comorbidity in a staging system, improved prognostic stratification is more likely to be demonstrated in the cancer patient with the higher survival rate. Conversely, the impact of the comorbid condition has been found to be more important in older patients than younger patients.[56]

Comorbidity Instruments

Comorbidity instruments can be classified into two groups depending on whether the data are of primary or secondary origin. Primary data are collected from physicians, nurses, or patients through direct contact or medical record review. Secondary data are collected from the administrative and financial databases maintained by hospitals, insurance companies, and state and federal agencies.

Primary Data

The following instruments have been developed to measure comorbidity based on primary data: the Kaplan-Feinstein Index (KFI), the Charlson Comorbidity Index (CCI), and the Index of Coexistent Disease (ICED).[57-61]

The KFI was developed from a study on comorbidity in patients with diabetes mellitus.[57] Specific diseases and conditions were classified into four groups according to the severity of organ decompensation and prognostic impact: none, mild, moderate, or severe. Conditions classified as severe comorbidity include congestive heart failure or myocardial infarction within past 6 months, recent stroke, and severely decompensated alcoholism (> one episode of alcoholic seizures or delirium tremens). Moderate comorbidity includes poorly controlled hypertension, old stroke with residual defect, and history of one episode of alcoholic seizure. Mild comorbidity includes mild hypertension, old myocardial infarction, and a "drinking problem" resulting in mild decompensation. The KFI has been used to study the impact of comorbidity in several cancers.[54, 62-68]

The CCI was created from a study of 1-year mortality rates among patients admitted to a medical unit at a teaching hospital. The CCI is a weighted index that incorporates the number and seriousness of comorbid diseases. The scoring system for this instrument assigns weights of 1, 2, 3, and 6 for specific diseases present on admission. A composite score is then calculated to represent the patient's overall prognostic status.[58]

The ICED (Greenfield and Apolone, unpublished data) predicts length of stay and resource utilization after hospitalization for patients undergoing surgical procedures. The ICED assesses the patient's status in two separate components: physiologic and functional burden. The scores from both categories are then used to calculate the overall burden of comorbidity.

Secondary Data

The second group of comorbidity instruments collects information from administrative and financial databases. These databases generally use the International Classification of Diseases, 9th revision, Clinical Modification system (ICD-9-CM).[59] The ICD-9-CM was created to trace the epidemiology of disease and associated mortality. Clinical modifiers were added to the strict epidemiologic taxonomy of the ICD-9 code to provide more clinically relevant information for research. Deyo and coinvestigators recently validated an automated version of the Charlson Index for use with Medicare inpatient claims and ICD-9-CM diagnostic codes.[69]

Problems arise in ICD-9-CM coding for several reasons.[70,71] Inaccuracies may result from poor coding techniques of medical record technicians. Investigators are often unable to determine whether comorbid conditions developed prior to or during the index hospitalization. The large number of codes allows the assignment of different codes to the same comorbid condition. Assigning different codes can have great impact on the determination of overall comorbidity. Studies that use the ICD-9-CM system as an instrument for coding comorbidity should be interpreted in the context of these potential limitations.

Comorbidity and Upper Aerodigestive Tract Cancer

Formal evaluation of the impact of comorbidity on cancer of the upper aerodigestive tract has been studied in larynx cancer.[54,63] Data from Piccirillo et al demonstrates the impact of the comorbidity on 5-year survival within tumor, node, metastasis (TNM) stage (Table 13–8).[72] The 5-year survival rate decreased when prognostic comorbidity was present, and this effect on survival remained within each TNM stage. By incorporating appropriate ratings of comorbidity and symptom severity, Piccirillo et al created a clinical-severity staging system, which reduced clinical heterogeneity within TNM stages and thereby improved prognostic stratification across the stage groupings (Table 13–9).[73]

Several studies have applied multivariate techniques to large patient populations in an attempt to identify prognostically significant factors. Mick et al performed a multivariate analysis on a group of patients with squamous cell carcinoma of the head and neck, and identified pretherapy weight loss, alcohol use, and N stage as independent predictors of survival.[74] Wolfensberger used Cox's proportional hazards model to screen 61 variables for prognostic significance in 800 patients with squamous cell carcinoma of the head and neck.[75] The majority of the 19 variables that were found to correlate with survival were tumor related (eg, site, T stage, node status, and the presence of metastases). Age greater than 70 years was the only host factor identified as prognostically significant. These studies demonstrate the utility of using multivariate analysis to examine the prognostic impact of a large number of variables on outcome. However, most fail to adequately examine the potential value of clinical variables.

Deleyiannis et al used the Surveillance, Epidemiology, End Results (SEER) database of western Washington state to identify the

Table 13–8. Impact of prognostic comorbidity on 5-year survival rates within TNM stages for patients with larynx cancer

Prognostic Comorbidity	TNM Stage* I	II	III	IV	Total
Absent, n/n (%)	59/71 (83)	31/41 (76)	25/38 (66)	8/19 (50)	123/166 (74)
Present, n/n (%)	1/6 (17)	1/7 (14)	2/7 (28)	0/7 (0)	4/27 (15)
Total, n/n (%)	60/77 (78)	32/48 (67)	27/45 (60)	8/23 (35)	127/193 (66)

*TNM — tumor, node, metastasis.
Source: Adapted from Piccirillo[72] with permission.

Table 13–9. Five-year survival rates in composite clinical-severity staging system

Stage	5-Year Survival,* n/n (%)
A	53/60 (88)
B	24/30 (80)
C	38/60 (63)
D	12/43 (28)
Total	127/193 (66)

*There is a 60% gradient in 5-year survival from group A to D.
Source: Adapted from Piccirillo and Feinstein[73] with permission.

features of alcohol use that are related to survival for head and neck cancer patients.[76] Alcoholism (relative risk, [RR] = 2.06; 95% confidence interval [CI] = 1.43–9.98) and a history of alcohol-related liver disease, pancreatitis, delirium tremens, or seizures (RR = 2.76; 95% CI = 1.69–4.49) were significantly associated with an increased risk of death, whereas abstinence (RR = 0.62; 95% CI = 0.39–0.97) was significantly associated with a decreased risk of death. An alcoholic-severity staging system was then developed that demonstrated a distinct prognostic gradient across stage for all sites of cancer (Figure 13–1). The author emphasizes that the classification system for alcohol use in this study identifies more prognostic information than the alcohol subsection of the KFI comorbidity instrument. The data show that abstinence, as well as alcohol abuse, has prognostic impact. Because there is a high level of alcohol use in patients with head and neck cancer, a comorbidity index that contains alcohol-specific components and is developed specifically for head and neck cancer should provide even greater prognostic information than previous comorbidity instruments.

Deleyiannis et al examined the impact of comorbidity and anemia on survival in hypopharyngeal cancer in a study of histologic invasion of the laryngeal framework.[77] Interestingly, after creating a two-level staging system (mild and severe illness) based on the presence or absence of anemia and comorbidity, the authors found that histologic invasion provided additional prognostic information only for patients in the mild category. This paper demonstrates that patient- and tumor-based factors both contain important prognostic information.

COST EFFECTIVENESS ANALYSIS

Bevan Yueh, MD

In an era of limited resources, surgical management is increasingly intertwined with cost containment. Head and neck surgeons are asked to maximize treatment outcomes such as quality of life while simultaneously minimizing consumption of financial resources.

As a result, in addition to standard measures such as mortality rates, functional status, and patient satisfaction, financial costs have become an important outcome variable. Although interested parties now agree to seek a balance between costs and therapeutic options, there is less accord over the placement of the fulcrum.[78] Cost analyses are helpful if they provide objective data with consistent methods, so that decision-makers can apply these data in a framework of relative costs.

Principles in Cost-effectiveness Research

A variety of excellent reviews on the principles of cost-effectiveness analysis have been published. They range from introductions of elementary concepts,[79,80] to critical assessments of the published literature,[81,82] to more formal discussions of methods[83] and new developments in the field.[84] A full review of the methods and principles of cost-effectiveness analysis is not the intent of this chapter; however, the following issues will be discussed: perspective of analysis, delineation of costs and benefits, discounting, and sensitivity analysis.

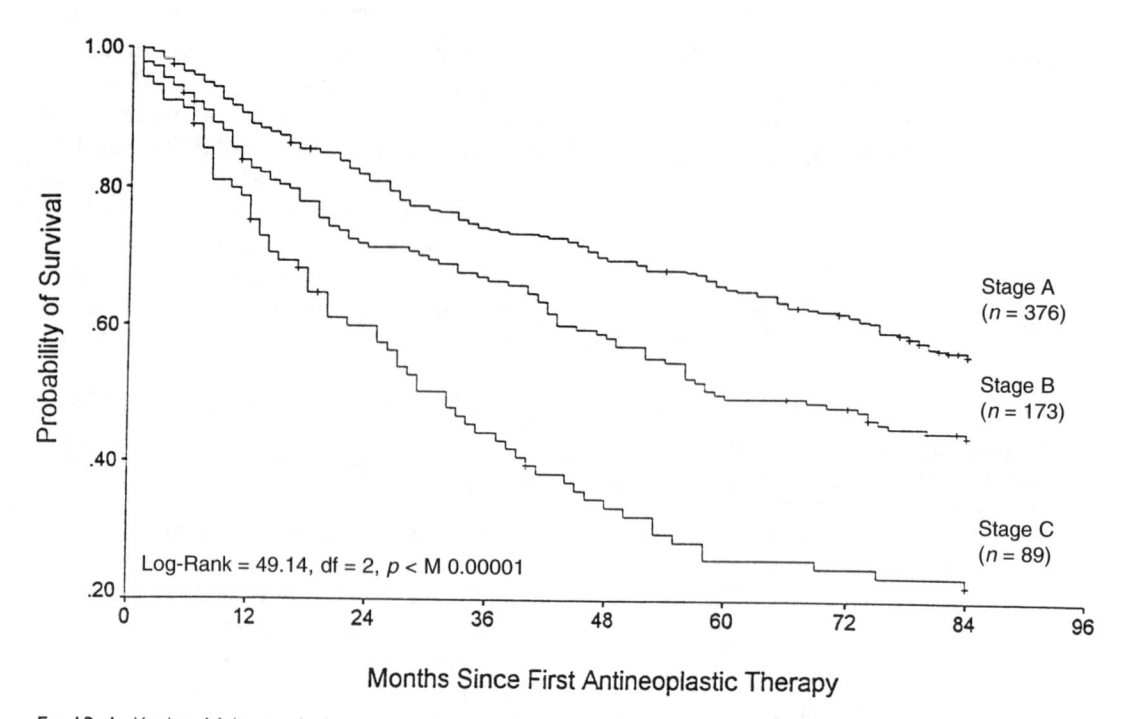

FIG 13-1. Kaplan–Meier survival curves for 7 years of follow-up for patients with head and neck cancer according to alcoholic severity stage. A three-level composite alcoholic severity staging system demarcated a distinct prognostic gradient for the entire study cohort. The categories of patients within each alcoholic severity stage were as follows: stage A (1) nonalcoholics and (2) abstinent alcoholics without a history of alcohol-related systemic health problems; stage B (1) abstinent alcoholics with a history of alcohol-related systemic health problems and (2) alcoholics currently drinking without a history of alcohol-related systemic health problems; and stage C, alcoholics currently drinking with a history of alcohol-related systemic health problems. Alcoholism was defined as having a MAST (Michigan Alcoholism Screening Test) score > 5 or a history of alcohol-related systemic health problems (eg, liver disease, pancreatitis, delirium tremens, or seizures due to alcohol). Abstaining and currently drinking refer to whether patients were drinking at the reference date, which was 1 year prior to the diagnosis of cancer. (This section is abstracted with permission of Rapid Science Publishers and the authors Pugliano FA, Piccirillo JF: The importance of comorbidity in staging upper aerodigestive tract cancer. *Current Opinion in Otolaryngol Head Neck Surg.* 1996;4:88–93.)

Perspective of Analysis

Costs incurred by patients are often different from those experienced by physicians, health organizations, or society at large. For example, the time spent recuperating from a laryngectomy is costly to the working patient and to society, but generally not to the hospital or insurer; similarly, costs borne by the hospital are unimportant to the patient. It may sometimes be appropriate to perform an analysis from more than one perspective. However, to see the costs in the proper context, the perspective that is adopted should be identified.

In many cases, authors discuss the costs of different therapies by comparing billing records. This may be inaccurate, because there are differences between *costs* and *charges*. Although the charges on a hospital bill represent the cost of the therapy for the patient, this is not the case for the hospital. From the hospital's perspective, the "cost" of medical care is theoretically "the value of the lost opportunity to use the resources in another way."[83]

Practically speaking, it may be easier to see that the "costs" of providing services to a patient are in general likely to be lower than the charges (in hospitals that plan to remain solvent). In addition, sometimes hospitals incur "costs" (eg, caring for the indigent) that are never directly billed to patients. Furthermore, charges for identical services may vary by patient, depending on the hospital's contract with the patient's managed care organization.

Delineation of Costs and Benefits

The explicit delineation of the costs and benefits to be measured, and the process used to measure them, are among the most challenging aspects of cost analysis. Almost all investigators consider the assessment of direct variable costs, such as operating room time, labor, or equipment, to be straightforward. Measures such as fixed costs (eg, administrative overhead), which are often overlooked, are also relatively easy to obtain. However, these items often account for only a fraction of the total cost. Indirect costs from resultant morbidity and mortality must be considered; the use of lost lifetime earnings as a proxy for such costs is problematic, as it implicitly places no value on the recently retired. Pain, suffering, inconvenience, and family burden are also real "costs" and difficult to quantify. Lost opportunity costs further add to the complexity.

Similarly, benefits must also be explicitly delineated. On occasion, benefits are measured in dollars. However, benefits can also be expressed with a variety of health measures, such as years of life saved, improvements in quality of life, or prevention of future adverse events. To compare the costs incurred by alternative treatments against benefits, the benefits need to be appraised with standardized techniques and measured with reproducible methods.

Discounting

For studies that take place over a period of years, the time effect on the value of money must also be taken into account. Given a choice between taking a sum of money now or tomorrow, it is wiser to take the money now, because it has investment potential. For example, $5000 invested today at a 5% annual rate of return grows to more than $8000 in 10 years. Therefore, the value of $5000 "invested" today in a head and neck reconstruction should not be considered equivalent to the $5000 "returned" in earnings 10 years hence. To estimate the value of future dollars in present terms, researchers use a "discount" rate. Figures of 5% to 6% are popular, but specific rates may vary depending on the scenario and the purpose of the analysis.[83]

Sensitivity Analysis

Sensitivity analysis is critical for testing the stability, or "robustness," of the conclusions in cost-effectiveness analyses. Because cost analyses generally make a number of assumptions about the values for a series of variables, it is important to know how dependent the conclusions are on what are essentially educated guesses.

For example, although efforts to estimate mortality rates, indirect costs, or discount rates in a study are based on the best available literature, it is extremely unlikely that there will be universal agreement on any particular value for these numbers. Sensitivity analysis is a process by which the assumptions are systematically varied to see whether the conclusions are affected.

Another use of sensitivity analysis is to identify the variables that have the greatest impact on the results. The values of some variables, no matter what is assumed, will have little effect on the conclusions. However, for other variables, even small changes in the assumed values may alter the results of the study. Valuable insight is gained by knowing which variables are most responsible for the outcome.

Definition of Cost-effectiveness

Authors have become accustomed to describing treatments that are either inexpensive or effective as "cost-effective," but neither use is technically correct. A true cost-effectiveness analysis presents summary information about treatment costs and associated outcomes simultaneously, usually as a ratio, where costs are placed in the numerator, and units of health effect (eg, extra years of life) are put in the denominator.[81] To clarify the confusion over this terminology, it is helpful to discuss the various types of cost analyses.

Cost-identification analyses simply aim to document the costs (or charges) of services and equipment. To provide meaningful contrasts, of course, cost-identification studies implicitly assume that the outcomes of each alternative are equivalent. When these assumptions cannot be made, cost-identification analyses are intended to be descriptive studies.

Cost-effectiveness studies are more sophisticated, because costs are assigned to a measure of health. (Because these health measures are usually desired utilities, these studies may also be called *cost-utility* analyses.) These health measures are generally nonmonetary, such as an added year of health, the ability to detect one additional thyroid neoplasm, or the prevention of a nosocomial infection. They may also include abstract concepts such as improved quality of life. Of course, because the "price" of an arbitrary health measure has only relative meaning, these results need to be compared with other alternatives, ideally with familiar and standardized methods.

One such popular measure is the "quality-adjusted life year" (QALY). The QALY takes into account not only extended survival but also the quality of life in those extra years. To use a hypothetical example, the sacrifice of a carotid artery may allow complete tumor extirpation and extend survival by 2 years, but the resultant hemiparesis might cause a 50% reduction in quality of life. The QALY would therefore be just 1 (= 0.5 ÷ 2.0) year.

It is important to note that any ratio in isolation has little meaning, unless it is presented in comparison with its alternatives. Knowing that chemotherapy (hypothetically) costs $40,000/QALY is of little use to a decision maker unless he or she is aware of the cost ratios for radiotherapy and for surgery. Some authors have argued for the presentation of cost-effectiveness ratios in marginal or incremental terms.[82,83]

Cost-benefit analyses can be even more complex, because both costs and benefits need to be expressed in units of currency. This necessitates a conversion of abstract health measures such as QALYs into dollars. These analyses have been used for relatively straightforward topics such as the evaluation of large population-based screening programs. However, cost-benefit analyses have not been applied yet for diseases in head and neck oncology, where benefits are not readily converted into units of currency.

Cost Analyses in Head and Neck Oncology

Cost analyses in head and neck surgery have largely been cost-identification efforts, and even these studies have been limited to the analysis of relatively simple topics, such as issues in the management of early glottic lesions[85,86] or for diagnostic algorithms.[87-91] We will list some of the existing cost analyses in the head and neck literature, and then conclude with a discussion of the challenges facing cost-effectiveness research in head and neck oncology.

Primary Treatment

Several authors have compared the costs of treating T1 glottic lesions with either radiation or surgery. Cragle et al pointed out the costs of therapy were less expensive with a surgical laser approach than with radiotherapy, with equivalent rates of cure.[85] Myers showed that the costs of managing patients with initial surgery rather than radiotherapy would result in average savings of approximately $3000 per patient in the long run.[86]

Other authors have emphasized the need to be aware of costs in treating tumors of the head and neck. Glenn et al discussed treatment options in a series of tumors of the retromolar trigone and estimated the costs of each alternative.[92] Hoffman et al have detailed the costs of evaluation and treatment of oral cavity carcinomas.[93]

Reconstructive Surgery

A recent cost-identification study by Miller et al compared hospital charges of free tissue transfer for oncologic, traumatic, and congenital indications.[94] They documented significantly higher charges in oncologic cases, with an average reconstruction "cost" of $37,400. Tsue et al have documented charges of similar magnitude in a comparison of free versus pedicled soft tissue transfer in oral cavity and oropharynx reconstruction: $41,122 for free tissue transfer and $37,160 for pedicled reconstruction.[95]

Diagnostic Tests

Shaha et al questioned whether the benefits of triple endoscopy justified its expense, pointing out that in a cohort of 140 patients, routine endoscopy, which averaged $1900, failed to detect any additional synchronous tumors.[87] This position was supported by Benninger et al, who argued for the use of multiple endoscopy only when symptoms were present.[89] They estimated that had selective endoscopy been used in 100 consecutive patients, approximately 33% of billings (charges) could have been saved.

Other cost-identification studies include one by Barlow et al, which questioned the routine use of chest radiographs after tracheotomy.[90] The replacement of rigid esophagoscopy by flexible fiberoptic examination was proposed by Glaws et al, on the basis of improved diagnostic sensitivity as well as cost (charge) savings of nearly $800 per examination.[91] Summers et al have suggested more inexpensive strategies for performing pre-operative parathyroid imaging.[88]

Other Studies

Several other authors have performed cost-identification studies on related topics. Blair et al argued that cost considerations should not dominate the decision to use prophylactic antibiotics in clean head and neck surgery.[96] Sartori et al compared the costs of percutaneous endoscopic gastrostomy and nasogastric tubes.[97] Cohen et al have shown decreased costs after institution of critical pathways for patients admitted for head and neck oncological surgery or chemotherapy.[98]

Challenges in Cost-effectiveness Analyses

A well done cost-effectiveness study on more complex head and neck oncological issues must overcome several formidable barriers. First, more data must be collected about the myriad of possible outcomes for an expanding list of treatment options. Quality of life and functional outcome data are particularly needed, especially for newer adjuvant therapy. Better financial data are needed as well; many hospital databases are not configured to reveal the actual costs of caring for its patients.

Second, the comparisons need to be standardized. Because case mix is usually different for individual hospitals, adjustments for disease severity are necessary to prevent biased comparisons. Variations in geographical practice patterns, training, and pay or mix also potentially confound these analyses. Outcomes need to be measured in standardized fashion as well, so that one QALY represents the same entity in Connecticut as it does in Washington, in women as well as men, and in the indigent as well as the well-to-do.

Finally, head and neck surgeons need to be educated about the methodological concerns in cost analysis research. For example, surgeons must become more adept at identifying costs, more able to recognize biased comparisons, and more comfortable with exploring outcomes beyond morbidity, mortality, and 5-year survival.

REFERENCES

1. Weymuller EA Jr. Moratorium on multi-institutional head and neck cancer trials. *Head Neck*. 1994;16(6):529–530.
2. Ferrans CE, Powers MJ: Psychometric assessment of the quality of life index. *Res Nursing Health*. 1992;15:29–38.

3. Cella DF, Tulsky DS. Quality of life in cancer: definition, purpose, and method of measurement. *Cancer Investig.* 1993;11(3):327–336.
4. Cella DF. Quality of life during and after cancer treatment. *Comprehensive Ther.* 1988;14(5):69–75.
5. Ferrans CE, Powers MJ. Quality of life index: development and psychometric properties. *ANS.* 1985;8(1):15–24.
6. Aaronson NK, Bullinger M, Ahmedzai S. A modular approach to quality-of-life assessment in cancer clinical trials. *Rec Results Cancer Res.* 1987;111:231–248.
7. Aaronson NK. Quality of life assessment in clinical trials: methodologic issues. *Controlled Clin Trials.* 1989;10:195S–208S.
8. Schipper H, Clinch J, McMurray A, Levitt M. Measuring the quality of life of cancer patients: the functional living index-cancer: development and validation. *J Clin Oncol.* 1984;2(5):472–483.
9. Gill TM, Feinstein AR. A critical appraisal of the quality of quality-of-life measurements. *JAMA.* 1994;272(8):619–626.
10. Patrick DL, Deyo RA. Generic and disease-specific measures in assessing health status and quality of life. *Medical Care.* 1989;27(3):S217–230.
11. Bergner M, Bobbitt RA, Carter WB, et al. The Sickness Impact Profile: development and final revision of a health status measure. *Medical Care.* 1981;19(8):787–805.
12. Bush J. General Health Policy Model/Quality of Well-being (QWB) Scale. In: Wenger NK, Mattson ME, Furber CD, et al, eds. *Assessment of Quality of Life in Clinical Trials of Cardiovascular Therapies.* New York: Lejack Publishing Inc; 1984.
13. Ware JE, Sherbourne CD. The MOS 36-item short-form health survey (SF-36) I. Conceptual framework and item selection. *Medical Care.* 1992;30(6):473–483.
14. Karnofsky DA, Burchenal JH. Clinical evaluation of chemotherapeutic agents in cancer. In: McLeod CM, ed. *Evaluation of Chemotherapeutic Agents.* New York, Columbia University Press; 1949.
15. Kihlgren M, Dubiel WT. Rehabilitation after aortic valve replacement with autologous fascia lata: a sociomedical study. *Ann Thoracic Surg.* 1977;24(4):346–351.
16. Sprangers MAG, Cull A, Bjordal K, et al. The European Organization for Research and Treatment of Cancer approach to quality of life assessment: guidelines for developing questionnaire modules. *Qual Life Res.* 1993;2:287–295.
17. Cella DF, Tulsky DS, Gray G, et al. The functional assessment of cancer therapy scale: development and validation of the general measure. *J Clin Oncol.* 1993;11:570–579.
18. Cella DF. Manual for the Functional Assessment of Cancer Therapy (FACT) Scales and the Functional Assessment of HIV (FAHI) Scale (Version 3). Chicago, IL: Rush-Presbyterian-St. Luke's Medical Center; 1994.
19. Hutchinson TA, Boyd NF, Feinstein AR. Scientific problems in clinical scales as demonstrated by the Karnofsky Index of Performance Status. *J Chron Dis.* 1979;32:661–666.
20. Schagg CC, Heinrich RL, Ganz PA. Karnofsky Performance Status revisited: reliability, validity and guidelines. *J Clin Oncol.* 1984;2:187–193.
21. Anderson JP, Bush JW, Berry CC. Classifying function for health outcome and quality-of-life evaluation, self-versus interviewer modes. *Medical Care.* 1986;24(5):454–470.
22. Nunnally JC. *Psychometric Theory.* New York: Mc-Graw-Hill; 1978.
23. Selby PJ, Chapman JAW, Etazadi-Amoli J, et al. The development of a method for assessing the quality of life of cancer patients. *Br J Cancer.* 1984;50:13–22.
24. Kramer MS, Feinstein AR. Clinical biostatistics: LIV. The biostatistics of concordance. *Clin Pharmacol Ther.* 1981;29:111–123.
25. Landis RJ, Koch GG. The measurement of observer agreement for categorical data. *Biometrics.* 1977;33:159–174.
26. Zubrod CG, Schneiderman M, Frei E, et al. Appraisal of methods for the study of chemotherapy of cancer in man: comparative therapeutic trail of nitrogen mustards and triethylene thiophosphoramide. *J Chronic Dis.* 1960;11:7–33.
27. American Joint Committee (AJC) on Cancer. *Manual for Staging of Cancer,* 4th ed. Philadelphia: Lippincott Co; 1992.
28. Spitzer WO, Dobson AJ, Hall J, et al. Measuring the quality of life of cancer patients, a concise QL-index for use by physicians. *J Chron Dis.* 1981;34:585–597.
29. Bergman B, Sullivan M, Sorenson S. Quality of life during chemotherapy for small cell lung cancer. II. A longitudinal study of the EORTC core quality of life questionnaire and comparison with the sickness impact profile. *Acta Oncol.* 1992;31(1):19–28.

30. List Ma, Ritter-Sterr C, Lansky SB. A performance status scale for head and neck cancer patients. *Cancer.* 1990;66:564–569.
31. Bjordal K, Kaasa S. Psychometric validation of the EORTC core quality of life questionnaire, 30-item version and a diagnosis-specific module for head and neck cancer patients. *Acta Oncol.* 1992;31(3):311–321.
32. Hassan SJ, Weymuller EAL. Assessment of quality of life in head and neck cancer patients. *Head Neck.* 1993;15:485–496.
33. Browman GP, Levine MN, Hodson DI, et al. The head and neck radiotherapy questionnaire: a morbidity/quality-of-life instrument for clinical trials of radiation therapy in locally advanced head and neck cancer. *J Clin Oncol.* 1993;11:863–872.
34. Harrison LB, Zelefsky MJ, Sessions RB, et al. Base-of-tongue cancer treated with external beam irradiation plus brachytherapy: oncologic and functional outcome. *Radiology.* 1992;184:267–270.
35. Harrison LB, Zelefsky MJ, Armstrong JG, et al. Performance status after treatment for squamous cell cancer of the base of tongue—a comparison of primary radiation therapy versus primary surgery. *Int J Radiat Oncol Biol Phys.* 1994;30:953–957.
36. Deleyiannis FW-B, Weymuller EA, Coltrera MD. Quality of life of disease-free survivors of advanced (Stage III or IV) oropharyngeal cancer. *Head Neck.* 1997;19:466–473.
37. Larson DL, Lindberg RD, Lane E, et al. Major complications of radiotherapy in cancer of the oral cavity and oropharynx a 10 year retrospective study. *Am J Surg.* 1983;146:531–536.
38. Harwood AR, Rawlinson E. The quality of life of patients following treatment for laryngeal cancer. *Int J Rad Onc Biol Phys.* 1983;9(3):335–338.
39. The Department of Veterans Affairs Laryngeal Cancer Study Group. Induction chemotherapy plus radiation in patients with advanced laryngeal cancer. *N Engl J Med.* 1991;324:1685–1690.
40. Forastiere AA. Cisplatin and radiotherapy in the management of locally advanced head and neck cancer. *Int J Rad Onc Biol Phys.* 1993;27(2):465–470.
41. Shirinian MH, Weber RS, Lippman SM, et al. Laryngeal preservation by induction chemotherapy plus radiotherapy in locally advanced head and neck cancer: The MD Anderson Cancer Center experience. *Head Neck.* 1994;16(1):39-44.
42. Urba SG, Forastiere AA, Wolf GT, et al. Intensive induction chemotherapy and radiation for organ presevation in patients with advanced resectable head and neck carcinoma. *J Clin Oncol.* 1994;12(5):946–953.
43. Velanovich V. Choice of treatment for stage I floor-of-mouth cancer a decision analysis. *Arch Otolaryngol Head Neck Surg.* 1990;116:951–956.
44. Teichgraeber J, Bowman J, Goepfert H. Functional analysis of treatment of oral cavity cancer. *Arch Otolaryngol Head Neck Surg.* 1986;112:959–965.
45. McConnel FMS, Teichgraeber JF, Alder RK. A comparison of three methods of oral reconstruction. *Arch Otolaryngol Head Neck Surg.* 1987;113:496–500.
46. Komisar A, Warman S, Danziger E. A critical analysis of immediate and delayed mandibular reconstruction using A-O plates. *Arch Otolaryngol Head Neck Surg.* 1989;115:830–833.
47. Komisar A. The functional result of mandibular reconstruction. *Laryngoscope.* 1990;100:364–374.
48. Urken ML, Buchbinder D, Weinberg H, et al. Functional evaluation following microvascular oromandibular reconstruction of the oral cancer patient: a comparative study of reconstucted and nonreconstructed patients. *Laryngoscope.* 1991;101:935–950.
49. McConnel FMS, Pauloski BR, Rademaker AW, et al. The functional results of primary closure verse flaps in oropharyngeal reconstruction: a prospective study of speech and swallowing outcomes. In: Proceedings of the Fourth International Conference on Head and Neck Cancer, July 28–August 1, 1996; Toronto, Canada. 797–807.
50. DeSanto LW, Olsen KD, Perry WC, Rohe DE, Keith RL. Quality of life after surgical treatment of cancer of the larynx. *Ann Otol Rhinol Laryngol.* 1995;104:763–679.
51. D'Antonio LL, Zimmerman GJ, Cella DF, Long SA. Quality of life and functional status measures in patients with head and neck cancer. *Arch Otolaryngol Head Neck Surg.* 1996;122:482–487.
52. List MA, D'Antonio LL, Cella DF, et al. The performance status scale for head and neck cancer patients and the functional assessment of cancer therapy—head and neck scale: a study of utility and validity. *Cancer.* 1996;77:2294–2301.
53. Feinstein AR. The pre-therapeutic classification of comorbidity in chronic disease. *J Chronic Dis.* 1970;23:455–469.

54. Piccirillo JF, Wells CK, Sasaki CT, Feinstein AR. New clinical severity staging system for cancer of the larynx five year survival rates. *Ann Otol Rhinol Laryngol.* 1994;103:83–92.
55. Weymuller EA Jr. Unpublished report to NCI. Clinical staging and operative reporting for multi-institutional trials in head and neck squamous cell carcinoma. Jan 1997.
56. Charlson M, Szatrowski TP, Peterson J, Gold J. Validation of a combined comorbidity index. *J Clin Epidemiol.* 1994;47:1245–1251.
57. Kaplan MH, Feinstein AR. The importance of classifying initial comorbidity in evaluating the outcome of diabetes mellitus. *J Chronic Dis.* 1974;27:387–404.
58. Charlson ME, Pompei P, Ales HL, MacKenzie CR. A new method of classifying prognostic comorbidity in longitudinal studies: development and validation. *J Chronic Dis.* 1987;40:373–383.
59. Israel RA: The International Classification of Disease: two hundred years of development. *Public Health Rep.* 1978;93:150–152.
60. Greenfield S, Apolone G, McNeil BJ, Cleary PD. The importance of coexistent disease in the occurrence of postoperative complications and one-year recovery in patients undergoing total hip replacement: comorbidity and outcomes after hip replacement. *Med Care.* 1993;31:141–154.
61. Greenfield S, Aronow HU, Elashoff RM, Watanbe D. Flaws in mortality data: the hazards of ignoring comorbid disease. *JAMA.* 1988;260:2253–2255.
62. Feinstein AR, Schimpff CR, Andrews JR Jr, Wells CK. Cancer of the larynx: a new staging system and a re-appraisal of prognosis and treatment. *J Chronic Dis.* 1977;30:277–305.
63. Clemens JD, Feinstein AR, Holabird N, Cartwright S. A new clinical-anatomic staging system for evaluating prognosis and treatment of prostatic cancer. *J Chronic Dis.* 1986;39:913–928.
64. Wells CK, Stoller JK, Feinstein AR, Horwitz RI. Comorbid and clinical determinants of prognosis in endometrial cancer. *Arch Intern Med.* 1984;144:2004–2009.
65. Feinstein AR. Clinical and intellectual causes of defective statistics for the prognosis and treatment of lung cancer. *Med Clin North Am.* 1967;51:549–562.
66. Feinstein AR, Schimpff CR, Hull EW. A reappraisal of staging and therapy for patients with cancer of the rectum. I. Development of two new systems of staging. *Arch Intern Med.* 1975;135:1441–1453.
67. Feinstein AR, Wells CK. Lung cancer staging: a critical evaluation. *Clin Chest Med.* 1982;3:291–305.
68. Feinstein AR, Wells CK. A clinical-severity staging system for patients with lung cancer. *Medicine* (Baltimore). 1990;69:1–33.
69. Deyo RA, Cherkin DC, Ciol MA. Adapting a clinical comorbidity index for use with ICD-9-CM administrative databases. *J Clin Epidemiol.* 1992;45:613–619.
70. Romano PS, Roos LL, Jollis JG. Adapting a clinical comorbidity index for use with ICD-9-CM administrative data: Differing perspectives. *J Clin Epidemiol.* 1993;46:1075–1079.
71. Romano PS, Roos LL, Jollis JG. Response: further evidence concerning the use of a clinical comorbidity index with ICD-9-CM administrative data. *J Clin Epidemiol.* 1993;46:1085–1090.
72. Piccirillo JF. The inclusion of comorbidity in a staging system for head and neck cancer. *Oncology.* 1995;9:831–836.
73. Piccirillo JF, Feinstein AR. Problems in the current TNM staging system for cancer. *Cancer.* 1996;77:834–842.
74. Mick R, Vokes EE, Weichselbaum RR, Panje WR. Prognostic factors in advanced head and neck cancer patients undergoing multimodality therapy. *Otolaryngol Head Neck Surg.* 1991;105:62–73.
75. Wolfensberger M. Using Cox's proportional hazards model for prognostication in carcinoma of the upper aero-digestive tract. *Acta Otolaryngol (Stockh).* 1992;112:376–382.
76. Deleyiannis FW-B, Thomas DB, Vaughn TL, Davis S. Alcoholism: Independent predictor of survival in patients with head and neck cancer. *J Natl Cancer Inst.* 1996;88:542–549.
77. Deleyiannis FW-B, Piccirillo JF, Kirchner JA. Relative prognostic importance of histologic invasion of the laryngeal framework by hypopharyngeal cancer. *Ann Otol Rhinol Laryngol.* 1996;105:101–108.
78. Young EW. The ethics of nontreatment of patients with cancers of the head and neck. *Arch Otolaryngol Head Neck Surg.* 1991;117(7):769.
79. Eddy DM. Clinical decision making: from theory to practice. Cost-effectiveness analysis. A conversation with my father. *JAMA.* 1992;267(12): 1669.
80. Eddy DM. Clinical decision making: from theory to practice. Cost-effectiveness analysis. Is it up to the task? *JAMA.* 1992;267(24):3342.

81. Doubilet P, Weinstein MC, McNeil BJ. Use and misuse of the term "cost effective" in medicine. *N Engl J Med*. 1986;314(4):253.
82. Udvarhelyi IS, Colditz GA, et al. Cost-effectiveness and cost-benefit analyses in the medical literature. Are the methods being used correctly? [see comments]. *Ann Intern Med*. 1992;116(3):238.
83. Eisenberg JM. Clinical economics: a guide to the economic analysis of clinical practices. *JAMA*. 1989;262:2879.
84. Russell LB, Gold MR, et al. The role of cost-effectiveness analysis in health and medicine. *JAMA*. 1996;276:1172.
85. Cragle SP, Brandenburg JH. Laser cordectomy or radiotherapy: cure rates, communication, and cost. *Otolaryngol Head Neck Surg*. 1993;108(6):648.
86. Myers EN, Wagner RL, Johnson JT. Microlaryngoscopic surgery for T1 glottic lesions: a cost-effective option [see comments]. *Ann Otol Rhinol Laryngol*. 1994;103(1): 28.
87. Shaha A, Hoover E, et al. Is routine triple endoscopy cost-effective in head and neck cancer? *Am J Surg*. 1988;155(6):750.
88. Summers GW, Dodge DL, Kammer H. Accuracy and cost-effectiveness of preoperative isotope and ultrasound imaging in primary hyperparathyroidism. *Otolaryngol Head Neck Surg*. 1989;100(3):210.
89. Benninger MS, Enrique RR, Nichols RD. Symptom-directed selective endoscopy and cost containment for evaluation of head and neck cancer. *Head Neck*. 1993;15(6):532.
90. Barlow DW, Weymuller E Jr, Wood DE. Tracheotomy and the role of postoperative chest radiography in adult patients. *Ann Otol Rhinol Laryngol*. 1994;103(9):665.
91. Glaws WR, Etzkorn KP, et al. Comparison of rigid and flexible esophagoscopy in the diagnosis of esophageal disease: diagnostic accuracy, complications, and cost. *Ann Otol Rhinol Laryngol*. 1996;105(4):262.
92. Glenn MG, Komisar A, Laramore GE. Cost-benefit management decisions for carcinoma of the retromolar trigone. *Head Neck*. 1995; 17(5):419.
93. Hoffman HT, Funk GF, et al. Cost analysis of treatment of oral cavity squamous cell carcinoma. *Otolaryngol Head Neck Surg*. 1995;113: 50. Abstract.
94. Miller MJ, Swartz WM, et al. Cost analysis of microsurgical reconstruction in the head and neck. *J Surg Oncol*. 1991;46(4):230.
95. Tsue TT, Desyatnikova SS, et al. Comparison of cost and function in reconstruction of the posterior oral cavity and oropharynx: free versus pedicled soft tissue transfer. *Arch Otolaryngol Head Neck Surg*. 1997;123:731–737.
96. Blair EA, Johnson JT, et al. Cost analysis of antibiotic prophylaxis in clean head and neck surgery. *Arch Otolaryngol Head Neck Surg*. 1995;121(3):269.
97. Sartori S, Trevisani L, et al. Cost analysis of long-term feeding by percutaneous endoscopic gastrostomy in cancer patients in an Italian health district. *Support Care Cancer*. 1996;4(1):21.
98. Cohen J, Stock M, et al. Critical pathways for head and neck surgery: development and implementation. *Arch Otolaryngol Head Neck Surg*. 1997;123:11.

Index

A

Accelerated fractionation
  caution regarding late toxicity of, 32–34
  moderately, 30
  treatment results of, 29
Accelerated radiation therapy for squamous cell carcinoma of head and neck, *see* Hyperfractionated or accelerated radiation therapy
Acoustic analysis of voice and speech, 101–102
Advanced head and neck cancer, cisplatin chemotherapy for, 59–68
Aerodigestive tract cancer, upper, *see* Upper aerodigestive tract cancer
Aerodynamic measures of voice and speech, 102
Aided esophageal voice as option, 112–113
Air charge, inhalation method of, 111–112
AL, *see* Artificial larynx, 108
Alaryngeal whisper, 108
Alloplastic fixation appliances, 138
American Joint Committee (AJC) on Cancer Performance Scales, 152, 153
Andy Gump deformity, 134
Anterior or lateral neck dissection
  with postoperative radiation therapy, results, 40
  without postoperative radiation therapy, results, 40–41
    floor of mouth, 40
    larynx (supraglottic, glottic, transglottic), 41
    lower gum/retromolar trigone, 40–41
Anterior surgical approaches to nasopharynx, 50–51
Anterior-symphyseal defects, 134
Anterolateral surgical approach to nasopharynx, 51–56
  clinical application and results, 52–55
    patients, 52–55
    results, 55
  complications and their management, 55–56
  surgical technique, 51–52
Apoptosis, 16–17
  bcl-2, 16
  definition of, 8
  p53 in apoptosis, 17
Artificial larynx (AL) use, 108–109
  pneumatic, 109
Aryepiglottic fold in false vocal cord, 80
Arytenoids, proper positioning of postoperatively, 93–94

B

Bcl-2, clinical correlation with in HNSCC, 16
Browman's HNRQ, 161

C

C-erbB-2, 19
Cancer-specific QOL questionnaires, 152–153
Candida Albicons, 113
Carcinogenesis of upper aerodigestive tract, 6–8
  oncogenes and tumor suppression genes, 7–8
Carcinoma, biology of, *see* Squamous cell carcinoma; Supraglottic carcinoma: Upper aerodigestive tract carcinoma
Cell cycle control, 9–14
Charlson-Comorbidity Index (CCI), 162, 163
Chemoradiation, concomitant, 64
Chemotherapy, *see* Cisplatin technique for advanced head and neck cancer
CHEP, *see* Cricohyoidoepiglottopexy
Children with head and neck cancer, management of, 4

CHP, *see* Cricohyoidopexy
Cisplatin chemotherapy for advanced head and neck cancer
  conclusions, 67–68
  laboratory evidence for cisplatin resistance, 59–60
  targeted supradose cisplatin technique, 60–67
Collagenase, 18–19
  c-erbB-2, 19
  stromolysin, 18–19
  type I collagenase, 18
  type IV collagenase, 18
    MMP–2, 18
    MMP–9, 18
Combination therapy for advanced head and neck cancer, 59
Communication assessment of voice and speech, 101
Comorbidity, importance of in staging upper aerodigestive tract cancer, 162–165
  and upper aerodigestive tract cancer, 164–165
  instruments, 163
    primary data, 163
    secondary data, 163–164
Concomitant chemoradiation, 64
Consonant injection, 110
Continuity defects of mandible, 134
Contraindications for SCPL
  with CHEP, 92
  with CHP, 91
Cost-effectiveness analysis in head and neck oncology
  cost-identification efforts, 168–169
    challenges in, 169
    diagnostic tests, 169
    other studies, 169
    primary treatment, 168–169
    reconstruction surgery, 169
  principles in research, 165–168
    definition of, 167–168
    delineation of costs and benefits, 167
    discounting, 167
    perspectives of analysis, 166–167
    sensitivity analysis, 167
Costochondral graft, 142–143
Costs of mandibular reconstruction, 144
Cricohyoidoepiglottopexy (CHEP), 83
  closure of, 94
  SCPLC with, 83, 88
    closure, 88–90, 94
    exposure, 88
    resection, 88
Cricohyoidopexy (CHP), 83, 84
  SCPL with
    closure, 86–88
    exposure, 84–85
    resection, 85–86
Cyclin D1 protein, 10–11
  p53, 11–13
  9p21, 13–14
Cytokeratins, 15

D

Decannulation, 95
Deep circumflex iliac artery (DCIA), 139
Dental reconstruction of mandibulectomy, 143

E

Early laryngeal cancer, management of, 3
Eastern Cooperative Oncology Group (ECOG), 152, 153
EGFR and TGF-#, 14
Endoscopic laser resection of laryngeal cancer
  development of, 73–74
  future directions, 81
  of stage I and stage II glottic cancer, 74–77
  summary, 81
  of supraglottic cancer, 77–81
Endoscopic removal of laryngeal cancer, 4
Esophageal voice as option after laryngectomy, 109–112
  TEP aided, 112–113
European Organization for Research and Treatment of Cancer (EORTC) scales, 148, 153, 155

F

Fixation of mandibular reconstruction, 140
Fixed mandibular implant (FMI), 143
Florida Laryngectomee Association, annual voice institutes of, 115
Functional Assessment of Cancer Therapy (FACT), 148, 153
Functional Living Index—Cancer (FLIC), 149, 153
Functional outcome following SCPL, optimizing, 92–95

G

Gastroesophageal reflux, 93
General versus disease-specific QOL, 148
Genetic alterations in HNSCC development, 7
Glossopharyngeal press, 110
Glottic cancer, endoscopic resection of stage I and stage II, 74–77

H

Head and neck cancer, functional assessment of patients treated for
  conclusions, 103
  eating, 102–103
  studies, 99–100
  voice and speech, 100–102
    acoustic analysis, 101–102
    aerodynamic measures, 102
    communication assessment, 101
    perceptual analysis, 100–101
Head and neck oncology, overview, 1–4
Head and Neck Radiotherapy Questionnaire (HNQR), 153, 155
Head and neck specific questionnaires, 153–156
Head and neck squamous cell carcinoma (HNSCC), 9
HER2/neu/c-erB-2, 14
Heterozygosity at segment of genome, 8
HNSCC, *see* Head and neck squamous cell carcinoma, 9
Humidifiers, 114
Hyperfractionated or accelerated radiation therapy for squamous cell carcinoma of head and neck, 2
  clinical experience with multiple fractions per day, 27–29
  conclusions, 32–34
    caution regarding late toxicity of accelerated fractionation, 32–34
    efficacy, 32
  convenience of, 25–26
  improvement in therapeutic ratio, 26–27
  patient comfort, 16
  treatment results, 29–32
    accelerated fractionation, 29, 30
    hyperfractionation, 29–32
Hyperfractionation, treatment results of, 29–32

I

ICD-9-CM, *see* International Classification of Diseases
Index of Coexistent Disease (ICED), 163
Indications and contraindications
  for SCPL with CHEP, 92
  for SCPL with CHP, 91
Inferior alveolar nerve (IAN), 133, 134
Inferior surgical approach to nasopharynx, 48–50
  transcervical, 50
  transpalatal, 48–50
Infrahyoid epiglottis, T1 suprahyoid carcinoma of, 80–81

Inhalation method of air charge, after laryngectomy, 111–112
Innovative treatment methods for eradicating laryngeal cancer, 3–4
Instruments, comorbidity, 163–164
Intergroup Rhabdomyosarcoma Study Group (IRS), 119
  clinical grouping, 120, 123
  studies, 125–126
Internal regulation of proliferation, cell cycle control, 9–14
  cyclin D1 protein, 10–11
  p53, 11–13
  9p21, 13–14
International Classification of Diseases, 163
  problems in coding, 164
Intraepithelial neoplasia, 6

K

Kaplan-Feinstein Index (KFI), 162, 163
Karnofsky Performance Status Scale for cancer, 148, 152, 153
Kinetics of tumor, 8

L

Laboratory evidence for cisplatin resistance, 59–60
Laryngeal cancer, endoscopic resection of
  development of endoscopic laser resection, 73–74
  endoscopic resection of stage I and stage II glottic cancer, 74–77
  endoscopic resection of supraglottic cancer, 77–81
  future directions, 81
  summary, 81
Laryngeal resistance, 102
Laryngectomy, oral communication after, 105–115
  consequences of surgery, 106
  fears associated with cancer and, 106
Larynx, cross-sectional view of, 79
Larynx cancer and hypopharynx, hyperfractionation of, 31
Larynx surgery, results without postoperative radiation therapy, 41
Laser excision of stage II glottic cancer, 77
Laser resection
  development of, 73–74
  for stage II glottic cancer, 75
Lateral-body defects, 134
Lateral surgical approach to nasopharynx, 47, 48
Likert Scales, 151, 152

List's Performance Status Scale for Head and Neck Cancer Patients, 153, 155
Lost cord clubs, for patient support, 114–115
Lower gum/retromolar trigone surgery, results without postoperative radiation therapy
   oral tongue, 40
   pyriform sinus, 41
Lymph node metastases, management of, 2–3
Lymphatic drainage from supraglottis, 93

M

Mandibular defect following ablative treatment for head and neck cancer, 4
Mandibular reconstruction, techniques for
   anatomy, 133–134
   complications, 143–144
   conclusions, 144
   continuity defects of mandible, 134
   costs, 144
   dental reconstruction, 143
   fixation of reconstruction, 140
   options for, 138
   oral soft tissue reconstruction, 137
   postoperative evaluation and management, 135–136
   preferred donor sites for vascularized osseous mandibular reconstruction, 139–140
     fibula, 139
     iliac crest, 139–140
     scapula, 140
   principles and technical goals of mandibular reconstruction, 135
   resection, 136–137
   timing and therapeutic options of reconstruction, 137–139
   TMJ reconstruction, 140–143
Medical Outcomes Study 36-item short-form health survey (SF-36), 148
Microlaryngeal suction, 78
MMP-2, 18
MMP-9, 18
Mouth Squeeze process, 110
Mouth floor surgery results without postoperative radiation therapy, 40
Multiple fractions per day, clinical experience with, 27–29
Mutations, 7

N

Nasopharyngeal carcinoma, 2–3
Nasopharyngectomy via anterolateral approach, 54–55
Nasopharynx, surgical approaches to
   anterior approaches, 50–51
   anterolateral approach, 51–56
     clinical application and results, 52–55
     complications and their management, 55–56
     surgical technique, 51–52
   comments, 56–57
   inferior approach, 48–50
     transcervical, 50
     transpalatal, 48–50
   lateral approach, 47, 48
Neck cancer, functional assessment of patients treated for, 99–104, see also Head and neck cancer
Neck dissection, selected
   goal of, 42–43
   types of, 43–44
     anterior or lateral, 44
     supraomohyoid, 43–44
Neck stage, results based on, 41
New York Heart Association Functional Classification, 148
Nominal standard dose formula (NSD), 25
Non-small cell lung cancer (NSCLC), 16
Nonparameningeal head and neck rhabdomyosarcoma, 127–128
   clinical features, 127
   therapeutic considerations, 127–128

O

Oncogenes and tumor suppression genes, 7–8
Oncologic rationale, indications and contraindications, 90–92
   indications and contraindications for SCPL with CHEP, 92
   indications and contraindications for SCPL with CHP, 91
   oncologic rationale of SCPL with CHEP, 91–92
   oncologic rationale of SCPL with CHP, 90–91
Optivox, 108
Oral and cutaneous soft tissue defects, 139
Oral communication after laryngectomy
   assistance from other devices, 113–114
     humidifiers, 114
     tracheostoma valve, 113–114
   options, 107–109
     alaryngeal whisper, 108
     artificial larynx use, 108–109
     pantomimed speech using oral gestures, 107–108
   patient support, lost cord clubs, 114–115
   pre- and postoperative consultation, 105–107
   standard esophageal voice as option, 109–112
     inhalation method of air charge, 111–112
     pumping methods of air intake, 110–111

TEP aided esophageal voice as option, 112–112
Oral soft tissue reconstruction, 137
Oral tongue, 40
Orbital rhabdomyosarcoma, 121–124
    clinical features of, 121
    therapeutic considerations, 122–124
Organ preservation
    protocols, 99–104
    therapeutic approach, 67
Oropharyngeal cancer, hyperfractionation of, 31
Osseocutaneous donor sites, 139
Osseus reconstruction, problems with, 144

P

p53, 11–13
    in apoptosis, 17
9p21, 13–14
Pantomimed speech using oral gestures, 107–108
Parameningeal rhabdomyosarcoma, 124–127
    clinical features, 124–125
    chemotherapy for, 126
    therapeutic considerations, 125–127
Patient support, lost cord clubs, 114–115
Peer-Support for Laryngectomized Persons, 114
Perceptual analysis of voice and speech, 100–101
Phonation threshold pressure (PTP), 102
Piccirillo's Head and Neck Tumor Outcome Measure, 153
Postoperative evaluation and management of mandibular reconstruction, 135–136
Postoperative radiation therapy
    suprahyoid dissection with, 38
    suprahyoid dissection without, 38
    supraomohyoid dissection with, 38–39
    supraomohyoid dissection without, 39–40
Practice Guidelines of American Society of Head and Neck Surgery, 84
Pre- and postoperative laryngectomy consultation, 105–107
Proliferation in upper aerodigestive tract carcinoma
    EGFR and TGF-α, 14
    HER2/neu/c-erB-2, 14
Proplast-Teflon TMJ implant, 143
Pumping methods of air intake, 110–111
Pyriform sinus, 41

Q

QOL, *see* Quality of life
Quality of life, after head and neck cancer, 4
Quality of Life (QOL) in head and neck cancer treatment
    cancer-specific QOL questionnaires, 152–153
    defining concept and content of, 148
    future, 162
    general versus disease-specific QOL, 148
    head and neck specific questionnaires, 153–156
    methodology, 148–150
        assessment, 150–151
        considerations for response scales and computation of overall QOL score, 151
        measurement, 149–150
        specific times of assessment, 151
    previous studies of QOL in head and neck cancer patients, 153
    statistical criteria for judging QOL questionnaires, 151–152
        reliability, 152
        responsibility, 152
        validity, 151
    studies and head and neck cancer QOL, 156–162
Quality of Life Index (QL-Index), 153
Quality of Well-Being Scale, 148
Quality-adjusted life year (QALY), 168
Questionnaire response and importance scales, 152

R

Radiation myelitis, incidence of, 33
Radiation therapy, postoperative
    suprahyoid dissection with, 38
    suprahyoid dissection without, 38
    supraomohyoid dissection with, 38–39
    supraomohyoid dissection without, 39–40
Radiation Therapy Oncology Group (RTOG), 162
Radical neck dissection for upper aerodigestive tract carcinoma
    clinical considerations, 41–44
    history of, 37–38
    results, 38–41
        anterior or lateral neck dissection with postoperative radiation therapy, 40
        anterior or lateral neck dissection without postoperative radiation therapy, 40–41
        results based on neck stage, 41
        suprahyoid dissection with postoperative radiation therapy, 38
        suprahyoid dissection without postoperative radiation therapy, 38
        supraomohyoid dissection with postoperative radiation therapy, 38–39
        supraomohyoid dissection without postoperative radiation therapy, 39–40
    summary, 44–45

Radiotherapy, very accelerated fractionation, 28, 29, 30
RADPLAT protocol, measuring patients treated in, 100–104
Ramus/condyle defects, 134
Resection of mandibular reconstruction, 136–137
Retinoids, 15–16
Rhabdomyosarcoma (RMS) of head and neck in children
   acute and delayed effects of therapy, 128–129
      acute complications, 129
      delayed effects, 129
   future directions, 129–130
   history on therapy, 119–120
   nonparameningeal head and neck rhabdomyo-sarcoma, 127–128
      clinical features, 127
      therapeutic considerations, 127–128
   orbital rhabdomyosarcoma, 121–124
      clinical features of, 121
      therapeutic considerations, 122–124
   parameningeal rhabdomyosarcoma, 124–127
      clinical features, 124–125
      therapeutic considerations, 125–127
RMS, see Rhabdomyosarcoma

S

SCPL, see Supracricoid partial laryngectomy
Severe mucositis, 129
Sickness Impact Profile (SIP), 148, 150
Silastic prosthesis, 112
Speech, TEP as procedure to facilitate, 110
Speech and voice, evaluating, 100–102
Split-course irradiation, 26
Squamous cell carcinoma of glottis, stage I, endoscopic laser excision of, 77
Squamous cell carcinoma of head and neck, see Hyperfractionated or accelerated radiation therapy
Squamous cell carcinoma (SCC) of upper aerodigestive tract (UADT), 59–60, see also Cisplatin chemotherapy
Stage I squamous cell carcinoma, 77
Stage II glottic cancer, endoscopic resection of, 74–77
Stage I glottic cancer, endoscopic resection of, 74–77
Statistical criteria for judging QOL questionnaires, 151–152
Sternohyoid, 84, 85
Strap musculature, 84, 87–88
Stromolysin, 18–19
Subglottic pressure, assessment of, 102
Superior laryngeal nerves (SLN), 93
Supracricoid partial laryngectomy (SCPL)
   oncologic rationale, indications and contraindications, 90–92
      indications and contraindications for SCPL with CHEP, 92
      indications and contraindications for SCPL with CHP, 91
      oncologic rationale of SCPL with CHEP, 91–92
      oncologic rationale of SCPL with CHP, 90–91
   optimizing functional outcome following supracricoid partial laryngectomy, 92–95
   summary, 95
   surgical technique, 84–90
      supracricoid partial laryngectomy with cricohyoidoepiglottopexy, 88
      supracricoid partial laryngectomy with cricohyoidopexy, 84–88
   types of, 83–84
Supradose cisplatin technique, targeted, 60–67
   advantages of over IV chemotherapy, 62–63
   clinical trials, 64
   follow-up, 65–67
   studies on, 61–62, 64
   thiosulfate and, 63
   toxicity and, 65
Supraglottic cancer, endoscopic resection of, 77–81
Supraglottic carcinoma, management of, 90–91
Supraglottic laryngectomies (SGLs), 84
Supraglottic resection, major steps in, 80
Suprahyoid dissection
   with postoperative radiation therapy, 38
   without postoperative radiation therapy, 38
Suprahyoid epiglottis, transection of, 79
Supraomohyoid dissection
   with postoperative radiation therapy, 38–39
   without postoperative radiation therapy, 39–40
Supraomohyoid selective neck dissection, 39
Surgical technique for SCPL, 84–90
   with cricohyoidoepiglottopexy, 88
      closure, 88–90
      exposure, 88
      resection, 88
   with cricohyoidopexy, 84–88
      closure, 86–88
      exposure, 84–85
      resection, 85–86
Surveillance, Epidemiology, and End Results Section of the National Cancer Institute (SEER), 119, 164–165

T

T1 carcinomas of infrahyoid epiglottis, 80
T1 suprahyoid epiglottic cancers, 80

Targeted chemoradiation, 3
Telangiectasia, severity of, 34
Temporo-mandibular joint (TMJ), 133, 134, 136
    Proplast-Teflon implant, 143
    reconstruction, 140–143
TEP, see Tracheoesophageal/pharyngeal puncture
TGF-α and EGFR, 14
Therapy for rhabdomyosarcoma, acute and delayed effects of, 128–129
    acute complications, 129
    delayed effects, 129
Timing and therapeutic options of mandibular reconstruction, 137–139
Tongue lock, 110
Tracheostoma valve, 113–114
Tracheostomy, 89, 95
Tracheoesophageal/pharyngeal puncture (TEP), 110
    aided esophageal voice as option, 112–113
    as procedure to facilitate speech, 110
Transcervical approach to nasopharynx, 50
Transoral CO_2 laser excision, 76
Transoral supraglottic resection, 74
Transpalatal approach to nasopharynx, 48–50
TruTone, 108–109
Tumor biology, principles of, 1–2
Tumor suppression genes and oncogenes, 7–8
Type I collagenase, 18
Type IV collagenase, 18
    MMP-2, 18
    MMP-9, 18

U

UADT, see Upper aerodigestive tract
University of Washington (UW) QOL Questionnaire, 153, 155, 157–161, 162
Upper aerodigestive tract, SCC of, 59–60
Upper aerodigestive tract carcinoma, biology of
    apoptosis, 16–17
        bcl-2, 16
        p53 in apoptosis, 17
    carcinogenesis, 6–8
        oncogenes and tumor suppression genes, 7–8
    differentiation, 14–16
        cytokeratins, 15
        retinoids, 15–16
    invasion and metastasis, 17–19
        collagenase, 18–19
        urokinase, 17
    pathology, 5–6
        intraepithelial neoplasia, 6
    proliferation, 8–14
        external regulation of proliferation, growth factors and signaling pathways, 14
        internal regulation of proliferation, cell cycle control, 9–14
    radical neck dissection for, 37–44
    summary, 19
    tumor kinetics, 8
Urokinase, 17

V

Vascularized osseus mandibular reconstruction, donor sites for, 139–140
    fibula, 139
    iliac crest, 139–140
    scapula, 140
Vascularized bone graft reconstruction, 141
Velvet-tipped suction, 78
Vertical partial laryngectomy (VPL), 76, 84
Vocal quality following SCPL, 95
Voice and speech, evaluating, 100–102
    acoustic analysis, 101–102
    aerodynamic measures, 102
    communication assessment, 101
    perceptual analysis, 100–101